Cesarean Section: Complications of Labor and Delivery

Cesarean Section: Complications of Labor and Delivery

Editor: Tianna Davis

AMERICAN
MEDICAL PUBLISHERS
www.americanmedicalpublishers.com

AMERICAN
MEDICAL PUBLISHERS
www.americanmedicalpublishers.com

Cataloging-in-Publication Data

Cesarean section : complications of labor and delivery / edited by Tianna Davis.
p. cm.
Includes bibliographical references and index.
ISBN 978-1-63927-151-1
1. Cesarean section. 2. Cesarean section--Complications. 3. Delivery (Obstetrics).
4. Obstetrics--Surgery. I. Davis, Tianna.
RG761 .C47 2022
618.86--dc23

American Medical Publishers,
41 Flatbush Avenue,
1st Floor, New York,
NY 11217, USA

ISBN 978-1-63927-151-1 (Hardback)

Contents

Preface

This book aims to highlight the current researches and provides a platform to further the scope of innovations in this area. This book is a product of the combined efforts of many researchers and scientists, after going through thorough studies and analysis from different parts of the world. The objective of this book is to provide the readers with the latest information of the field.

Cesarean section or C-section refers to the use of surgery to aid the delivery of a baby. It is performed when a vaginal delivery puts the baby or the mother at risk. Cases of obstructed labor, problems with the umbilical cord or placenta, high blood pressure, twin pregnancy or breech birth can present risks to the delivery. The surgery is performed depending on the shape of the mother's pelvis and the history of previous C-section. Cesarean section can be performed under regional anesthesia or general anesthesia. Regional anesthesia offers advantages such as absence of risks of pulmonary aspiration of gastric contents and prevention of persistent post operative pain for long duration. General anesthesia may however be necessary in severe fetal distress, or when patients experience heavy uncontrolled breathing. The procedure is associated with risks of incisional hernias that may require surgical correction, postoperative adhesions and wound infections. This book discusses the fundamentals as well as modern approaches of cesarean section. It provides insight into the complications of labor and delivery which will be crucial for the management of pregnancy and childbirth. This book includes contributions of experts and scientists which will provide innovative insights into this procedure.

I would like to express my sincere thanks to the authors for their dedicated efforts in the completion of this book. I acknowledge the efforts of the publisher for providing constant support. Lastly, I would like to thank my family for their support in all academic endeavors.

Editor

1

The impact of caesarean section on breastfeeding initiation, duration and difficulties in the first four months postpartum

Amy J. Hobbs[1*], Cynthia A. Mannion[2], Sheila W. McDonald[3], Meredith Brockway[2] and Suzanne C. Tough[1,3]

Abstract

Background: The caesarean section (c-section) rate in Canada is 27.1 %, well above the 5–15 % of deliveries suggested by the World Health Organization in 2009. Emergency and planned c-sections may adversely affect breastfeeding initiation, milk supply and infant breastfeeding receptivity compared to vaginal deliveries. Our study examined mode of delivery and breastfeeding initiation, duration, and difficulties reported by mothers at 4 months postpartum.

Methods: The All Our Babies study is a prospective pregnancy cohort in Calgary, Alberta, that began in 2008. Participants completed questionnaires at <25 and 34–36 weeks gestation and approximately 4 months postpartum. Demographic, mental health, lifestyle, and health services data were obtained. Women giving birth to singleton infants were included ($n = 3021$). Breastfeeding rates and difficulties according to mode of birth (vaginal, planned c-section and emergency c-section) were compared using cross-tabulations and chi-square tests. A multivariable logistic regression model was created to examine the association between mode of birth on breastfeeding duration to 12 weeks postpartum.

Results: More women who delivered by planned c-section had no intention to breastfeed or did not initiate breastfeeding (7.4 % and 4.3 % respectively), when compared to women with vaginal births (3.4 % and 1.8 %, respectively) and emergency c-section (2.7 % and 2.5 %, respectively). Women who delivered by emergency c-section were found to have a higher proportion of breastfeeding difficulties (41 %), and used more resources before (67 %) and after (58 %) leaving the hospital, when compared to vaginal delivery (29 %, 40 %, and 52 %, respectively) or planned c-sections (33 %, 49 %, and 41 %, respectively). Women who delivered with a planned c-section were more likely (OR = 1.61; 95 % CI: 1.14, 2.26; $p = 0.014$) to discontinue breastfeeding before 12 weeks postpartum compared to those who delivered vaginally, controlling for income, education, parity, preterm birth, maternal physical and mental health, ethnicity and breastfeeding difficulties.

Conclusions: We found that when controlling for socio-demographic and labor and delivery characteristics, planned c-section is associated with early breastfeeding cessation. Anticipatory guidance around breastfeeding could be provided to women considering a planned c-section. As well, additional supportive care could be made available to lactating women with emergency c-sections, within the first 24 hours post birth and throughout the early postpartum period.

Keywords: Caesarean section, Mode of birth, Vaginal delivery, Breastfeeding, Postpartum

* Correspondence: hobbs.aj@gmail.com
[1]Cumming School of Medicine, Department of Community Health Sciences, University of Calgary, TRW Building 3rd Floor, 3280 Hospital Drive NW, Calgary, Alberta T2N 4Z6, Canada
Full list of author information is available at the end of the article

Background

The rate of caesarean section (c-section) in Canada has increased from 17.6 % in 1995 to 27.1 % in 2012 [1]. Although worldwide consensus on the optimal rate of c-section is variable [2], the World Health Organization (WHO) [3] suggests 5–15 % of all live births, far below current c-section rates in Canada. C-sections are associated with poor maternal and infant health outcomes [4–6], such as higher incidences of maternal infection and uterine haemorrhage, and infant respiratory distress and hypoglycaemia [6, 7]; all of which may adversely impact breastfeeding success.

Researchers have shown that women who deliver by c-section delivery are less likely to breastfeed, or delay breastfeeding initiation [8–14]. Breastfeeding within the first hour post-delivery has been cited as an important predictor of continued breastfeeding [15–17]. An early study by Rowe-Murray and Fisher (2002), found that babies born via c-section were less likely to be have skin-to-skin contact immediately after birth and were more likely not to have attempted breastfeeding within the first 24 h post delivery [8]. Skin-to-skin contact has been suggested to improve breastfeeding initiation, maintenance and duration [18]. Delays in breastfeeding initiation accompanying c-section delivery are associated with maternal/infant separation, reduced suckling ability, decreased infant receptivity, and insufficient milk supply, which are predictive of shortened breastfeeding duration [8, 12–14, 19–23].

Breastfeeding is associated with infant health benefits, such as fewer childhood illnesses, lower blood pressure and cholesterol levels, lower prevalence of obesity, and improved intelligence as adults [24, 25]. Maternal benefits of breastfeeding include faster involution of the uterus and lower risk of haemorrhage after birth, in addition to lower a lower lifetime incidence of type II diabetes, and breast and ovarian cancer [26]. These studies have suggested that the benefits of breastfeeding act in a dose response relationship, whereby increasing breastfeeding duration results in more infant health benefits [24–26]. Since it has been established that breastfeeding confers several long-term maternal and infant benefits, it is important to understand the impact of c-section delivery on breastfeeding initiation, and duration.

Health Canada [27] and the WHO [16] recommend that all infants should be breastfed exclusively for the first six months of life, and continue breastfeeding up to and beyond two years of age. Perinatal Health Indicators for Canada (2013) state that breastfeeding initiation rates in Canada remain at approximately 87 % (2005–2010) [28]. However, the 2008 Perinatal Health Report found that only 53.9 % of babies were still breastfeeding at 6 months of age [29]. The rate of exclusive breastfeeding at 6 months has slowly increased from 20.3 % in 2005 to 25.9 % in 2010 [28],but the rate is still low. Only three of the 13 provinces and territories in Canada have designated facilities that meet the WHO Baby Friendly Hospital Initiative (BFI) guidelines [30]; thus, improvements in this area could help to meet the national and international breastfeeding recommendations [16, 27].

Research comparing the effect of c-section delivery to vaginal delivery on breastfeeding duration document conflicting results and often lack adequate sample sizes to support their findings [20, 31–33]. Pérez-Escamilla et al. (1996) indicated that c-section delivery did not affect breastfeeding duration if women initiated breastfeeding from birth and maintained breastfeeding for at least four weeks postpartum, [32]. However, Brown & Jordan (2013) contradict these results reporting that mothers who gave birth via c-section were more likely to discontinue breastfeeding compared to those who gave birth vaginally [33]. The Ontario Mother and Infant Study, by Watt et al (2012), found no differences between c-section and vaginal deliveries on breastfeeding initiation or duration to 6 weeks postpartum [14]. However, this study found that emergency c-sections and assisted vaginal deliveries were associated with an increased likelihood of initiation and duration of breastfeeding, when compared to planned c-section and unassisted vaginal birth [14]. Watt et al. (2012) acknowledged that these results were unexpected and suggested further research to explore all modes of delivery and impact on breastfeeding [14].

In addition, studies have found that the type of c-section, either emergency or planned, influences breastfeeding outcomes [3, 14, 22, 34]. A meta-analysis performed by Prior et al. (2012) pooling 48 studies ($n = 553{,}306$) found that women who delivered by planned c-section were less likely to initiate any breastfeeding; whereas emergency c-section delivery had no significant impact on initiation. The authors found no association between any type of c-section delivery and exclusive breastfeeding up to six months [31]. However, the authors of this meta-analysis acknowledge that the clarity of the association between mode of birth and several breastfeeding outcomes is limited given that it was not the primary outcome of most of the studies included and that there was evidence of heterogeneity between studies, often resulting from small sample sizes and unadjusted point estimates from individual studies.

Guidelines by the WHO BFI [16] state that keeping mother and baby together for at least the first hour post birth leads to improved initiation and duration of breastfeeding [34, 35]. Although findings support that both emergency and planned c-section affect breastfeeding initiation and duration, the direction of the association among studies is inconclusive and warrants further exploration of breastfeeding, stratified by type of c-section. Our large population-based study examined the effect of planned or emergency c-section and vaginal delivery of singletons, comparing breastfeeding initiation, duration, and difficulties in the early postpartum period, while taking into account for key indicators of breastfeeding success.

Methods

Study design

The All Our Babies (AOB) study is a prospective community-based pregnancy cohort in Calgary, Alberta, that began in 2008. Participants completed questionnaires before 25 weeks gestation, 34–36 weeks gestation, and at approximately 4 months (12–16 weeks) postpartum (questionnaires provided in Additional file 1). Further details about the design and methods of the AOB study have been previously published [36]. The AOB collected information during pregnancy on participant's pregnancy history, health service utilization, demographics, lifestyle, mental, psychosocial and physical health, life events, quality of life, work status, and breastfeeding. Questions about the mode of birth and breastfeeding intention were collected from the pregnancy questionnaire at 34–36 weeks gestation and assessment of breastfeeding outcomes was collected in the questionnaire completed between 12–16 weeks postpartum. Only women giving birth to a singleton infant were included in this study ($n = 3021$). The AOB study was approved by the Child Health Research Office and the Conjoint Health Research Ethics Board of the Faculties of Medicine, Nursing, and Kinesiology at the University of Calgary. Informed consent was obtained from the study participants at the time of recruitment, who were also provided copies for their records.

Exposure and outcome variables

The main exposure variable of mode of birth was based on maternal self-reported response to the question "How was your baby delivered?" Responses were classified into three levels: emergency c-section (including both before and after the onset of labour), planned c-section, or vaginal delivery. The AOB study validated that maternal recall of the type of birthing method was high when compared to the details in the medical charts [37]. Since medical charts in Calgary and the AOB questionnaire do not distinguish between different types of vaginal delivery, spontaneous, assisted, and instrumental vaginal births were classified together. Breastfeeding outcomes were characterized by maternal reported breastfeeding intention, initiation (e.g., on first attempt, within the first 24 h, prior to leaving the hospital), difficulties (e.g., latching, reports of sore nipples, perceived lack of milk supply), and lactation support sought after discharge. Breastfeeding success was based upon self-reports by breastfeeding mothers in response to two questions: "Were you able to successfully breastfeed on your first attempt?" and "Were you able to breastfeed before you went home from the hospital?" Breastfeeding duration was categorized based on maternal reports of "any breastfeeding" between birth and the data collection time point at 12–16 weeks postpartum. According to breastfeeding status at this time point, we characterized women either as having breastfed for greater than 12 weeks or as having breastfed for 12 weeks or less (early cessation). As the questionnaire asked mothers about any breastfeeding at this time point, we were unable to distinguish between exclusive breastfeeding, or if babies were feeding at the breast versus being offered breast milk with a bottle.

Data analysis

All data were analyzed using the Statistical Package for Social Science (SPSS Inc. Version 19.0, Chicago, Illinois, USA). Descriptive statistics (means, standard deviation (SD), frequencies, and percentages) were used to characterize the sample and describe breastfeeding and labour and delivery variables. Bivariate associations between demographic, breastfeeding, and labour and delivery variables and mode of birth (vaginal, planned c-section and emergency c-section) were examined using cross-tabulations and Pearson chi square tests.

Multivariable logistic regression was used to examine the association between mode of birth and dichotomized breastfeeding duration, controlling for confounding variables. Significance of covariates was assessed via backwards selection, with comparison to the crude model to assess for confounding whereby all covariates with a p-value of <0.05 were retained in the final adjusted model. Potential confounders were assessed in the multivariable model and included: income (<\$60,000 or ≥ \$60,000), education (≤ high school or at least some post-secondary), previous birth (yes or no), preterm birth (yes or no), postpartum maternal physical health (SF-12 physical component summary score), postpartum maternal mental health (SF-12 mental component summary score), ethnicity (Caucasian or non-Caucasian, breastfeeding difficulties (≤1 difficulty or > 1 difficulty). Only participants with available data were included in the analyses.

This research adhered to the STROBE guidelines for observational studies [38] (checklist added as Additional file 2).

Results

Table 1 shows demographic and labour and delivery characteristics of the sample of women with singleton infants ($n = 3021$). Of these, 2279 (75 %) delivered vaginally and 739 (25 %) delivered via c-section.Surgical deliveries included 15 % ($n = 438$) emergency c-sections, and 10 % ($n = 301$) planned c-sections. The mean age of the sample was 32 years (SD: 4.4). The majority of the women in our sample were married, highly educated, Caucasian and born in Canada.

Table 1 Comparison of demographic and labour and delivery characteristics between vaginal deliveries, emergency c-sections and planned c-sections

Characteristic	Full Sample $N = 3021^1$	Vaginal $N = 2279^a$	Emergency c-section $N = 438^a$	Planned c-section $N = 301^a$	*P*-value
	n (%)	*n* (%)	*n* (%)	*n* (%)	
Demographics					
Maternal age at delivery					
Mean (SD)	31.7 (4.4)	31.5 (4.4)	31.8 (4.5)	33.3 (4.4)	< 0.001
Marital status					
Married/Common Law	2855 (95.3)	2150 (95.2)	409 (93.6)	293 (98.7)	0.006
Other	141 (4.7)	109 (4.8)	28 (6.4)	4 (1.3)	
Education					
High school or less	297 (9.9)	222 (9.8)	44 (10.1)	30 (10.1)	0.998
Some or completed university/college	2233 (74.5)	1683 (74.5)	327 (74.8)	222 (74.5)	
Some or completed grad school	467 (15.6)	354 (15.7)	66 (15.1)	46 (15.4)	
Ethnicity					
Caucasian	2385 (79.6)	1822 (80.6)	327 (75.0)	233 (78.7)	0.026
Non-Caucasian	610 (20.4)	438 (19.4)	109 (25.0)	63 (21.3)	
Income					
< $60,000	471 (16.2)	352 (16.1)	80 (18.8)	39 (13.6)	0.164
≥ $60,000	2434 (83.8)	1838 (83.9)	345 (81.2)	248 (86.4)	
Born in Canada					
Yes	2368 (78.9)	1809 (80.0)	323 (73.9)	233 (78.2)	0.017
No	632 (21.1)	453 (20.0)	114 (26.1)	65 (21.8)	
Labour and delivery					
Parity					
No previous births	1458 (48.9)	1094 (48.6)	304 (69.9)	60 (20.3)	< 0.001
≥1 previous birth	1524 (51.1)	1155 (51.4)	131 (30.1)	235 (79.7)	
Gestational age					
< 37 weeks	211 (7.0)	146 (6.5)	55 (12.7)	10 (3.4)	< 0.001
≥ 37 weeks	2784 (93.0)	2117 (93.5)	379 (87.3)	285 (96.6)	
Small for gestational age[b]					
Yes	300 (10.6)	227 (10.5)	51 (12.6)	22 (8.0)	0.152
No	2537 (89.4)	1927 (89.5)	353 (87.4)	254 (92.0)	

[a]Due to missing values, the denominator changes across variables
[b]Small for Gestational Age defined as <10th percentile for weight-for-gestational age [47]

Significant associations were found across mode of birth compared to parity ($p<0.001$) and gestational age ($p<0.001$). Of the emergency c-section births, approximately 70 % ($n = 304$) were nulliparous compared to 49 % $n = 1094$) of vaginal births and 20 % ($n = 60$) of planned c-sections. Conversely, the majority of women who delivered by planned c-section (80 %, $n = 235$) were multiparous. Although 93 % ($n = 2784$) of the sample delivered at full term (≥ 37 weeks gestation), preterm deliveries were found in 13 % ($n = 55$) of women who delivered by emergency c-section, versus a smaller proportion of vaginal births (6.5 %, $n = 146$) and planned c-section (3.4 %, $n = 10$).

Breastfeeding outcomes according to mode of birth are summarized in Table 2. The majority of the sample, regardless of delivery mode, intended to breastfeed (96 %, $n = 2846$) and initiated breastfeeding (98 %, $n = 2954$). Mode of birth was significantly associated with both planning to breastfeed ($p = 0.003$) and breastfeeding initiation ($p = 0.012$). Women who had a planned c-section, had a higher percentage of those who did not plan to or initiate breastfeeding (7.4 % and 4.3 %, respectively).

Our study found associations between mode of birth and a successful first attempt at breastfeeding ($p<0.001$),

Table 2 Comparison of breastfeeding success and outcomes between vaginal deliveries, emergency c-sections and planned c-sections

Characteristic	Vaginal $N = 2279^{a}$ n (%)	Emergency c-section $N = 438^{a}$ n (%)	Planned c-section $N = 301^{a}$ n (%)	*P*-value
Planned to breastfeed				
Yes	2157 (96.6)	415 (96.3)	274 (92.6)	0.003
No	75 (3.4)	16 (3.7)	22 (7.4)	
Initiated breastfeeding				
Yes	2239 (98.2)	427 (97.5)	288 (95.7)	0.012
No	40 (1.8)	11 (2.5)	13 (4.3)	
Breastfed within 24 h				
Yes	2158(96.9)	392(92.7)	282(97.9)	<0.001
No	69(3.1)	31(7.3)	6(2.1)	
Successful first attempt				
Yes	1677(75.6)	256(60.6)	214(74.3)	<0.001
No	542(24.4)	167(39.4)	74(25.7)	
Successful when leaving hospital				
Yes	1908(90.7)	343(82.7)	263(92.3)	<0.001
No	196(9.3)	72(17.3)	22(7.7)	
Seen LC before leaving hospital				
Yes	862 (40.0)	284 (67.1)	141 (49.3)	<0.001
No	1294 (60.0)	139 (32.9)	145 (50.7)	
Sought additional support after leaving hospital				
Yes	1138 (51.9)	245 (57.8)	117 (40.6)	<0.001
No	1055 (48.1)	179 (42.2)	171 (59.4)	
Difficulties with baby (baby having trouble latching or having a sleepy baby)				
Yes	1016 (44.6)	236 (53.9)	135 (44.9)	0.002
No	1263 (55.4)	202 (46.1)	166 (55.1)	
Discomfort (swollen breasts, sore nipples, or painful breasts)				
Yes	1468 (64.4)	245 (55.9)	182 (60.5)	0.002
No	811 (35.6)	193 (44.1)	119 (39.5)	
Other difficulties (not producing enough milk, flat or inverted nipples)				
Yes	658 (28.9)	180 (41.1)	98 (32.6)	<0.001
No	1621 (71.1)	258 (58.9)	203 (67.4)	

[a]Due to missing values, the denominator changes across variables

breastfeeding within the first 24 h ($p<0.001$), and success with breastfeeding when leaving the hospital ($p<0.001$). Almost 40 % ($n = 167$) of women who had an emergency c-section were unable to successfully breastfeed their baby on the first attempt compared to approximately 25 % of women who either delivered vaginally ($n = 542$) or by planned c-section ($n = n = 74$). A higher proportion of women who delivered by emergency c-section did not successfully breastfeed within the first 24 h of birth (7.3 %, $n = 31$), when compared to vaginal births (3.1 %, $n = 69$) and planned c-sections (2.1 %, $n = 6$). Of the women who had an emergency c-section, 7.3 % ($n = 31$) reported not being able to successfully breastfeed within the first 24 h post delivery, and 17 % ($n = 72$) of the women were less likely to breastfeed prior to being discharged from the hospital.

Of the women who initiated breastfeeding ($n = 2954$), 62 % ($n = 1832$) reported having more than one difficulty with breastfeeding. For the women in our study, there were significant differences across mode of birth and breastfeeding difficulties with baby (e.g., latching or a sleepy baby) ($p = 0.002$), personal discomfort with breastfeeding (e.g., sore nipples, swollen breasts) ($p<0.001$), and other difficulties (e.g., perceived low milk supply or having flat or inverted nipples) ($p<0.001$). More than half of the women (54 %, $n = 236$) who delivered by emergency c-section, reported having had breastfeeding difficulties with baby and 41 % ($n = 180$) had described other difficulties. Conversely, approximately 45 % of women who delivered either vaginally (n=1016) or by planned c-section ($n = 135$) reported difficulties with baby and only around 30 % (vaginally $n = 658$ or planned c-section $n = 98$) reported other difficulties with breastfeeding.

The women in our sample were asked about breastfeeding supports accessed in and out of the hospital. Mode of birth was associated with seeing a lactation consultant in hospital ($p<0.001$) and seeking additional support from a breastfeeding clinic or visiting a health care provider after discharge ($p<0.001$). Approximately 67 % ($n = 284$) of women who delivered by emergency c-section saw a lactation consultant and 58 % ($n = 245$) found additional supportive care after discharge. Conversely, about 41 % ($n = 117$) of women who had a planned c-section sought additional breastfeeding support upon discharge from the hospital.

Eighty-three percent ($n = 2391$) of women were still breastfeeding at >12 weeks postpartum. Women who had an emergency or planned c-section were more likely to have stopped breastfeeding at 12 weeks ($p = 0.02$). A multivariable logistic regression model (Table 3) was created to assess breastfeeding duration up to 12 completed weeks postpartum adjusting for income, education, parity, preterm birth, postpartum maternal physical and mental health, ethnicity and number of breastfeeding difficulties. Using vaginal delivery as the reference group, mode of birth remained a significant independent predictor for breastfeeding cessation at or prior to 12 weeks postpartum ($p = 0.014$).

In an unadjusted analysis, women who delivered by emergency c-section were more likely to discontinue breastfeeding ≤12 weeks postpartum (OR=1.35; 95 % CI: 1.03, 1.76; $p = 0.029$), when compared to those who delivered vaginally; there was no significant difference between planned c-sections and vaginal birth. However, in

Table 3 Unadjusted and adjusted logistic regression model of mode of delivery on breastfeeding duration to 12-weeks postpartum

Independent variable	Unadjusted OR (95 % CI)	Adjusted OR (95 % CI)
Mode of birth[a]		–[b]
Emergency caesarean	1.35 (1.03, 1.76)[b]	1.22 (.91, 1.62)[a]
Planned caesarean	1.33 (0.97, 1.82)[a]	1.61 (1.14, 2.26)[b]
Low income	1.61 (1.25, 2.06)[c]	1.58 (1.19, 2.09)[b]
Lower education	2.14 (1.61, 2.85)[c]	1.82 (1.31, 2.53)[c]
No previous birth	1.38 (1.13, 1.68)[b]	1.42 (1.13, 1.77)[b]
Preterm birth	1.66 (1.18, 2.33)[b]	1.54 (1.06, 2.23)[b]
Maternal physical health	0.96 (0.95, 0.98)[c]	.96 (0.94, 0.98)[c]
Maternal mental health	0.99 (0.98, 1.00)[b]	.99 (0.97, 0.99)[b]
Caucasian	1.49 (1.14, 1.95)[b]	1.67 (1.25, 2.22)[c]
≥ 1Breastfeeding difficulty	2.09 (1.67, 2.61)[c]	1.82 (1.43, 2.31)[c]

[a]≥0.05; [b]<0.05;[c]<0.001
[a]Reference group set as vaginal delivery

the adjusted multivariable logistic regression model (Table 3), women who had a planned c-section were more likely to have early cessation of breastfeeding (≤12 weeks) (OR=1.61; 95 % CI: 1.14, 2.26; $p = 0.006$) when compared to those who delivered vaginally. There was no significant difference in breastfeeding cessation between women who had an emergency c-section and women who delivered vaginally in the adjusted analysis. Covariate patterns and resulting confounding structure in the multivariable model explains the change in magnitude of the effect estimates and the reversal in the association between the levels of exposure in mode of birth in the unadjusted versus adjusted analysis. An important confounder in the adjusted model was parity as it was strongly associated with both early breastfeeding cessation and mode of birth (Table 1 and Table 3); a significantly higher proportion of multiparous women were found among those who delivered by planned c-section (80 %, $n = 235$), compared to vaginal (51 %, $n = 1155$)) or emergency deliveries (30 %, n=131) (p<0.0001).

Discussion

Our findings demonstrate that planned c-sections are associated with reduced breastfeeding success in the first 4 postpartum months, when compared to vaginal births. In particular, we have successfully added to the growing evidence that planned c-sections negatively affect breastfeeding initiation and duration.

All of the Calgary area hospitals support breastfeeding but may not have a specific breastfeeding protocol instituted, nor are they BFI accredited. Each hospital in Calgary has a lactation consultant and post discharge breastfeeding resources with physician and nursing support available. In our study, women who delivered via c-section were more likely to report breastfeeding difficulties when compared to women having had vaginal deliveries. Brown and Jordan (2013) found similar findings; women in their study who delivered via c-section also had more problems with latching, positioning and more pain when compared to those women with vaginal birth [33].

In our study, women who had an emergency c-section were more likely to have had an unsuccessful first breastfeeding attempt, were unable to breastfed their baby within the first 24 h, and were unable to breastfeed upon leaving the hospital. Zanardo et al. (2010) found similar results, reporting that women who delivered via emergency c-section were more likely not to have been able to breastfeed their baby at delivery or at discharge [39]. It has been hypothesized that the maternal and fetal stress response associated with complications during delivery, particularly related to c-sections, may be related to increased difficulty and early cessation in breastfeeding during the early postpartum period [14, 33]. Lactogenesis may be equally affected by the insult of abdominal surgery in both planned and emergency c-sections, although the notion of an "emergency" may invoke a greater or prolonged maternal stress response.

Our data showed that women with planned c-sections were more likely to indicate they did not intend to breastfeed and therefore did not initiate it compared to those with other delivery modes. This concurs with a large meta-analysis that found an association between a lower likelihood of initiation of breastfeeding and planned c-sections [31]. Although our study did not analyze maternal or medical reasons for planned c-section, reasons for planned c-section coupled with no intention to breastfeed should be explored given that the rate of planned c-sections has been rising since the year 2000 [1, 28]. The Canadian Maternity Experiences Survey in 2008 reported that of all 6,421 women who completed the survey, 26 % delivered by c-section and 13.5 % of all c-sections were planned [29]. Of those planned c-sections, the majority (86.9 %) were planned for medically indicated reasons [29]. The Canadian Perinatal Surveillance System acknowledged that c-section rates are increasing and recognize that c-sections on maternal request could be part of this growing burden [21]. However, a study by Hutton and Kornelsen (2012) found that in British Columbia, one of the provinces with the highest rates of c-section delivery, very few women requested c-sections with no medical indication and concluded that the increased rate of c-section delivery in Canada may not be related to maternal choice [40]. Similarly, a review of 17 articles on the topic of maternal decision making found that only a small portion of women requested c-sections for non-medically indicated reasons in each study [41]. However, the studies included in this review were susceptible to a high risk of bias due to small sample sizes, warranting further studies specifically investigating maternal decision making surrounding requested c-section deliveries for non-medical indication.

Lower breastfeeding initiation and increased difficulties with breastfeeding in women with c-section deliveries may be related to a physiologic influence on lactogenesis [42, 43]. A study by Evans et al. (2003) found that breast milk transfer among women with c-sections was significantly lower in the first 5 days postpartum, compared to women with vaginal births [42]. Similarly, Scott and Binns (2007) found that delayed onset of lactation was significantly higher in mothers that delivered via c-section compared to those that delivered vaginally [43]. It is postulated that the hormonal pathway that stimulates lactogenesis is disrupted by c-section delivery, either from maternal stress or decreased oxytocin secretion, and can hinder milk production [34, 39, 42, 44]. Late preterm infants, those born between 34 and 36 6/7 weeks gestation, often have a multitude of issues including disorganized sucking skills, lower birth weight and low level of alertness, all of which can adversely affect breastfeeding initiation [34, 45]. Since planned c-sections are performed prior to the onset of labour and before 40 weeks gestation, it is possible that physiological reasons are responsible for the decreased likelihood or troubled breastfeeding initiation. In response, the American College of Obstetricians and Gynecologists (2013) recommended that c-sections performed prior to onset of labour should not be conducted prior to 39 weeks unless medically indicated [46].

When controlling for other variables potentially associated with breastfeeding, we found that planned c- section predicts early breastfeeding cessation, defined as weaning at or prior to 12 weeks. Although Zanardo et al. (2013) found that c-section delivery was associated with lower rates of exclusive breastfeeding at 6 months, no difference between planned versus emergency c-sections was found [19]. Women who had planned c-sections in our study were less likely to intend to breastfeed or initiate breastfeeding, and less likely to seek lactation support. Although we controlled for parity in our multivariable model, the bivariate associations with mode of birth and breastfeeding intention and initiation may be related to the other factors such as variable infant feeding choices or return to work. Multiparous women may have had a previous challenging breastfeeding experience and chose not to breastfeed. Previous breastfeeding experiences in women are known to impact future decisions surrounding breastfeeding. Although this study did not look at prior experiences with breastfeeding, women who have had difficult breastfeeding experiences with prior births may require particular attention to promote future positive breastfeeding experiences. More targeted interventions towards women planning on c-section delivery from the perinatal period and into the postpartum time, may encourage breastfeeding initiation and continuation of breastfeeding.

As our study found that women who have emergency c-sections were more likely to have difficulties with breastfeeding and to seek additional lactation support, focused education surrounding breastfeeding techniques and encouragement to these mothers could be given immediately post birth in order to provide the appropriate anticipatory guidance to reduce difficulties. In Canada, there are few hospitals that have breastfeeding practices that adhere to these standards set by the BFI. We recommend that health care professionals should be aware that those women who have delivered via c-section may require more supportive care immediately post-delivery and in the early postpartum period. In particular, our study identified that those who delivered via emergency c-section may require access to lactation consultation and other supports for breastfeeding. These supports could be made available in the immediate post-partum period in order to encourage breastfeeding within 1 h post birth and ensure successful breastfeeding within the first 24 h, as recommended by the BFI and many research studies as being indicative of long term breastfeeding success [15–17]. As women who delivered via emergency c-section were more likely not to have successfully breastfed before leaving the hospital, the postpartum home visit presents an ideal opportunity to provide additional breastfeeding assessments and support to overcome any difficulties for these women.

Limitations

Our study reflects the demographics of urban Calgary (predominately caucasion, highly educated and of a higher SES); however, generalizability to other populations should be interpreted with this in mind. Due to the nature of the questionnaire, the outcome variable in this study looked at maternal self-reports of any breastfeeding and did not explore the relationship between mode of birth and exclusive breastfeeding. As the majority of the variables used in these analyses were assessed via questionnaire at 4 months, we were unable to assess variations in health status over the entire postpartum period. It would be interesting to further explore how variations in maternal physical or mental health are associated with each mode of birth and if there is a relationship with breastfeeding. Additionally, there could be some residual confounding related to the obstetric factors that we were unable to control for given content contained in the questionnaire. In particular, further analysis, through medical chart review, looking at how the complications during labour and delivery could impact and possibly confound the relationship between mode of birth and breastfeeding success and duration. Since mode of birth was based on maternal self-report, it is possible that there was misclassification between emergency and planned deliveries. However, a recent validation study conducted by the AOB confirmed that maternal recall of delivery method (vaginal, emergency c-section, or planned c-section) was high when compared to electronic medical chart records [37]. Also, this study did not distinguish between the type of vaginal birth (assisted versus spontaneous), and some instrumental deliveries can be challenging. This would attenuate responses and underestimate the positive effect that an uncomplicated vaginal delivery has on breastfeeding initiation, and duration.

Conclusion

Our study suggests that c-sections are associated with more breastfeeding difficulties, greater use of resources, and shorter breastfeeding duration compared to vaginal deliveries. Planned c-sections coupled with no intention of breastfeeding may be an emerging trend among women that requires further exploration. As planned c-section delivery may be associated with lower intention to and initiate breastfeeding as well as early cessation of breastfeeding, health care provider support and counselling in order to provide anticipatory guidance surrounding breastfeeding could be given prenatally to pregnant mothers and families considering a planned c-section. As well, additional supportive care made available to lactating women with emergency c-sections during the immediate to early postpartum period would be recommended in order to ensure early success with breastfeeding.

Abbreviations

AOB: all our babies; c-section: caesarean section; WHO: World Health Organization.

Competing interests

The authors declare that they have no competing interests.

Authors' contributions

SCT is responsible for the overall integrity, progress, questionnaire development and timely completion of the AOB study. AJH, CAM and SWM were responsible in the design for this study. AJH and MB performed the literature review. SWM performed the statistical analysis. AJH drafted and revised the manuscript. All authors contributed to data interpretation, read and approved the final manuscript.

Acknowledgements

We are extremely grateful to the participants involved in the All Our Babies cohort, and to the All Our Babies staff and research team. We are extremely grateful to the investigators, co-ordinators, research assistants, graduate and undergraduate students, volunteers, clerical staff, and managers. The University of Calgary has provided trainee salary support. Alberta Innovates Health Solutions provided funding towards this cohort and salary support for Suzanne Tough.

Author details

[1]Cumming School of Medicine, Department of Community Health Sciences, University of Calgary, TRW Building 3rd Floor, 3280 Hospital Drive NW, Calgary, Alberta T2N 4Z6, Canada. [2]Faculty of Nursing, University of Calgary, 2800 University Way NW, Calgary, AB T2N1N4, Canada. [3]Cumming School of Medicine, Department of Paediatrics, University of Calgary, 2888 Shaganappi Trail NW, Calgary, Alberta T3B 6A8, Canada.

References

1. Canadian Institutes for Health Information. Health Indicators 2013. Ottawa: CIHI; 2013.
2. Monitoring emergency obstetric care: A handbook, World Health Organization. Monitoring emergency obstetric care: A handbook. Geneva: World Health Organization; 2009.
3. McDonald SD, Pullenayegum E, Chapman B, Vera C, Giglia L, Fusch C, Foster G. Prevalence and predictors of exclusive breastfeeding at hospital discharge. Obstetrics Gynecology. 2012;119(6):1171–9.
4. Zhou YB, Li HT, Zhu LP, Liu JM. Impact of cesarean section on placental transfusion and iron-related hematological indices in term neonates: a systematic review and meta-analysis. Placenta. 2014;35(1):1–8.
5. Bodner K, Wierrani F, Grunberger W, Bodner-Adler B. Influence of the mode of delivery on maternal and neonatal outcomes: a comparison between elective cesarean section and planned vaginal delivery in a low-risk obstetric population. Arch Gynecol Obstet. 2011;283(6):1193–8.
6. Wax JR. Maternal request cesarean versus planned spontaneous vaginal delivery: maternal morbidity and short term outcomes. Semin Perinatol. 2006;30(5):247–52.
7. Karlstrom A, Lindgren H, Hildingsson I. Maternal and infant outcome after caesarean section without recorded medical indication: findings from a Swedish case-control study. BJOG. 2013;120(4):479–86. discussion 486.
8. Rowe-Murray HJ, Fisher JRW. Baby friendly hospital practices: cesarean section is a persistent barrier to early initiation of breastfeeding. Birth (Berkeley, Calif). 2002;29(2):124–31.
9. Chapman DJ, Perez-Escamilla R. Identification of risk factors for delayed onset of lactation. J Am Diet Assoc. 1999;99(4):450–4. quiz 455-456.
10. Dewey KG, Nommsen-Rivers LA, Heinig MJ, Cohen RJ. Risk factors for suboptimal infant breastfeeding behavior, delayed onset of lactation, and excess neonatal weight loss. Pediatrics. 2003;112(3 Pt 1):607–19.
11. Lawson K, Tulloch MI. Breastfeeding duration: prenatal intentions and postnatal practices. J Adv Nurs. 1995;22(5):841–9.
12. Patel RR, Liebling RE, Murphy DJ. Effect of operative delivery in the second stage of labor on breastfeeding success. Birth (Berkeley, Calif). 2003;30(4):255–60.
13. Regan J, Thompson A, DeFranco E. The influence of mode of delivery on breastfeeding initiation in women with a prior cesarean delivery: a population-based study. Breastfeeding Med. 2013;8:181–6.
14. Watt S, Sword W, Sheehan D, Foster G, Thabane L, Krueger P, Landy CK. The effect of delivery method on breastfeeding initiation from the The Ontario Mother and Infant Study (TOMIS) III. J Obstetric Gynecol Neonatal Nursing. 2012;41(6):728–37.
15. Meedya S, Fahy K, Kable A. Factors that positively influence breastfeeding duration to 6 months: a literature review. Women Birth. 2010;23(4):135–45.
16. World Health Organization. Baby-Friendly Hospital Initiative: Revised, updated and expanded for integrated care. Section 1: Background and implementation. Geneva: United Nations Children's Fund; 2009.
17. Fund UNC's. Global Strategy for Infant and Young Child Feeding. Geneva: World Health Oganization; 2003.
18. Moore ER, Anderson GC, Bergman N, Dowswell T. Early skin-to-skin contact for mothers and their healthy newborn infants. Cochrane Database Syst Rev. 2012;5:CD003519.
19. Zanardo V, Pigozzo A, Wainer G, Marchesoni D, Gasparoni A, Di Fabio S, Cavallin F, Giustardi A, Trevisanuto D. Early lactation failure and formula adoption after elective caesarean delivery: cohort study. Archives Disease Childhood Fetal Neonatal Edition. 2013;98(1):F37–41.
20. Pérez-Ríos N, Ramos-Valencia G, Ortiz AP. Cesarean delivery as a barrier for breastfeeding initiation: the Puerto Rican experience. J Hum Lact. 2008;24(3):293–302.
21. Chalmers B, Kaczorowski J, Darling E, Heaman M, Fell DB, O'Brien B, Lee L. Maternity Experiences Study Group of the Canadian Perinatal Surveillance S:

Cesarean and vaginal birth in canadian women: a comparison of experiences. Birth (Berkeley, Calif). 2010;37(1):44–9.
22. Ahluwalia IB, Li R, Morrow B. Breastfeeding practices: does method of delivery matter? Maternal Child Health J. 2012;16 Suppl 2:231–7.
23. MacMullen NJ, Dulski LA. Factors related to sucking ability in healthy newborns. J Obstetric Gynecol Neonatal Nursing. 2000;29(4):390–6.
24. Horta BL, Bahl R, Martines JC, Victora CG: Evidence on the long-term effects of breastfeeding: Systematic reviews and meta-analyses. In. Geneva, Switzerland: World Health Organization; 2007.
25. Victora CG, Horta BL, Loret de Mola C, Quevedo L, Pinheiro RT, Gigante DP, Goncalves H, Barros FC. Association between breastfeeding and intelligence, educational attainment, and income at 30 years of age: a prospective birth cohort study from Brazil. Lancet Glob Health. 2015;3(4):e199–205.
26. Ip S, Chung M, Raman G, Chew P, Magula N, DeVine D, Trikalinos T, Lau J: Breastfeeding and maternal and infant health outcomes in developed countries. Evid Rep Technol Assess (Full Rep) 2007(153):1-186. http://www.ncbi.nlm.nih.gov/pubmed/17764214.
27. Infant Feeding: Food and Nutrition. http://www.hc-sc.gc.ca/fn-an/nutrition/infant-nourisson/index-eng.php. Accessed on 31 July 2013.
28. Public Health Agency of Canada. Perinatal Health Indicators for Canada 2013: A Report of the Canadian Perinatal Surveillance System. In. Ottawa; 2013
29. Public Health Agency of Canada. Canadian Perinatal Health Report. Ottawa: Canadian Perinatal Surveillance System; 2008.
30. Venter K: The Baby-Friendly Initiative (BFI) in Canada: Status Update. In. Edited by Canada BCf. Drayton Valley, AB. Canada:; 2012.
31. Prior E, Santhakumaran S, Gale C, Philipps LH, Modi N, Hyde MJ. Breastfeeding after cesarean delivery: a systematic review and meta-analysis of world literature. Am J Clin Nutrition. 2012;95(5):1113–35.
32. Pérez-Escamilla R, Maulén-Radovan I, Dewey KG. The association between cesarean delivery and breast-feeding outcomes among Mexican women. Am J Public Health. 1996;86(6):832–6.
33. Brown A, Jordan S. Impact of birth complications on breastfeeding duration: an internet survey. J Adv Nurs. 2013;69(4):828–39.
34. Riordan J, Wambach K. Breastfeeding and human lactation. 4th ed. Sudbury: Mass.: Jones and Bartlett Publishers; 2010.
35. DiGirolamo AM, Grummer-Strawn LM, Fein SB. Effect of maternity-care practices on breastfeeding. Pediatrics. 2008;122:S43–49.
36. McDonald SW, Lyon AW, Benzies KM, McNeil DA, Lye SJ, Dolan SM, Pennell CE, Bocking AD, Tough SC. The All Our Babies pregnancy cohort: design, methods, and participant characteristics. BMC Pregnancy Childbirth. 2013;13(1):S2.
37. Bat-Erdene U, Metcalfe A, McDonald SW, Tough SC. Validation of Canadian mothers' recall of events in labour and delivery with electronic health records. BMC Pregnancy Childbirth. 2013;13(1):S3.
38. von Elm E, Altman DG, Egger M, Pocock SJ, Gotzsche PC, Vandenbroucke JP: The Strengthening the Reporting of Observational Studies in Epidemiology (STROBE) statement: guidelines for reporting observational studies. Lancet (London, England) 2007;370(9596):1453–57.
39. Zanardo V, Svegliado G, Cavallin F, Giustardi A, Cosmi E, Litta P, Trevisanuto D. Elective cesarean delivery: does it have a negative effect on breastfeeding? Birth (Berkeley, Calif). 2010;37(4):275–9.
40. Hutton EK, Kornelsen J. Patient-Initiated Elective Cesarean Section of Nulliparous Women in British Columbia, Canada. Birth (Berkeley, Calif). 2012; 39(3):175–82.
41. McCourt C, Weaver J, Statham H, Beake S, Gamble J, Creedy DK. Elective cesarean section and decision making: a critical review of the literature. Birth (Berkeley, Calif). 2007;34(1):65–79.
42. Evans KC, Evans RG, Royal R, Esterman AJ, James SL. Effect of caesarean section on breast milk transfer to the normal term newborn over the first week of life. Arch Dis Child Fetal Neonatal Ed. 2003;88(5):F380–2.
43. Scott JA, Binns CW, Oddy WH. Predictors of delayed onset of lactation. Matern Child Nutr. 2007;3(3):186–93.
44. Hyde MJ, Mostyn A, Modi N, Kemp PR. The health implications of birth by Caesarean section. Biol Rev. 2012;87(1):229–43.
45. Radtke JV. The paradox of breastfeeding-associated morbidity among late preterm infants. J Obstetric Gynecologic Neonatal Nursing. 2011;40(1):9–24.
46. Carlander AK, Edman G, Christensson K, Andolf E, Wiklund I. Contact between mother, child and partner and attitudes towards breastfeeding in relation to mode of delivery. Sex Reprod Healthc. 2010;1(1):27–34.
47. Battaglia FC, Lubchenco LO. A practical classification of newborn infants by weight and gestational age. J Pediatr. 1967;71(2):159–63.

Definitions, measurements and prevalence of fear of childbirth

C. Nilsson[1,2*], E. Hessman[3], H. Sjöblom[3], A. Dencker[2], E. Jangsten[2], M. Mollberg[2], H. Patel[2], C. Sparud-Lundin[2], H. Wigert[2] and C. Begley[4,2]

Abstract

Background: Fear of Childbirth (FOC) is a common problem affecting women's health and wellbeing, and a common reason for requesting caesarean section. The aims of this review were to summarise published research on prevalence of FOC in childbearing women and how it is defined and measured during pregnancy and postpartum, and to search for useful measures of FOC, for research as well as for clinical settings.

Methods: Five bibliographic databases in March 2015 were searched for published research on FOC, using a protocol agreed a priori. The quality of selected studies was assessed independently by pairs of authors. Prevalence data, definitions and methods of measurement were extracted independently from each included study by pairs of authors. Finally, some of the country rates were combined and compared.

Results: In total, 12,188 citations were identified and screened by title and abstract; 11,698 were excluded and full-text of 490 assessed for analysis. Of these, 466 were excluded leaving 24 papers included in the review, presenting prevalence of FOC from nine countries in Europe, Australia, Canada and the United States. Various definitions and measurements of FOC were used. The most frequently-used scale was the W-DEQ with various cut-off points describing moderate, severe/intense and extreme/phobic fear. Different 3-, 4-, and 5/6 point scales and visual analogue scales were also used. Country rates (as measured by seven studies using W-DEQ with ≥85 cut-off point) varied from 6.3 to 14.8%, a significant difference (chi-square = 104.44, d.f. = 6, $p < 0.0001$).

Conclusions: Rates of severe FOC, measured in the same way, varied in different countries. Reasons why FOC might differ are unknown, and further research is necessary. Future studies on FOC should use the W-DEQ tool with a cut-off point of ≥85, or a more thoroughly tested version of the FOBS scale, or a three-point scale measurement of FOC using a single question as 'Are you afraid about the birth?' In this way, valid comparisons in research can be made. Moreover, validation of a clinical tool that is more focussed on FOC alone, and easier than the longer W-DEQ, for women to fill in and clinicians to administer, is required.

Keywords: Fear of childbirth, Systematic review, Prevalence, W-DEQ, FOBS, Request for caesarean section

Background

Being pregnant and giving birth are described as a transition phase, or an existential threshold that childbearing women have to cross [1]. Childbirth is an experience with many dimensions, multifaceted and unique for each woman, still strongly influenced by her social context [2]. Women's expectations and experiences of pregnancy and birth are both positive and negative in nature, involving feelings of joy and faith but also worries, anxiety and fears. Despite the fact that maternity care in high income countries is safe, fear of childbirth is a common problem affecting women's health and wellbeing before and during pregnancy, as well as after childbirth. Fear of childbirth has consequences for women's relationships with their baby, partner and family [3], and often leads to requests for caesarean section (CS) by women striving for control in an exposed situation [4–7].

During the last few decades there has been a growing research interest in women's fear of childbirth. For some

* Correspondence: christina.nilsson@hb.se
[1]Faculty of Caring Science, Work Life and Social Welfare, University of Borås, S-501 90 Borås, Sweden
[2]Institute of Health and Care Sciences, The Sahlgrenska Academy at University of Gothenburg, Box 457, -405 30 Gothenburg, SE, Sweden
Full list of author information is available at the end of the article

women, the fear only relates to childbirth, but for others fear occurs in relation to other types of anxiety also [3, 8]. Fear of parturition is not new, and was described by the French psychiatrist Louis Victor Marcé (1858) [9]. The term 'fear of childbirth' (FOC) was characterised in 1981 in a population of Swedish pregnant women, defined as: "a strong anxiety which had impaired their [the women's] daily functioning and wellbeing" [10, p. 265]. In addition, a more moderate fear was described as a significant anxiety, which did not interfere with the women's daily life [10]. Later, during the 1990s, studies from Finland defined FOC as a health issue for a pregnant woman related to an anxiety disorder or a phobic fear including physical complications, nightmares and concentration problems, as well as demands for caesarean section [11]. The term 'clinical FOC' describes a "disabling fear that interferes with occupational and domestic functioning, as well as social activities and relationships", and in some cases even reaches the classification for a specific phobia according to the DSM IV [3, p. 141]. The label "tokophobia" is also used [12, 13], characterised as an "unreasoning dread of childbirth" in women, a "specific and harrowing condition" [12, p. 83] including a "pathological dread" and "avoidance of childbirth" [13, p. 506]. Moreover, FOC is strongly related to the increasing caesarean section (CS) rates in Western countries, as being a common cause for women requesting a surgical birth [14, 15].

In early studies, the prevalence of FOC for pregnant women in Scandinavia was reported as 20%, with approximately 5–10% women experiencing intense fear [10]. The prevalence in Europe seems to vary between countries, from 1.9–14% [16], while Australia indicates higher rates of around 30% [17], leaving questions on possible cultural differences in FOC, or differing definitions. However, the variations in prevalence can also depend on the measures used; these can vary from fear being self-defined by women, or self-reported via different questionnaires, or estimated through measurement of physiological indices such as stress hormones in childbirth [3, 18, 19].

For women lacking experience of childbirth (so called primary tokophobia or FOC), their fears may date from adolescence or early adulthood, where experiences of others' fearful responses to childbirth or a history of anxiety disorders could be important [8, 12, 13]. Secondary tokophobia or FOC is related to the event of birth, and is usually linked to fears developed after a previous negative or traumatic experience of childbirth, sometimes related to posttraumatic stress disorder (PTSD) [3, 8, 11–13]. Tokophobia is also described as a symptom of prenatal depression [12, 13]. However, the research on FOC has been criticised for constructing women's fear as a medical category, having too pathological an approach that searches for errors in women, instead of examining possible causes of women's fear within maternity care itself [20, 21].

To summarise, the research field is extensive, complex, and difficult to survey without any consensus on definitions. The concept "fear of childbirth" seems to be used as a broad label for all kinds of anxiety and fears that women experience in relation to pregnancy and childbirth. Relevant questions are: How common is FOC? Are there any cross cultural differences? Which measures are pertinent? What is FOC? There is a need for systematic reviews on FOC to be able to direct future research on developing optimal care and effective treatment for women fearing childbirth and to identify factors that reduce, as well as increase, women's fears. Therefore, as a first step, we conducted a systematic review of all studies demonstrating a prevalence of FOC. The aims of this review were to identify the prevalence of FOC in childbearing women and how it is defined and measured during pregnancy and postpartum, and to search for useful measures of FOC, for research as well as for clinical settings.

Methods

Inclusion criteria

Types of participants

Participants were childbearing women (defined as the period covering pregnancy, labour and birth, and the first year postpartum).

Types of studies

Surveys, cross-sectional studies, experimental and quasi-experimental studies (where the control group could provide data), observational studies, systematic reviews, and meta-analyses, were eligible for inclusion.

Types of outcome

The primary outcome was prevalence of fear of childbirth, where this was defined clearly by study authors. Papers measuring fear during labour were excluded. Many studies used the same population (i.e., a number of PhD students accessed the same population at the same time and conducted different studies, but reported the same prevalence). We only included studies that were the first to report prevalence in a population and at similar time points. Studies reporting the same prevalence, on the same population or on a sub-sample (less representative, were excluded.

Search and selection strategy

A search strategy was developed and reviewed for accuracy, by one member not involved in its development (CS-L), using the Peer Review of Electronic Search Strategies (PRESS) criteria [22]. No restrictions were applied to years searched, but papers included were limited to English and Swedish publications only. We searched electronic bibliographic databases of The Cochrane Library, PubMed, Scopus, PsycINFO and CINAHL from their inception dates, in March 2015, using the agreed search strategy as described in Additional file 1.

Selection of studies

Studies were selected for inclusion from the papers identified, by team members working in pairs, using the above criteria. Any disagreements were resolved by a third member.

Quality assessment of included studies

The Effective Public Health Practice Project (EPHPP) quality assessment tool [23] was chosen to assess methodological quality of all studies included. Components of study design and methods assessed by this tool include selection and allocation bias, confounding, blinding, methods of data collection, withdrawals/drop-outs and analysis and intervention integrity. As some dimensions of the EPHPP (e.g. the sections on confounding and intervention integrity) are not relevant for reviews of non-intervention studies, the tool did have some shortcomings. For example, following discussion, it was agreed by the team to rate all cross-sectional studies (single cohort) as moderate, to avoid studies of otherwise good quality being excluded. Despite these problems, the tool was useful, especially for identifying 'Weak' experimental studies and excluding them. An overall quality rating was assigned to each study following assessment, of Strong (where no weak ratings were assigned), Moderate (one weak rating) or Weak (two or more weak ratings). An a priori decision was made that studies receiving a 'Weak' global rating score would be excluded from analysis. Team members in pairs assessed the quality of included studies. Any disagreements were discussed and resolved by consensus, or by a third member of the review team if necessary. In addition, as one of the team-members was co-author in some of the studies, those were assessed by other members of the review team.

Data extraction and analysis

Using a pre-designed data extraction form, data on prevalence, definitions and measurements were extracted independently by each member of the four review teams and checked for accuracy by the other reviewer.

Due to the differing types of studies, it was seldom possible to combine results into a meta-analysis. A narrative synthesis was provided instead.

Results

Results of search and selection strategy

In total, 18,464 citations were identified using the search strategy designed. After removing duplicates, 12,188 unique citations were screened by title and abstract and 11,698 excluded. Full-text papers of the remaining 490 citations were read and 354 of these were subsequently excluded, leaving 136 for inclusion (Fig. 1).

Methodological quality of included studies

The 136 papers were assessed and 76 were rated as "Weak", and therefore excluded. The main reasons for "Weak" ratings were that the samples were unlikely to be representative of the population and the data collection tools were either not tested for validity, or there was insufficient information on their testing. This resulted in 60 papers meeting the inclusion criteria for this review (Fig. 1). At data extraction stage, however, it was clear that, for nine of the papers, no prevalence data could be identified [24–32], for six others, the whole sample of women had FOC [33–38], 11 papers were qualitative [39–49], and 10 papers had double reporting or reported the prevalence of a subsample of a population already included in the review [50–59]; these were excluded leaving a total of 24 papers for inclusion, based on data from 23 study populations (two papers [60, 61] presented FOC during pregnancy and postpartum, based on the same population) (Fig. 1 and Table 1). Thirteen of these had been rated as methodologically "Strong" and 11 were rated as "Moderate" (Table 1).

Description of studies

The studies had been conducted in twelve countries, with Sweden emerging as the country with the most research into FOC (Table 1). Ten papers (reporting on nine studies) were from Sweden (one of which also included a cohort of women from Australia), two from Norway, four from Finland, two from Denmark, two from the United States of America, and one each from Canada, Australia, Switzerland, and Croatia. One study had included data from six countries: Belgium, Norway, Iceland, Denmark, Estonia, and Sweden [62]. The majority (n = 20) had collected data using either postal or self-completed and personally returned surveys, one in the post-natal period, 16 in the antenatal period and six at both time periods. Two studies used telephone interviews, one in the third trimester of pregnancy and 1 month after birth [63] and the second in early and late pregnancy [64]. One study used a randomised controlled trial methodology and we used the data from the population screened by W-DEQ to identify FOC in early pregnancy, prior to trial entry [65].

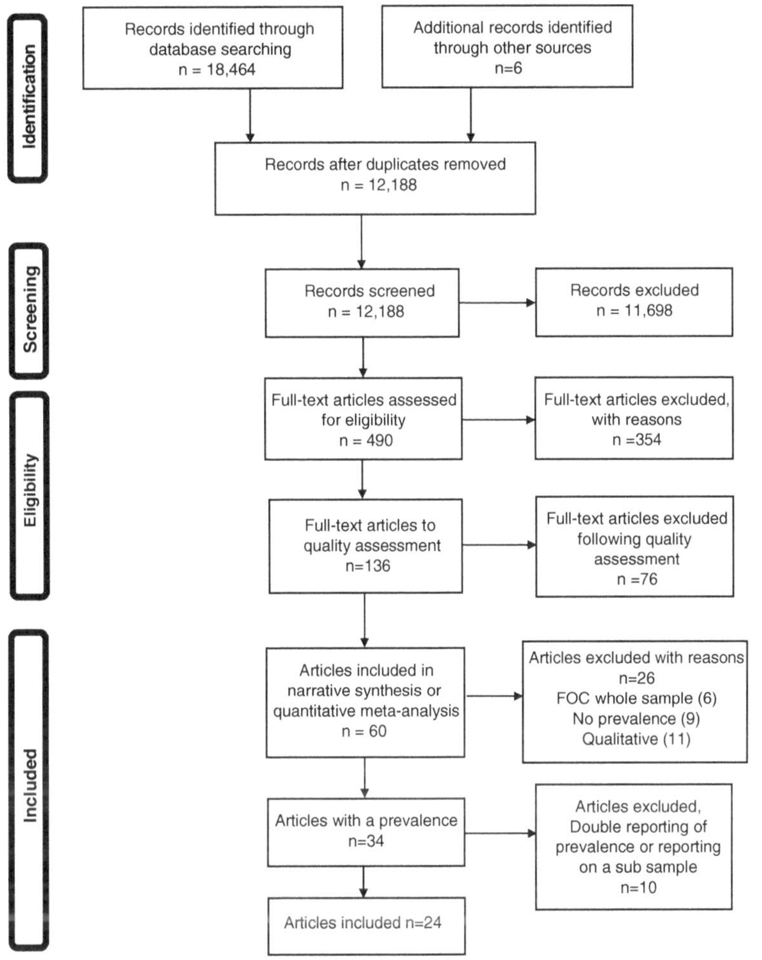

Fig. 1 Prisma flow chart Single file. Prisma flow-diagram of the search and selection process

One study [66] used a retrospective analysis of a national database to gather data on FOC, defined according to ICD code 099.80 (Table 1). Sample sizes ranged from 200 to 788,317.

Eight papers were published based on studies using the same population, with surveys administered at four time-points, and care has been taken to ensure that rates have not been double-counted. Of these eight papers we only included three [60, 61, 67]; the others were excluded due to repeated prevalence reporting or because they reported on a subsample of a previously reported population [50–54]. Hildingsson et al. 2010 [60] included 1212 women and presented the results for FOC in mid-pregnancy, and Nilsson et al. [61] used the same sample, but presented the results for FOC in women 1 year after birth (n = 763). Haines et al. [67] took a subset of 386 women from the full population, who had attended one regional hospital, and recruited 122 Australian women also. As a VAS was used for the response format, these results are presented separately and are not merged with any other.

Definitions and measurements of FOC used by included studies

Eleven papers used the W-DEQ questionnaire, an instrument specifically designed to measure fear of labour and birth (Table 2). It consists of a 33-item questionnaire, and can be scored from 0 to 165 [68]. Various different cut-off points are used to define 'severe fear of birth,' from scores of '66 or greater' to 'greater than 100,' which makes comparison of prevalence difficult.

The authors of two papers [64, 69] used a 3-point scale to measure fear/anxiety about birth, in answer to similar questions relating to FOC (Table 2). The three response options were variously expressed as: "no, I am not afraid/not at all;" "yes, I am a bit afraid/yes, a little;" "yes, I am very afraid/yes, a lot," respectively, which were deemed suitable to merge (Table 2). Their

Table 1 Characteristics of included studies on Fear of Childbirth

First author, year of publication [reference number]	EP-HPP rating	Aim of study	Study design	Population	Sample size (response rate, %)	Country
Adams 2012 [80]	S	To assess the association between FOC and duration of labour	Prospective cohort study, using postal survey at 32 weeks	All women scheduled to give birth at a University hospital Nov 2008-April 2010	2206 (63.0)	Norway
Elvander 2013 [63]	M	To estimate the effects of different levels of fear of birth and mode of delivery on birth experience 1 month after birth	Prospective study, using telephone interviews in the third trimester of pregnancy and 1 month after birth	Nulliparous English and Spanish-speaking women aged 18–35, with a single fetus, who birthed >34 weeks', recruited in a variety of ways, in 2009–2011	3005 (NA) Number eligible not mentioned	USA
Eriksson 2005 [71]	S	To investigate and compare experiential factors associated with childbirth-related fear in women (and men)	Cross-sectional observational study, using postal survey 14–26 months postnatal. FOC was assessed retrospectively	All women who had a baby in a University hospital, March 1997–March 1998	410 (73.5)	Sweden
Fabian 2004 [73]	M	To investigate the attendance rate at childbirth and parenthood education classes // and describe the characteristics of women who did not attend	Cohort study using a postal questionnaire in early pregnancy and at 2 months postpartum	All women attending 97% of all antenatal clinics in Sweden for 1 week in May and September 1999, and January 2000	2546 (55.0)	Sweden
Fenwick 2009 [77]	M	To investigate levels of pre- and postpartum of childbirth fear in a cohort of childbearing women and explore the relationship to birth outcomes	A prospective correlation design using postal surveys at 36 weeks' gestation and 6 weeks' postpartum	All women (English-speaking with a single healthy fetus) attending antenatal clinic at a tertiary hospital, September 2005–March 2006	401 (43.0)	Australia
Geissbuehler 2002 [69]	M	To examine the intensity and type of childbirth fears among pregnant women in the 2nd-3rd trimester // to consider whether birth preparation influences childbirth anxiety	Cross-sectional, self-administered survey in 24th–28th weeks	All women booked to give birth in a large hospital, November 1991–October 1999	8528 (79.1)	Switzerland
Haines 2011 [67]	S	To examine the prevalence of childbirth-related fear (CBRF) in two rural populations (Sweden and Australia) and to pilot a short easy-to-administer tool	Cross-sectional study, using postal survey at 18 weeks gestation	Women undergoing routine ultrasound at 17–19 weeks at a regional Swedish hospital during 2007 and women booked booked at 18–20 weeks in an Australian regional hospital, year not described	509 (NA) (Sweden: $n = 386$ and Australia: $n = 123$) Number eligible not mentioned	Sweden and Australia
Hall 2009 [85]	S	To explore women's levels of childbirth fear, sleep deprivation, anxiety, and fatigue and their relationships during the 3rd trimester of pregnancy	Cross-sectional using surveys at term in a convenience sample at 35–39 weeks	English speaking low-risk women at 35–39 weeks gestation from May 2005–July 2007	650 (NA) Number eligible not mentioned	Canada

Table 1 Characteristics of included studies on Fear of Childbirth *(Continued)*

First author, year of publication [reference number]	EP-HPP rating	Aim of study	Study design	Population	Sample size (response rate, %)	Country
Heimstad 2006 [78]	M	To estimate prevalence of FOC in a defined area in Norway and to study the possible relationship between FOC and psychosocial background, degree of anxiety and abuse	Cross-sectional study, using postal questionnaires at 18–20 weeks	All pregnant women scheduled for a routine ultrasound at a University Hospital, June 2001–August 2002	1452 (54.2)	Norway
Hildingsson 2010 [60]	S	To describe and study background characteristics, feelings and support in relation to thoughts about childbirth in mid-pregnancy	Cross-sectional study, using self-administered surveys at 17–19 weeks	All pregnant women who had a routine ultrasound at three hospitals in one region, year 2007	1212 (51.4)	Sweden
Jespersen 2014 [81]	S	To assess the association between FOC and emergency caesarean section	Prospective cohort study using 2 questionnaires; at 37 weeks gestation and at admission to labour ward	All nulliparous, pregnant low risk women in spontaneous labour at 4 major university hospitals, 3 country hospitals and 2 local district departments, May 2004–July 2005	2598 (71.1)	Denmark
Jokić-Begić 2014 [82]	S	To examine the role of demographic variables, expected pain level, trait anxiety and anxiety sensitivity in FOC among nulliparous and multi-parous women in the last trimester of pregnancy	Cross-sectional/single cohort study using one questionnaire in 8th–9th months of pregnancy	Pregnant women attending at a perinatal clinic at one University hospital in Zagreb, Jan-May 2012	200 (67.6)	Croatia
Laursen 2008 [64]	M	To describe the association between FOC and social, demographics and psychological factors in healthy nulliparous women with uncomplicated pregnancies	Population-based prospective cohort study (pre-post design), using telephone interviews at 16 and 32 weeks	All nulliparous women with uncomplicated pregnancies, 1997–2003	30,480 (approx. 30%)	Denmark
Lowe 2000 [74]	M	To test whether the theoretically predicted inverse relationship between childbirth self-efficacy and fear exists, and to characterize specific personality attributes associated with women who express low or high FOC	Cross-sectional cohort study (secondary analysis), using the Childbirth Attitudes Questionnaire distributed in the third trimester and returned by post	Nulliparous women enrolled in childbirth education classes, year for data collection not described	280 (NA) Number eligible not mentioned	USA
Lukasse 2014 [62]	M	To assess the prevalence of severe FOC and investigate the association between severe FOC and selected background variables	Cohort study, using a self-completed survey in pregnancy at varying times	Pregnant women attending antenatal care in 6 countries between March 2008–August 2010	6870; 828 (B) 585 (I), 1252 (D) 896 (E) 2351 (N) 958 (S)	Belgium, Norway, Iceland, Denmark Estonia Sweden

Table 1 Characteristics of included studies on Fear of Childbirth *(Continued)*

First author, year of publication [reference number]	EP-HPP rating	Aim of study	Study design	Population	Sample size (response rate, %)	Country
					(NA)	
Nieminen 2009 [79]	M	Investigate the prevalence of intense FOC, association between the level of FOC and gestational age, the risk factors for intense FOC in primi and multiparous, and risk factors associated with preference for caesarean section	Cross-sectional, using a self-completed survey in pregnancy	All Swedish speaking primi and multiparous women in four districts, September–October 2006	1635 (98.3)	Sweden
Nilsson 2012 [61]	S	To explore FOC during pregnancy and 1 year after birth and its association with birth experience and mode of birth	A population based prospective longitudinal survey (pre and post design), using postal surveys in mid and late pregnancy, 2 months and 1 year postpartum	All pregnant women who had a routine ultrasound at three hospitals in one region, year 2007 (Same population as in Hildingsson 2010)	763 (86)	Sweden
Poikkeus 2006 [75]	M	To compare the prevalence and predictors of severe FOC and pregnancy related anxiety in groups of assisted reproduction treatment (ART) and spontaneously conceiving women with singleton pregnancies	Prospective longitudinal study with cohort (ART) and matched control (consecutive enrolment) groups, using a self-completed survey at 20 weeks	ART group = 367, and consecutive controls = 379, year 1999	746 (86.6)	Finland
Rouhe 2015 [65]	S	To assess effects of psycho-education versus conventional care during pregnancy in women with FOC	All nulliparous women at time of routine ultrasound at 11–13 weeks. 371 women with severe FOC participated in an RCT using psycho-education as relaxation (6 sessions during pregnancy, one postnatal) and conventional care by community nurses Questionnaires completed twice during pregnancy and/or 3 months postpartum	4575 screened by W-DEQ for severe FOC during routine ultra-sonography at 11–13 weeks. Those with scores >100 were included in the trial, in October 2007–August 2009	4575 (NA) Number eligible not mentioned	Finland
Räisänen 2014 [66]	S	To identify risk factors for FOC and evaluate relation between FOC and adverse perinatal outcomes	Cohort register study, using The Finnish Medical Birth Register, with FOC defined according to ICD – code 099.80	All singleton births during 1997–2010	788,317 (100?)	Finland

Table 1 Characteristics of included studies on Fear of Childbirth *(Continued)*

First author, year of publication [reference number]	EP-HPP rating	Aim of study	Study design	Population	Sample size (response rate, %)	Country
Söderqvist 2004 [83]	S	To investigate association between traumatic stress symptoms and FOC in late pregnancy	Cohort using self-completed survey at week 32	Consecutive recruitment of pregnant women visiting hospital in Kalmar and Linköping, in 1997	951 (48.2)	Sweden
Ternström 2014 [72]	S	To investigate the prevalence of childbirth-related fear in early pregnancy among Swedish and foreign-born women living in Sweden	Cross-sectional study of a total population attending ultrasound screening, using a self-completed questionnaire at 17–20 weeks	University hospital, 615 women screened during routine ultra-sonography, and asked to participate, year not described	606 (96.2)	Sweden
Waldenström 2006 [70]	M	To investigate the prevalence of FOC in a nationwide sample and its association with subsequent rates of CS and overall experience of childbirth	A longitudinal national cohort study, using postal survey at 16 weeks gestation and 2 months postpartum	All pregnant women invited to participate at 16th week gestation and at 2 months postpartum, 3 weeks: May and September 1999 and January 2000	2662 (97.0)	Sweden
Zar 2002 [84]	S	To investigate the prevalence of extreme FOC and anxiety disorders in late pregnancy	Prospective study using postal survey at week 28–30 and interview at 32 weeks	Pregnant women from a country hospital were invited to participate, during 8 months, year not described	506 (82.5)	Sweden

M Moderate, *S* Strong, *EPHPP* Effective Public Health Practice Project, *FOC* Fear Of Childbirth, *CS* Caesarean Section

definition of severe FOC was thus "yes, I am very afraid/yes, a lot." Laursen et al. [64] measured FOC in both early and late pregnancy, but as the other authors, Geissbuehler and Eberhard [69], measured FOC in late pregnancy only, a combination of the late pregnancy rates was made.

A question with a four-point response scale was used in a study of a Swedish population, reported by Hildingsson et al. [60], and Nilsson et al. [61], with all their data coming from the same cohort of women and using similar questions relating to FOC; "to what extent do you experience worries and fear?", With the addition of "when thinking of coming births" in the questionnaire 1 year after birth (Table 2). The authors dichotomised the scale into 'no fear' and 'fear'. 'No fear' was described variously as 'not at all + very little' and 'not at all + somewhat', and 'fear' was described as 'a lot + very much' and 'a great deal + very much' (Table 2).

The remaining papers used a heterogeneous mix of various scales for measurement, none of which could be combined. Elvander et al. [63] graded fear on a 5-point scale, where women answered 6 questions on feeling: 'nervous,' 'worried,' 'fearful,' 'relaxed,' 'terrified,' and 'calm,' in relation to their impending birth. Scores were divided into 3 categories: 6–13 (low fear), 14–20 (intermediate fear) and 21–30 (high fear, their definition of FOC). Waldenström et al. [70] also assessed FOC on a 5-point rating scale using the single question: "How do you feel when thinking about labour and birth?" Women ticking the "very negative" response alternative were defined as having childbirth related fear. Eriksson et al. [71] graded fear on a 6-point scale, from "no fear at all" to "very high fear." Intense fear was defined as four or above and agreement with the statement that "childbirth-related fear influences your daily life in a negative sense" (Table 2).

Two studies [67, 72] used the Fear of Birth (FOBS) visual analogue scale but with different cut-off points (>50 and ≥60), so results could not be merged. The FOBS scale consists of one question – "How do you feel right now about the approaching birth?"- graded by marking two 100 mm visual analogue scales, which are anchored with the words "calm/worried" and "no fear/strong fear" [67].

Fabian et al. [73] asked women to answer one question on whether they had attended, or felt they needed to attend, a clinic for counseling in relation to FOC, to which they answered 'yes' or 'no'. Lowe et al. [74] used a 15 item Childbirth Attitudes Questionnaire (high fear = 1 Standard Deviation above mean) and Poikkeus et al. [75] used a revised version of the Fear-of-Childbirth questionnaire, developed by Saisto et al. [76], and pregnancy anxiety scale. Total scores equal to or higher than the 90th percentile in the revised Fear-of-Childbirth questionnaire (total scores ≥6 and pregnancy anxiety scale, total scores ≥30) were considered "severe fear" and "severe pregnancy related anxiety" (Table 2). None of these results could be combined.

The majority of studies took measurements at only one time point or at varying times throughout pregnancy without comparing rates from different times. Laursen et al. [64] found rates in early pregnancy to be 2308 out of 30,480 (7.6%), similar to rates in late pregnancy, of 2245 out of 30,480 (7.4%). Postpartum rates of FOC were measured in only two studies [61, 77]. Due to differing measurement times and tools, no comparisons could be made but postpartum rates did not seem to differ greatly from those in the antenatal period (Table 2).

Prevalence

The prevalence of FOC varied, which may be due, in part, to the differing measurement scales. The most common scale was the W-DEQ, used in 11 studies, with four different cut-off points (some papers used more than one point). Three studies [65, 78, 79] used a cut-off point of greater than or equal to 100, with rates varying from 5.5 to 8.1%, giving an average 'very severe' FOC rate of 7.1% (536 out of 7531). A cut-off of greater than or equal to 85 in seven studies [62, 79–84] two cut-off levels gave FOC rates of 7.5% (165 out of 2206) to 15.5% (254 out of 1635), giving an average 'severe' rate of FOC of 11.1% (1545 out of 14,163) (Table 2). The final two studies using W-DEQ had cut-off points of greater than or equal to 66 [85] or 71 [77], which gave rates of 'moderate' FOC of 24.9 - 26.2% (Table 2).

The two studies using a 3-point scale [64, 69] had merged "extreme fear" FOC rates of 7.0% (2707 out of 38,801). The data collection using the dichotomised 4-point scale had rates (based on the same population) of 14% [60], in mid pregnancy, and 15.1% 1 year after birth [61] (Table 2).

Rates for the studies using 5- and 6-point scales [70, 71] varied considerably from 3.6 to 22.9%, and the 5-point scale was based on the question "How do you feel when thinking about labour and birth?" with the response "very negative" deemed to equate to FOC [70], which may not be accurate. Rates for all other prospective studies varied from 11 to 31.1%; the register study based on data from medical records [66] showed a rate of 28,960 out of 788,317 (3.7%) (Table 2).

Comparison of country rates

Rates of severe FOC in each country (as measured by seven studies using W-DEQ with ≥85 cut-off point) were combined, the average taken for each country, and then compared. The average rates varied from 6.3% in Belgium to 14.8% in Estonia, a significant

Table 2 Measurement tools used, prevalence, and parity in Fear of Childbirth studies

First author, year of publication, [reference number]	Measurement tools used, in descending order of cut-off point	Level of FOC	Time point of FOC	Prevalence, % (95% CI)	Number	Parity group[a]
	W-DEQ					
Rouhe 2015 [65]	W-DEQ, with score ≥ 100	Very severe FOC	Early pregnancy	8.1 (7.3–8.9)	371/4575	1
Heimstad 2006 [78]	W-DEQ score > 100 W-DEQ > 95	'Serious FOC; of clinical importance'	Mid pregnancy	5.5 (4.3–6.8) 7.3 (5.9–8.8)	72/1321 96/1321	2
Nieminen 2009 [79]	W-DEQ score ≥ 100 W-DEQ score ≥ 85	Very intense FOC Intense FOC	Pregnancy (various times)	5.7 (4.6–6.9) 15.6 (13.8–17.4)	93/1635 254/1635	2
Adams 2012 [80]	W-DEQ score ≥ 85	'High fear'	At 32 weeks	7.5 (6.4–8.7)	165/2206	2
Jespersen 2014 [81]	W-DEQ score ≥ 85	Severe FOC	At 37 weeks	9.0 (7.8–10.2)	207/2310	1
Jokić-Begić 2014 [82]	W-DEQ score ≥ 85	FOC	Late pregnancy	11.5 (7.4–16.8)	23/200	2
Lukasse 2014 [62]	W-DEQ score ≥ 85	Severe FOC	In pregnancy (various times)	11.2 (total population in six countries) [b] (10.5–12.0) Belgium: 6.3 (4.7–8.2) Iceland: 8.4 (6.3–10.9) Denmark: 9.2 (7.6–10.9) Norway: 11.8 (10.5–13.2) Sweden: 14.8 (12.6–17.2) Estonia: 14.8 (12.6–17.3)	Total: 769/6870 B: 52/828 I: 49/585 D: 115/1252 N: 278/2351 S: 142/958 E: 133/896	2
Söderqvist 2004 [83]	W-DEQ score ≥ 85	Severe FOC	Late pregnancy	13.5 (11.4–15.8)	127/942	2
Zar 2002 [84]	W-DEQ score ≥ 85	Severe FOC	Late pregnancy	11.1 (8.5–14.1)	56/506	2
Fenwick 2009 [77]	W-DEQ score ≥ 71	'High level of fear'	Late pregnancy 6 weeks postpartum	26.2 (21.9–30.8) 22.4 (17.3–28.1)	105/401 55/246	2
Hall 2009 [85]	W-DEQ score ≥ 66	'High fear'	Late pregnancy	24.9 (21.6–28.4)	162/650	2
	Fear of Birth scale (FOBS)					
Haines 2011 [67]	Fear of Birth Scale (FOBS) score > 50.	Elevated level of FOC	Mid-pregnancy	Sweden: 31.1 (26.5–36.0) Australia: 29.5 (21.6–38.4)	119/383 36/122	2
Ternström 2014 [72]	Fear of Birth Scale (FOBS) score > =60.	Childbirth related fear (CBRF)	Mid-pregnancy	22.1 (18.9–25.6)	134/606	2
	Various scales to measure FOC					
Elvander 2013 [63]	First Baby Study Birth Anticipation Scale score 21–30	High fear	Late pregnancy	20.3 (18.9–21.8)	611/3005	1
Lowe 2000 [74]	Childbirth Attitudes Questionnaire, 1 Standard Deviation above mean	High fear	Late pregnancy	19.3 (14.8–24.4)	54/280	1
Poikkeus 2006 [75]	Revised Fear-of-Childbirth questionnaire, total score ≥ 6	Severe fear	Mid pregnancy	11.0 (8.8–13.5)	82/746	2
	Single item question – 3 point Likert response scale					
Geissbuehler 2002 [69]	'Are you anxious or afraid about the birth?', answer by 'Yes, very afraid'	FOC	Late pregnancy	5.3 (4.8–5.8)	450/8528	2

Table 2 Measurement tools used, prevalence, and parity in Fear of Childbirth studies *(Continued)*

First author, year of publication, [reference number]	Measurement tools used, in descending order of cut-off point	Level of FOC	Time point of FOC	Prevalence, % (95% CI)	Number	Parity group[a]
Laursen 2008 [64]	'Are you anxious about the course of the upcoming delivery?' answered with 'A lot'	FOC	Early pregnancy Late pregnancy	7.6 (7.3–7.9) 7.4 (7.1–7.7)	2308/30,480 2245/30,480	1
	Single item question – 4 point Likert response scale					
Hildingsson 2010 [60]	'How do you feel when thinking about labour and birth?' answered with: 'A lot/very much'	Childbirth related fear	Mid pregnancy	14.0 (12.1–16.1)	170/1212	2
Nilsson 2012 [61]	'To what extent do you experience worries and fear?' answered with: 'A great deal/very much' [c]	FOC	1 year after childbirth	15.1 (12.6–17.9)	115/761	2
	Single item question – 5/6 point Likert response scale					
Eriksson 2005 [71]	A statement 'Childbirth-related fear influences my daily life in a negative sense' with a 6-point Likert scale	Intense fear	Assessed retrospectively	22.9 (18.9–27.3)	94/410	2
Waldenström 2006 [70]	A question: 'How do you feel when thinking about labour and birth?'answered by 'Very negative'	Childbirth related fear	Early pregnancy	3.6 (3.0–4.4)	97/2662	2
	Miscellaneous					
Fabian 2004 [73]	Yes to a question on whether they had attended/needed to attend a clinic for counseling because of FOC	FOC	Early pregnancy	15.4 (14.0–16.9)	385/2503	2
Räisänen 2014 [66]	Register study. FOC defined according to ICD – code 099.80	FOC	Pregnancy	3.7 (3.6–3.7)	28,960/ 788,317	2

VAS Visual Analogue Scale, *FOC* Fear Of Childbirth
[a]Parity group 1 = nulli/primiparous women only, 2 = both primi- and multiparous women
[b]Significant difference in country rates (chi-square = 55.5, d.f. = 5, $p < 0.0001$)
[c]Same study population as in Hildingsson 2010

difference in the seven countries (chi-square = 104.44, d.f. = 6, $p < 0.0001$) (Table 3).

Discussion

W-DEQ gave an average 'very severe' (greater than or equal to 100) FOC rate of 7.1%, severe (greater than or equal to 85) rate of 11.1%, and a 'moderate' rate of 25.3 - 26.2% (greater than or equal to 66 or 71). Merged rates from two studies [64, 69] using a question with a 3-point response scale and similar questions on fear (Table 2) had an average "extreme fear" rate in early pregnancy of 7%, very similar to the "very severe" rates measured by W-DEQ. The study using a similar question with a dichotomised 4-point Likert response scale (Table 2) had a rate in early pregnancy of 14.0% for fear or strong fear of childbirth [60].

Once W-DEQ cut-off points went below 85, or other scales had more than three (or four) points, the rates increased and also varied considerably from the average seen at the cut-off ≥85. This might indicate that using the W-DEQ tool with a cut-off point of ≥85, or a measurement of FOC using a single question such as 'Are you afraid about the birth?', with three responses such as 'no, I am not afraid; yes, I am a bit afraid; yes, I am very afraid' [69] would measure FOC equally but that needs further testing.

Rouhe et al. [86] have previously compared FOC levels in 1348 women using the 33-item W-DEQ scale (with a cut-off point of ≥85) with a one-item VAS scale, and a cut-off point of 5. Although there was some correlation they found it not to be as accurate as the W-DEQ, but pronounced it suitable for initial screening. Haines et al.

Table 3 Prevalence of FOC in different countries, measured by W-DEQ (cut-off ≥85)

First author, year of publication	Prevalence	Country total	Average country prevalence
Lukasse 2014	142 out of 958 (14.8%)	Sweden	579 out of 4041 (14.3%)
Nieminen 2009	254 out of 1635 (15.5%)[a]		
Söderqvist 2004	127 out of 942 (13.5%)		
Zar 2002	56 out of 506 (11%)		
Adams 2012	165 out of 2206 (7.5%)	Norway	443 out of 4557 (9.7%)
Lukasse 2014	278 out of 2351 (11.8%)		
Jespersen 2014	207 out of 2310 (9.0%)	Denmark	322 out of 3562 (9.0%)
Lukasse 2014	115 out of 1252 (9.2%)		
Jokić-Begić 2014		Croatia	23 out of 200 (11.5%)
Lukasse 2014		Belgium	Belgium: 52 out of 828 (6.3%)
		Iceland	Iceland: 49 out of 585 (8.4%)
		Estonia	Estonia: 133 out of 896 (14.8%)

[a]Calculation performed by review authors

[87] also compared the W-DEQ scale (using a cut-off point of ≥85) with the Fear of Birth scale (FOBS), a two-item VAS scale, involving 1410 women. Results showed a strong correlation. However, the FOBS's cut-off point was 54, approximately equivalent to the cut-off of 5 used in their work examined here [67], which resulted in quite high FOC rates.

Using the question with a four-point Likert response scale appeared to over-estimate FOC rates, especially when results were dichotomised so that 'extreme fear' was merged with more moderate fear. Dichotomising results before analysis appears to be common, but ultimately does not produce useful results if a true measure of severe FOC is the main aim.

Rates of severe FOC, measured in the same way, varied in different countries from 6.3 to 14.8%. These results are new as, although one study in this review involved measuring FOC in six countries, no paper has analysed data from all seven countries where FOC has been measured. Reasons why FOC might differ in different countries are unknown, and further research in this field is required. One reason may be poor translation, or insufficient testing of the translated version of W-DEQ, both problems highlighted by previous authors [77, 88]. Another possible explanation is that some factors may remain unidentified when measuring with W-DEQ. For instance most scales measuring fear of childbirth do not consider important dimensions such as fear of abandonment by staff during birth [89], fear of medical interventions, loss of autonomy and control, as well as fear of mistreatment and obstetrical violence [90]. In addition, the W-DEQ scale assesses a range of emotions about labour and birth, where fear is only one emotion among many others. However, despite its shortcomings, the W-DEQ has been highlighted in a recent systematic review on validated instruments used for measuring women's childbirth experiences as, currently, the best, most used and validated tool to measure FOC [91]. Culture-specific aspects in relation to fear of childbirth have been recognised in medicalised birth cultures, where young adults prefer CS over vaginal birth, and negative impressions of birth through visual media can be an important factor for generating fear [92, 93]. Moreover, traditions surrounding birth, women's rights, how antenatal and maternity care is organised, CS rates, and which professions (midwives, GPs, obstetricians) are involved in pregnant and childbearing women's care, could all influence women's fear of childbirth.

As FOC has been shown in a large systematic review and meta-analysis to be strongly associated with post-traumatic stress disorder [94], simple and early diagnosis and intervention for women with severe FOC is recommended. Antenatal education, a relatively cheap and cost-effective intervention has been shown to decrease fear of childbirth [95, 96], as has cognitive behavioural therapy, although the sample size was small [97]. We therefore also examined the published tools to see which might be most useful in the clinical area. As shorter tools have greater clinical utility than the W-DEQ, a comparison between W-DEQ and a measurement of FOC using a single question with three or four responses (that are not dichotomised before analysis) would be useful in making decisions as to how best to measure FOC swiftly and accurately in the clinical location. A comparison between W-DEQ and the FOBS scale, possibly after further testing using a higher cut-off point, would also be very useful to the research and maternity care communities.

Conclusions

Rates of severe FOC, measured in the same way, varied in different countries. Reasons why FOC might differ are unknown, and further research is necessary. Using the W-DEQ tool with a cut-off point of ≥85, or a measurement tool using a single question with three responses, are consistent in measuring levels of severe FOC. Research comparing W-DEQ and a measurement tool using a single question with three responses, or four responses that are not dichotomised before analysis, would be useful to both the research and clinical communities. Similarly, continued and further testing of the FOBS scale, especially using a higher cut-off point to separate out "severe" FOC from more moderate levels, could prove beneficial to clinicians.

Validation of a simpler tool like the FOBS or a single question is required as there is a need for a tool that is easy and quick for women to fill in, as not all clinicians have time to administer the longer W-DEQ. Newly-developed, untested scales cannot easily be compared with other studies, and should not be used in clinical practice without further testing.

We recommend that future studies on FOC should use either the W-DEQ tool with a cut-off point of ≥85, or a more thoroughly tested version of either the FOBS scale with a higher cut-off point, or a single question such as 'Are you afraid about the birth?' with a three- or un-dichotimised four-point Likert response scale. In this way, valid comparisons can be made between countries and other studies.

Further research is also needed into reasons why FOC might differ in different countries and whether care for women with FOC needs to be made culturally specific. Measurement of FOC needs to include aspects such as fear of abandonment by staff during birth, fear of medical interventions, loss of autonomy and control, as well as fear of mistreatment and obstetrical violence. This more focused research agenda to guide future studies will result in more meaningful results that can be used to improve care provided for all women with fear of childbirth.

Abbreviations

CS: Caesarean section; FOBS: Fear of birth scale; FOC: Fear of childbirth; VAS: Visual analogue scale; W-DEQ: The Wijma delivery expectancy/experience questionnaire

Acknowledgements

Not applicable

Funding

There is no funding to report for this study.

Authors' contributions

All authors contributed to the protocol. CN coordinated the review process. CS-L peer-reviewed the search strategy. CN developed the search string and conducted the searches with EH and HS. CN, AD, EJ, CS-L, MM, HP, HW, CB, independently selected papers for inclusion, assessed the quality of the included studies and extracted data. EH and HS documented the Prisma flow diagram. CB performed the data analysis. CB and AD made the Tables. CN wrote the background section. CB wrote the methodology and findings sections. All authors contributed to the discussion and read and commented on the manuscript during the writing process. All authors read and approved the final manuscript.

Authors' information

Not applicable

Consent for publication

Not applicable

Competing interests

The authors CB and CS-L are members of the BMC Pregnancy and Childbirth Editorial Board.

Author details

[1]Faculty of Caring Science, Work Life and Social Welfare, University of Borås, S-501 90 Borås, Sweden. [2]Institute of Health and Care Sciences, The Sahlgrenska Academy at University of Gothenburg, Box 457, -405 30 Gothenburg, SE, Sweden. [3]Biomedical Library, Gothenburg University Library at University of Gothenburg, Box 416, -405 30 Gothenburg, SE, Sweden. [4]Chair of Nursing and Midwifery, School of Nursing and Midwifery,Trinity College Dublin, 24, D'Olier St. Dublin 2, Dublin, Ireland.

References

1. Höjeberg P. Tröskelkvinnor: barnafödande som kultur [Threshold women: Childbirth as culture]. Carlsson: Stockholm; 2000.
2. Larkin P, Begley CM, Devane D. Women's experiences of labour and birth: an evolutionary concept analysis. Midwifery. 2009;25(2):e49–59.
3. Wijma K. Why focus on 'fear of childbirth'? J Psychosom Obstet Gynecol. 2003;24(3):141–3.
4. Bewley S, Cockburn J. Responding to fear of childbirth. Lancet. 2002; 359(9324):2128–9.
5. Storksen HT, Garthus-Niegel S, Adams SS, Vangen S, Eberhard-Gran M. Fear of childbirth and elective caesarean section: a population-based study. BMC Pregnancy childbirth. 2015;15:221.
6. Stützer PP, Berlit S, Lis S, Schmahl C, Sütterlin M, Tuschy B. Elective caesarean section on maternal request in Germany: factors affecting decision making concerning mode of delivery. Arch Gynecol Obstet. 2017; 295(5):1151–6.
7. Fuglenes D, Aas E, Botten G, Øian P, Kristiansen IS. Why do some pregnant women prefer cesarean? The influence of parity, delivery experiences, and fear. Am J Obstet Gynecol. 2011;205(1):45. e41-45.e49
8. Handelzalts JE, Becker G, Ahren M-P, Lurie S, Raz N, Tamir Z, Sadan O. Personality, fear of childbirth and birth outcomes in nulliparous women. Arch Gynecol Obstet. 2015;291(5):1055–62.
9. Marcé L-V: Traité de la folie des femmes enceintes, des nouvelles accouchées et des nourrices : et considérations médico-légales qui se rattachent à ce sujet / par le Dr L.-V. Marcé: J.-B. Baillière et fils (Paris); 1858.
10. Areskog B, Uddenberg N, Kjessler B. Fear of childbirth in late pregnancy. Gynecol Obstet Investig. 1981;12(5):262–6.
11. Saisto T, Halmesmaki E. Fear of childbirth: a neglected dilemma. Acta Obstet Gynecol Scand. 2003;82(3):201–8.
12. Hofberg K, Brockington I. Tokophobia: an unreasoning dread of childbirth. A series of 26 cases. Br J Psychiatry. 2000;176(JAN):83–5.

13. Hofberg K, Ward MR. Fear of pregnancy and childbirth. Postgrad Med J. 2003;79(935):505–10. quiz 508-510
14. Vogel JP, Betran AP, Vindevoghel N, Souza JP, Torloni MR, Zhang J, Tuncalp O, Mori R, Morisaki N, Ortiz-Panozo E, et al. Use of the Robson classification to assess caesarean section trends in 21 countries: a secondary analysis of two WHO multicountry surveys. Lancet Glob Health. 2015;3(5):e260–70.
15. European perinatal health report: The health and care of pregnant women and babies in Europe in 2010. Paris: Euro Peristat European comission; 2013.
16. Ayers S. Fear of childbirth, postnatal post-traumatic stress disorder and midwifery care. Midwifery. 2014;30(2):145–8.
17. Haines HM, Rubertsson C, Pallant JF, Hildingsson I. The influence of women's fear, attitudes and beliefs of childbirth on mode and experience of birth. BMC Pregnancy Childbirth. 2012;12:55.
18. Klabbers GA, JAvB H, MAvdH M, AJJM V. Severe fear of childbirth: its features, assesment, prevalence, determinants, consequences and possible treatments. Psychol Topics. 2016;25(1):107–27.
19. Alehagen S, Wijma B, Wijma K. Fear of childbirth before, during, and after childbirth. Acta Obstetricia & Gynecologica Scandinavica 2006;85:56–62.
20. Liljeroth P. Rädsla inför förlossningen : ett uppenbart kliniskt problem? Konstruktionen av förlossningsrädsla som medicinsk kategori [fear before delivery – an obvious clinical problem? The construction of fear of childbirth as a medical category]. Ekonomisk-statsvetenskapliga fakulteten vid Åbo Akademi: Åbo; 2009.
21. Walsh D. Birthwrite. Fear of labour and birth. Br J Midwifery. 2002;10(2):78.
22. Sampson M, McGowan J, Cogo E, Grimshaw J, Moher D, Lefebvre C. An evidence-based practice guideline for the peer review of electronic search strategies. J Clin Epidemiol. 2009;62(9):944–52.
23. EPHPP Quality Assessment tool for Quantitative Studies [http://www.ephpp.ca/tools.html].
24. Garthus-Niegel S, von Soest T, Knoph C, Simonsen TB, Torgersen L, Eberhard-Gran M. The influence of women's preferences and actual mode of delivery on post-traumatic stress symptoms following childbirth: a population-based, longitudinal study. BMC Pregnancy Childbirth. 2014;14:191.
25. Garthus-Niegel S, von Soest T, Vollrath ME, Eberhard-Gran M. The impact of subjective birth experiences on post-traumatic stress symptoms: a longitudinal study. Archives Women's Mentl Health. 2013;16(1):1–10.
26. Hildingsson I, Rådestad I, Rubertsson C, Waldenström U. Few women wish to be delivered by caesarean section. BJOG: Int J Obstet Gynaecol. 2002; 109(6):618–23.
27. Karlstrom A, Radestad I, Eriksson C, Rubertsson C, Nystedt A, Hildingsson I. Cesarean section without medical reason, 1997 to 2006: a Swedish register study. Birth (Berkeley, Calif). 2010;37(1):11–20.
28. Melender HL. Experiences of fears associated with pregnancy and childbirth: a study of 329 pregnant women. Birth (Berkeley, Calif). 2002;29(2):101–11.
29. Saisto T, Ylikorkala O, Halmesmaki E. Factors associated with fear of delivery in second pregnancies. Obstet Gynecol. 1999;94(5 Pt 1):679–82.
30. Schwartz L, Toohill J, Creedy DK, Baird K, Gamble J, Fenwick J. Factors associated with childbirth self-efficacy in Australian childbearing women. BMC Pregnancy Childbirth. 2015;15(1):465.
31. Stjernholm YV, Petersson K, Eneroth E. Changed indications for cesarean sections. Acta Obstet Gynecol Scand. 2010;89(1):49–53.
32. Takegata M, Haruna M, Matsuzaki M, Shiraishi M, Okano T, Severinsson E. Antenatal fear of childbirth and sense of coherence among healthy pregnant women in Japan: a cross-sectional study. Arch Women's Ment Health. 2014;17(5):403–9.
33. Nerum H, Halvorsen L, Sorlie T, Oian P. Maternal request for cesarean section due to fear of birth: can it be changed through crisis-oriented counseling? Birth (Berkeley, Calif). 2006;33(3):221–8.
34. Rouhe H, Salmela-Aro K, Gissler M, Halmesmaki E, Saisto T. Mental health problems common in women with fear of childbirth. BJOG : Int J Bbstetrics Gynaecol. 2011;118(9):1104–11.
35. Ryding EL, Persson A, Onell C, Kvist L. An evaluation of midwives' counseling of pregnant women in fear of childbirth. Acta Obstet Gynecol Scand. 2003;82(1):10–7.
36. Sjogren B. Fear of childbirth and psychosomatic support. A follow up of 72 women. Acta Obstet Gynecol Scand. 1998;77(8):819–25.
37. Sjogren B, Thomassen P. Obstetric outcome in 100 women with severe anxiety over childbirth (structured abstract). Acta Obstet Gynecol Scand. 1997;76:948–52.
38. Sydsjo G, Angerbjorn L, Palmquist S, Bladh M, Sydsjo A, Josefsson A. Secondary fear of childbirth prolongs the time to subsequent delivery. Acta Obstet Gynecol Scand. 2013;92(2):210–4.
39. Eriksson C, Jansson L, Hamberg K. Women's experiences of intense fear related to childbirth investigated in a Swedish qualitative study. Midwifery. 2006;22(3):240–8.
40. Faisal I, Matinnia N, Hejar AR, Khodakarami Z. Why do primigravidae request caesarean section in a normal pregnancy? A qualitative study in Iran. Midwifery. 2014;30(2):227–33.
41. Fenwick J, Staff L, Gamble J, Creedy DK, Bayes S. Why do women request caesarean section in a normal, healthy first pregnancy? Midwifery. 2010; 26(4):394–400.
42. Fisher C, Hauck Y, Fenwick J. How social context impacts on women's fears of childbirth: a western Australian example. Soc Sci Med. 2006;63(1):64–75.
43. Nilsson C, Bondas T, Lundgren I. Previous birth experience in women with intense fear of childbirth. J Obstet, Gynecol, Neonatal. 2010;39(3):298–309.
44. Nilsson C, Lundgren I. Women's lived experience of fear of childbirth. Midwifery. 2009;25(2):e1–9.
45. Ramvi E, Tangerud M. Experiences of women who have a vaginal birth after requesting a cesarean section due to a fear of birth: a biographical, narrative, interpretative study. Nursing Health Sci. 2011;13(3):269–74.
46. Ryding EL, Wijma K, Wijma B. Experiences of emergency cesarean section: a phenomenological study of 53 women. Birth (Berkeley, Calif). 1998;25(4):246–51.
47. Salomonsson B, Bertero C, Alehagen S. Self-efficacy in pregnant women with severe fear of childbirth. J Obstet, Gynecol Neonatal Nursing. 2013;42(2):191–202.
48. Lyberg A, Severinsson E. Fear of childbirth: mothers' experiences of team-midwifery care - a follow-up study. J Nurs Manag. 2010;18(4):383–90.
49. Melender HL. Fears and coping strategies associated with pregnancy and childbirth in Finland. J Midwifery Women's Health. 2002;47(4):256–63.
50. Larsson B, Karlstrom A, Rubertsson C, Hildingsson I. The effects of counseling on fear of childbirth. Acta Obstet Gynecol Scand. 2015;94(6): 629–66.
51. Hildingsson I, Nilsson C, Karlström A, Lundgren I. A longitudinal survey of childbirth-related fear and associated factors. J Obstet, Gynecol Neonatal Nurs. 2011;40(5):532–43.
52. Hildingsson I. Swedish couples' attitudes towards birth, childbirth fear and birth preferences and relation to mode of birth - a longitudinal cohort study. Sex Reprod Healthc. 2014;5(2):75–80.
53. Karlstrom A, Nystedt A, Johansson M, Hildingsson I. Behind the myth–few women prefer caesarean section in the absence of medical or obstetrical factors. Midwifery. 2011;27(5):620–7.
54. Karlstrom A, Nystedt A, Hildingsson I. A comparative study of the experience of childbirth between women who preferred and had a caesarean section and women who preferred and had a vaginal birth. Sex Reprod Healthc. 2011;2(3):93–9.
55. Hall WA, Stoll K, Hutton EK, Brown H. A prospective study of effects of psychological factors and sleep on obstetric interventions, mode of birth, and neonatal outcomes among low-risk British Columbian women. BMC Pregnancy Childbirth. 2012;12:78.
56. Stoll KH, Hall W. Childbirth education and obstetric interventions among low-risk canadian women: is there a connection? J Perinat Educ. 2012;21(4):229–37.
57. Laursen M, Johansen C, Hedegaard M. Fear of childbirth and risk for birth complications in nulliparous women in the Danish National Birth Cohort. BJOG : Int J Obstet Gynaecol. 2009;116(10):1350–5.
58. Ryding EL, Lukasse M, Parys AS, Wangel AM, Karro H, Kristjansdottir H, Schroll AM, Schei B. Fear of childbirth and risk of cesarean delivery: a cohort study in six European countries. Birth (Berkeley, Calif). 2015;42(1):48–55.
59. Eriksson C, Westman G, Hamberg K. Content of childbirth-related fear in Swedish women and men - analysis of an open-ended question. J Midwifery Women's Health. 2006;51(2):112–8.
60. Hildingsson I, Thomas J, Karlström A, Olofsson RE, Nystedt A. Childbirth thoughts in mid-pregnancy: prevalence and associated factors in prospective parents. Sex Reprod Healthc. 2010;1(2):45–53.
61. Nilsson C, Lundgren I, Karlström A, Hildingsson I. Self reported fear of childbirth and its association with women's birth experience and mode of delivery: a longitudinal population-based study. Women Birth. 2012; 25(3):114–21.
62. Lukasse M, Schei B, Ryding EL. Prevalence and associated factors of fear of childbirth in six European countries. Sex Reprod Healthc. 2014;5.
63. Elvander C, Cnattingius S, Kjerulff KH. Birth experience in women with low, intermediate or high levels of fear: findings from the first baby study. Birth: Issues Perinatal Care. 2013;40(4):289–96.

64. Laursen M, Hedegaard M, Johansen C. Fear of childbirth: predictors and temporal changes among nulliparous women in the Danish National Birth Cohort. BJOG. 2008;115(3):354–60.
65. Rouhe H, Salmela-Aro K, Toivanen R, Tokola M, Halmesmaki E, Saisto T. Life satisfaction, general well-being and costs of treatment for severe fear of childbirth in nulliparous women by psychoeducative group or conventional care attendance. Acta obstetricia et gynecologica Scandinavica 2015;94(5): 527–33.
66. Raisanen S, Lehto SM, Nielsen HS, Gissler M, Kramer MR, Heinonen S. Fear of childbirth in nulliparous and multiparous women: a population-based analysis of all singleton births in Finland in 1997-2010. BJOG. 2014;121(8): 965–70.
67. Haines H, Pallant JF, Karlström A, Hildingsson I. Cross-cultural comparison of levels of childbirth-related fear in an Australian and Swedish sample. Midwifery. 2011;27(4):560–7.
68. Wijma K, Wijma B, Zar M. Psychometric aspects of the W-DEQ; a new questionnaire for the measurement of fear of childbirth. J Psychosom Obstet Gynaecol. 1998;19:84–97.
69. Geissbuehler V, Eberhard J. Fear of childbirth during pregnancy: a study of more than 8000 pregnant women. J Psychosom Obstet Gynecol. 2002;23(4):229–35.
70. Waldenström U, Hildingsson I, Ryding EL. Antenatal fear of childbirth and its association with subsequent caesarean section and experience of childbirth. BJOG. 2006;113(6):638–46.
71. Eriksson C, Westman G, Hamberg K. Experiential factors associated with childbirth-related fear in Swedish women and men: a population based study. J Psychosom Obstet Gynecol. 2005;26(1):63–72.
72. Ternstrom E, Hildingsson I, Haines H, Rubertsson C: Higher prevalence of childbirth related fear in foreign born pregnant women - Findings from a community sample in Sweden. Midwifery 2014;31(4):445–40.
73. Fabian HM, Rådestad IJ, Waldenström U. Characteristics of Swedish women who do not attend childbirth and parenthood education classes during pregnancy. Midwifery. 2004;20(3):226–35.
74. Lowe NK. Self-efficacy for labor and childbirth fears in nulliparous pregnant women. J Psychosom Obstet Gynaecol. 2000;21(4):219–24.
75. Poikkeus P, Saisto T, Unkila-Kallio L, Punamaki RL, Repokari L, Vilska S, Tiitinen A, Tulppala M. Fear of childbirth and pregnancy-related anxiety in women conceiving with assisted reproduction. Obstet Gynecol. 2006;108(1):70–6.
76. Saisto T, Salmela-Aro K, Nurmi JE, Könönen T. E H: a randomized controlled trial of intervention in fear of childbirth. Obstet Gynecol. 2001;98(5):820–6.
77. Fenwick J, Gamble J, Nathan E, Bayes S, Hauck Y. Pre- and postpartum levels of childbirth fear and the relationship to birth outcomes in a cohort of Australian women. J Clin Nurs. 2009;18(5):667–77.
78. Heimstad R, Dahloe R, Laache I, Skogvoll E, Schei B. Fear of childbirth and history of abuse: implications for pregnancy and delivery. Acta Obstet Gynecol Scand. 2006;85(4):435–40.
79. Nieminen K, Stephansson O, Ryding EL. Women's fear of childbirth and preference for cesarean section - a cross-sectional study at various stages of pregnancy in Sweden. Acta Obstet Gynecol Scand. 2009;88(7):807–13.
80. Adams SS, Eberhard-Gran M, Eskild A. Fear of childbirth and duration of labour: a study of 2206 women with intended vaginal delivery. BJOG : an international journal of obstetrics and gynaecology. 2012;119:1238-46.
81. Jespersen C, Hegaard HK, Schroll A-M, Rosthøj S, Kjærgaard H. Fear of childbirth and emergency caesarean section in low-risk nulliparous women: a prospective cohort study. J Psychosom Obstet Gynecol. 2014; 35(4):109–15.
82. Jokić-Begić N, Žigić L, Radoš SN. Anxiety and anxiety sensitivity as predictors of fear of childbirth: different patterns for nulliparous and parous women. J Psychosom Obstet Gynecol. 2014;35(1):22–8.
83. Soderquist J, Wijma K, Wijma B. Traumatic stress in late pregnancy. J Anxiety disord. 2004;18(2):127–42.
84. Zar M, Wijma K, Wijma B. Relations between anxiety disorders and fear of childbirth during late pregnancy. Clin Psychol Psychother. 2002;9(2):122–30.
85. Hall WA, Hauck YL, Carty EM, Hutton EK, Fenwick J, Stoll K. Childbirth fear, anxiety, fatigue, and sleep deprivation in pregnant women. J Obstet Gynecol Neonatal Nurs. 2009;38(5):567–76.
86. Rouhe H, Salmela-Aro K, Halmesmäki E, Saisto T. Fear of childbirth according to parity, gestational age, and obstetric history. BJOG Int J Obstet Gynaecol. 2009;116(1):67–73.
87. Haines HM, Pallant JF, Fenwick J, Gamble J, Creedy DK, Toohill J, Hildingsson I. Identifying women who are afraid of giving birth: a comparison of the fear of birth scale with the WDEQ-A in a large Australian cohort. Sex Reprod Healthc. 2015;6(4):204–10.
88. Johnson R, Slade P. Does fear of childbirth during pregnancy predict emergency caesarean section? BJOG Int J Obstet Gynaecol. 2002;109(11):1213–21.
89. Roosevelt L, Low LK. Exploring fear of childbirth in the United States through a qualitative assessment of the Wijma delivery expectancy questionnaire. J Obstet Gynecol Neonatal Nurs. 2016;45(1):28–38.
90. Bohren MA, Vogel JP, Hunter EC, Lutsiv O, Makh SK, Souza JP, Aguiar C, Saraiva Coneglian F, Diniz ALA, Tunçalp Ö et al: The Mistreatment of Women during Childbirth in Health Facilities Globally: A Mixed-Methods Systematic Review (The Mistreatment of Women during Childbirth: A Systematic Review). 2015, 12(6):e1001847.
91. Nilvér H, Begley C, Berg M. Measuring women's childbirth experiences: a systematic review for identification and analysis of validated instruments. BMC Pregnancy Childbirth. 2017;17:203.
92. Stoll K, Hall W, Janssen P, Carty E. Why are young Canadians afraid of birth? A survey study of childbirth fear and birth preferences among Canadian University students. Midwifery. 2014;30(2):220–6.
93. Thomson G, Stoll K, Downe S, Hall WA. Negative impressions of childbirth in a north-West England student population. J Psychosom Obstet Gynaecol. 2017;38(1):37–44.
94. Ayers S, Bond R, Bertullies S, Wijma K. The aetiology of post-traumatic stress following childbirth: a meta-analysis and theoretical framework. Psychol Med. 2016;46(6):1121–34.
95. Karabulut Ö, Coşkuner Potur D, Doğan Merih Y, Cebeci Mutlu S, Demirci N. Does antenatal education reduce fear of childbirth? Int Nurs Rev. 2016;63(1):60–7.
96. Serçekuş P, Başkale H. Effects of antenatal education on fear of childbirth, maternal self-efficacy and parental attachment. Midwifery. 2016;34:166–72.
97. Nieminen K, Andersson G, Wijma B, Ryding EL, Wijma K. Treatment of nulliparous women with severe fear of childbirth via the internet: a feasibility study. J Psychosom Obstet Gynaecol. 2016;37(2):37–43.

3

Women's decision-making processes and the influences on their mode of birth following a previous caesarean section in Taiwan

Shu-Wen Chen[1,2*], Alison M. Hutchinson[1,3], Cate Nagle[4] and Tracey K. Bucknall[1,5]

Abstract

Background: Vaginal birth after caesarean (VBAC) is an alternative option for women who have had a previous caesarean section (CS); however, uptake is limited because of concern about the risks of uterine rupture. The aim of this study was to explore women's decision-making processes and the influences on their mode of birth following a previous CS.

Methods: A qualitative approach was used. The research comprised three stages. Stage I consisted of naturalistic observation at 33-34 weeks' gestation. Stage II involved interviews with pregnant women at 35-37 weeks' gestation. Stage III consisted of interviews with the same women who were interviewed postnatally, 1 month after birth. The research was conducted in a private medical centre in northern Taiwan. Using a purposive sampling, 21 women and 9 obstetricians were recruited. Data collection involved in-depth interviews, observation and field notes. Constant comparative analysis was employed for data analysis.

Results: Ensuring the safety of mother and baby was the focus of women's decisions. Women's decisions-making influences included previous birth experience, concern about the risks of vaginal birth, evaluation of mode of birth, current pregnancy situation, information resources and health insurance. In communicating with obstetricians, some women complied with obstetricians' recommendations for repeat caesarean section (RCS) without being informed of alternatives. Others used four step decision-making processes that included searching for information, listening to obstetricians' professional judgement, evaluating alternatives, and making a decision regarding mode of birth. After birth, women reflected on their decisions in three aspects: reflection on birth choices; reflection on factors influencing decisions; and reflection on outcomes of decisions.

Conclusions: The health and wellbeing of mother and baby were the major concerns for women. In response to the decision-making influences, women's interactions with obstetricians regarding birth choices varied from passive decision-making to shared decision-making. All women have the right to be informed of alternative birthing options. Routine provision of explanations by obstetricians regarding risks associated with alternative birth options, in addition to financial coverage for RCS from National Health Insurance, would assist women's decision-making. Establishment of a website to provide women with reliable information about birthing options may also assist women's decision-making.

Keywords: Vaginal birth after caesarean (VBAC), Repeat caesarean section (RCS), Mode of birth, Decision-making, Qualitative research, Risk evaluation

* Correspondence: chensw1119@gmail.com
[1]Deakin University, Faculty of Health, School of Nursing and Midwifery, Geelong, Australia
[2]National Taipei University of Nursing and Health Science, School of Nursing, Taipei, Taiwan
Full list of author information is available at the end of the article

Background

Previous caesarean sections (CS) account for a significant proportion of the high rates of repeat caesarean section (RCS) reported in high income countries [1–3]. While vaginal birth after caesarean (VBAC) is a safe intervention [4], there has been a dramatic decline in VBAC because of concerns about uterine rupture and perinatal death [5]. This is despite evidence that the rates of uterine rupture and perinatal death are relatively low [4]. According to findings from a systematic review of 203 studies, once a woman has experienced a CS, she has a baseline risk for uterine rupture in subsequent pregnancies that is estimated at 3 per 1000 [4]. For women choosing VBAC in a subsequent pregnancy, this baseline risk increases to 4.7 per 1000, compared with 0.3 per 1000 for women choosing RCS. Of concern, however, is that RCS is associated with an increased risk of adverse maternal and neonatal outcomes [6], and has a major economic impact on health care [7].

Several factors influence women's decision-making regarding birth mode. Historically, it has been reported that, associated with the notion of "once a caesarean, always a caesarean", obstetricians recommended RCS to women who had had a previous CS [8]. Higher preference for CS has been reported in women with previous CS [9]. While perceptions of safety were a common reason for caesarean section by maternal request (CSMR) without medical indication [10], evidence demonstrates inconsistent findings in maternal and neonatal risks [11]. Caesarean sections by maternal request (CSMR) were associated with higher rates of infection and length of hospital stay and neonatal respiratory morbidity, compared to planned vaginal birth [11]. Knowledge about birth options influences a woman's ability to make decisions regarding mode of birth. In a survey to explore how information women received in pregnancy affected their childbirth preferences, all ($n = 34$) women who chose a VBAC felt involved in the decision-making, while almost 20% ($n = 28$) of women who underwent a RCS reported not being involved in decision-making [12]. Women also use relevant information from previous birthing experiences to inform a birth decision [13]. According to findings of a qualitative study, 13 Australian women who had a VBAC reported that their previous caesarean experience was unacceptable to them and resulted in an unexpected extended recovery. These experiences reinforced their desire for a subsequent vaginal birth [14]. Fear of birth was related to previous negative birth experience [15]. Additionally, social context has been found to increase women's fears of birth, such as 'fear of the unknown', 'horror stories' and 'general fear for the well-being of the baby' [16]. In some countries, hospitals restrict access to VBAC based on the capabilities of the service and limitations of VBAC guidelines [17, 18].

Taiwan has high RCS rates [19]. In 2015, a total of 216,229 babies were born in Taiwan; 35.67% ($n = 77,144$) of babies were born by CS; that is, more than one in three women delivered by CS. Of all births, RCS accounted for 14.16% ($n = 30,622$) [19]. High RCS rates are associated with extremely low rates of practicing midwives in Taiwan. In 2016, of all births, 99.89% ($n = 215,983$) of babies were delivered by obstetricians while 0.06% ($n = 126$) of babies were born with midwives' assistance [19]. Between 1951 and 1971, a midwife was the main health professional to assist women during birth. With cultural vicissitudes and the concomitant rise of medicalisation within health services, numerous organisations adopted obstetrician-provided maternal care in Taiwan [20], similar to North America. Obstetricians are the primary providers of prenatal care for most childbearing women. An obstetrician is present for the birth, and nurses provide intrapartum and postnatal care [21]. As a result of the high CS rates, the Taiwan government reconsidered the role of midwives [22]. Midwifery education was recommenced and the midwifery qualification was advanced to undergraduate level in 1996 and then to a graduate level in 2000 [22].

Previous CS is ranked as the top reason for RCS in Taiwan [23]. While increasing VBAC is an efficient way to lower CS rates in Taiwan [24], the prevalence of VBAC was less than 0.37% ($n = 806$) in 2016 [19]. Although studies from high income countries have indicated that women's choice of RCS was related to: individual preferences [9]; safety [25]; insufficient information about various modes of birth [12–14]; health professionals' advice [26] and limitations of guideline and policy [18], these findings may not explain the phenomenon of extremely low VBAC rates in Taiwan. In particular, Taiwan has a different social context from high income countries. Studies conducted in high income countries have focussed on either health professionals' views or women's perspectives, but little is known about how cultural context and practice patterns influence women's decisions. More importantly, a number of quantitative studies have been conducted to examine factors related to CS in Taiwan [27–30]. However, qualitative research to explore decision-making regarding mode of birth in Taiwanese women who have had a previous CS, has not been undertaken. To redress this gap, the present study aimed to explore Taiwanese women's decision-making processes and the influences on their mode of birth following a previous CS.

Methods

Study design

Using a qualitative approach, the research encompassed three stages. Stage 1 consisted of naturalistic observation of obstetric consultations to understand how obstetricians assisted women to make their birth choices. Stage 2 involved interviews with pregnant women to explore their perceptions of the influences on their preferences for mode of birth. Stage 3 consisted of interviews in the postnatal period with the same women who were interviewed in Stage 2. The purpose of the Stage 3 interviews was to capture women's reflections about the influences on their decisions regarding mode of birth, and the relationship between their decisions and the actual birth mode outcome.

Setting and participants

The study was conducted in a private, tertiary teaching medical centre in northern Taiwan. At the hospital, there were between 350 and 450 births per month and the CS rate varied between 34% and 38%, consistent with Taiwan's overall CS rates [19]. A purposive sampling approach was used in this study. Pregnant women who had undergone a previous CS were eligible to be included. Inclusion criteria were: women who were aged 18-45 years of age, fluent in Mandarin or English, 30-32 weeks' gestation, and had experienced a previous CS. Exclusion criteria included women with a multiple pregnancy, a previous classic CS or myomectomy, and/or high-risk pregnancies (for example, women who had risk factors such as threatened premature labour, hypertension, heart disease, diabetes, epilepsy, or another pre-existing medical problem).

Data collection and procedures

Data collection included observation, in-depth interviews and field notes. Non-participant observation (the complete observer) was used in order to avoid influencing participants' decisions. The aim of observation is to seek detailed knowledge of the multiple dimensions of life within the natural setting and to understand participants' taken-for-granted meanings and rules from the perspective of those being observed [31, 32]. Instead of covert observation, where participants are unaware they are being observed, overt observation was used to study naturally occurring behaviour of participants [31]. Prior to observation, written consent from the obstetricians for the observation was obtained. Each woman participant was invited to participate and informed about how they would be observed and the purpose behind the observation. Interested participants provided written consent for observation of the consultation with the obstetrician.

Interviews were the main method for data collection. Interviews seek to describe the meaning of central themes in the life of the subjects. The main task in interviewing is to understand the meaning of the interviewees [33]. Interviews are particularly useful for obtaining the story behind a participant's experiences. The interviewer pursues in-depth information around the topic [34]. Two interviews of women were conducted to elicit their perspectives, preferences regarding birth choice before and birth reflections afterwards. A semi-structured interview guide was used for the interview to cover key issues for women participants.

Ethics approval was obtained from the university and hospital Human Research Ethics Committee. Prior to commencement, participants gave written informed consent for participation and the audio-recording of the interviews. The researcher invited eligible women to participate in the study when they attended the registration counter for their prenatal examination at the 33-34 weeks' gestation visit in the Outpatient Department of Obstetrics and Gynaecology. Interactions between the consulting obstetrician and the pregnant woman were observed and field notes were recorded.

A prenatal interview with the woman was scheduled to coincide with the woman's next visit to the obstetrician. The formal face-to-face interview was held at 35-37 weeks' gestation when the women visited their obstetrician. The quiet waiting room of the Outpatient Department of Obstetrics and Gynaecology was used to conduct the interview while the women waited for their obstetrician appointment. Interviews commenced with a key question, "Could you tell me what is your birth plan regarding mode of birth?" (Additional file 1) Following the provision (before the birth of the child) of signed consent for the postnatal interview, and at approximately 1 month after birth, a mobile text message requesting a postnatal interview was issued to the women to confirm their intention to participate in the interview. The face-to-face interviews were conducted in the waiting room of the Outpatient Department of Obstetrics and Gynaecology or the Neonatal Department after the postnatal women attended their routine follow-up postnatal appointment. The key opening question, "Could you tell me what influenced your decision about mode of birth?" (Additional file 1) guided the conversation. The procedure and recruitment process is illustrated (Fig. 1).

Interviews were transcribed verbatim in Chinese from the digital audio-recording as soon as was practicable after the interview. Once the interviews were transcribed, the researcher verified the transcripts by listening to the recording repeatedly. Two bilingual teachers who were Chinese and had masters' degrees in Taiwan assisted the researcher to translate interviews from Chinese to English.

Data analysis

The constant comparative analytic method of grounded theory informed data analysis [35, 36]. Data gathering, analysis and construction proceeded concurrently and coding and memo writing started soon after collection of the first interview and field notes [37]. N-Vivo 10

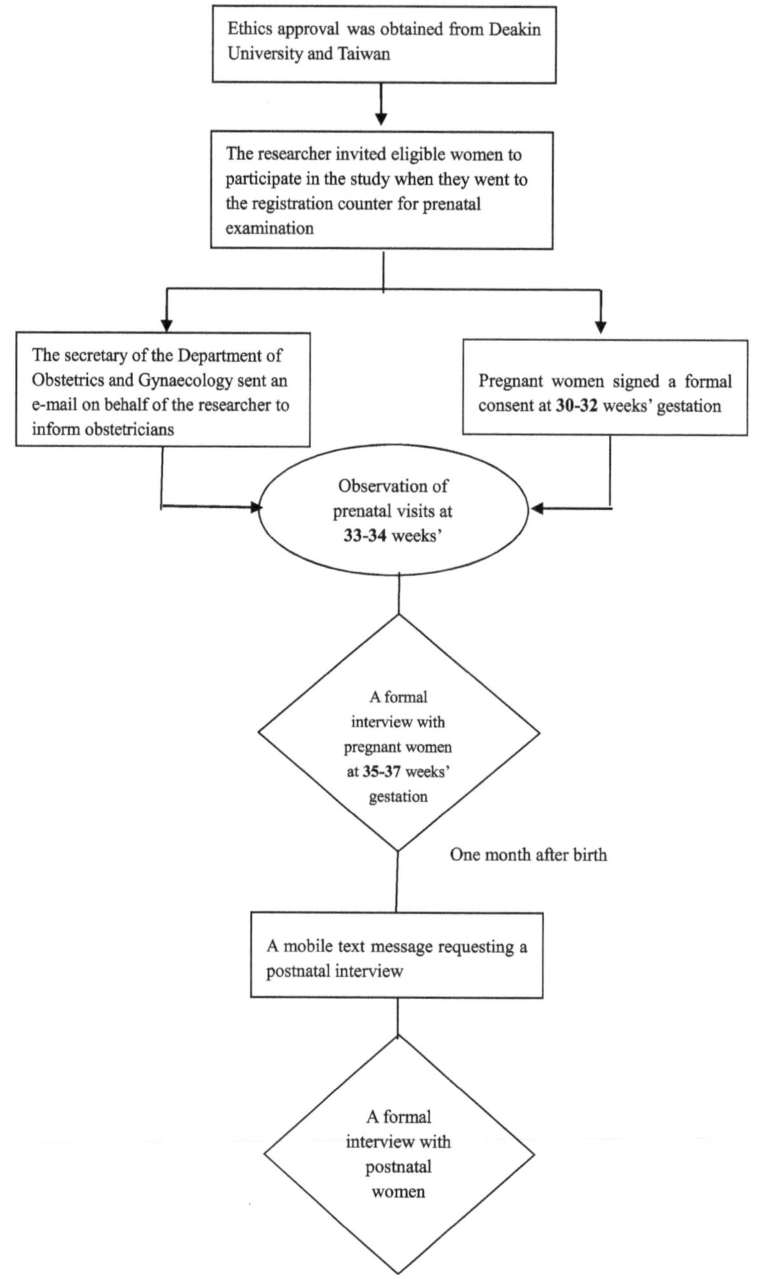

Fig. 1 Flow diagram of the recruitment procedure

software package was used for data coding and retrieval, organization and presentation. The four criteria of credibility, confirmability, dependability and transferability were employed to evaluate the trustworthiness of this qualitative research [38]. To ensure credibility, multiple strategies were used: open-ended interviews; field notes; observation and demographic information to build triangulation. The principal researcher who collected data specialised in teaching obstetric nursing, and has worked with students in delivery rooms for over 10 years. The prolonged engagement and extensive experience working with this population was important to establishing credibility with potential participants. Triangulation strategies were also used to reduce the effect of research bias to establish confirmability, including reflexive field notes and observation. Raw data, data analysis products and data reconstruction products were provided to the research team for verification. To ensure dependability, naturalistic observation and individual interview data were compared to examine the consistency of data (cross-validating data). Additionally, the research team discussed and came to consensus on the categories and theming during the stages of analysis. To ensure transferability, the study provides clear and detailed description of the data collection procedure and the process of analysis, as well as the findings. This detailed description will provide other researchers with the opportunity to assess the relevance to their own setting of the knowledge that is generated.

Results

A total of 24 pregnant women agreed to participate in the study and provided signed consent. Three women were excluded from the study including two women who transferred to another hospital located in southern Taiwan and one woman who miscarried before the prenatal interview. In total, nine obstetricians and 21 pregnant women participated in the study. Women completed a survey to provide their demographic characteristics (Table 1).

Table 1 Demographic characteristics of women ($N = 21$)

Characteristics	Number	Percent
Age group (years)		
26-30	3	14.3
31-35	8	38.1
36-40	7	33.3
41-45	3	14.3
Nationality		
Taiwanese	20	95.2
Chinese	1	4.8
Education (highest level achieved)		
High school	11	52.3
College	2	9.5
Undergraduate	6	28.6
Postgraduate	2	9.5
Professional		
Business	4	19.0
Health	3	14.3
Housewife	5	23.8
Other	9	42.9
Income $AUD/month		
< 500	6	28.6
501-1000	4	19.0
1001-1500	2	9.5
1501-2000	6	28.6
> 2000	3	14.3
Religion		
Buddhist	9	42.9
Taoism	7	33.3
Christian	2	9.5
Atheist	3	14.3
Obstetric data		
Parity		
Two	18	85.7
Three	3	14.3
Reasons for primary CS		
Prolonged labour	8	38.1
Foetal distress	3	14.3
Mal-presentation	4	19.1
Preeclampsia	2	9.5
Other	4	19.0

Observation of consultation between obstetricians and pregnant women

Of the 21 pregnant women who participated in the study, only nine were observed during the consultation with their obstetrician. A total of 12 pregnant women were not observed because their obstetricians did not agree to participate in the study. Interactions between obstetricians and pregnant women were observed during consultations in the Outpatient Department of Obstetrics and Gynaecology, when women were 33-34 weeks' gestation. Observational data were recorded and field notes were collected. During the consultation, women seldom asked questions. In most consultations obstetricians provided women with routine antenatal examinations such as checking the foetal heart beat and measuring the fundal height of the uterus. They did not provide any counselling regarding mode of birth. On average, each consultation was completed within 5-8 min.

Pregnant women's interviews

Ensuring the safety of the mother and baby was the overriding theme that emerged from the interviews with pregnant women. Two sub-themes within this overriding theme emerged: Influences on women's decision making and decision-making processes of women. Across these sub-themes, six categories were developed from thirteen sub-categories (Table 2).

Ensuring the safety of mother and baby

Women were concerned about their health and their baby's wellbeing. Most women in this study regarded the health and wellbeing of mothers and babies as the first consideration when making a decision regarding mode of birth. Two sub-themes were reflected in this theme: influences on women's decision-making and the decision-making processes of women.

Influences on women's decision-making

Previous birth experience Women's previous birth experience was the most frequently cited individual factor that affected women's decisions. Often women who had

Table 2 Categories and themes synthesized to core theme, ensuring the safety of mother and baby

Core theme	Ensuring the safety of mother and baby	
Themes	Categories	Sub-categories
Influences on women's decision-making	Previous birth experience	Positive experience Negatives experience
	Evaluation of mode of birth	Positive evaluation Negative evaluation
	Concern about the risks of vaginal birth	Uterine rupture Labour pain
	Current pregnancy situation	Foetal presentation Foetal size
	Informative resources	Obstetrician's recommendations The experience of significant others Impact of internet
	Health insurance	National Health Insurance Private insurance
Decision-making processes of women	Searching for information Listening obstetricians' professional judgment Evaluating alternatives Making a decision regarding mode of birth	

a positive birth experience for their previous birth opted for the same mode of birth for the subsequent birth. Conversely, women selected a different mode of birth if they had negative experiences during the previous birth.

Positive experience

Three women were confident in having a VBAC, based on their previous vaginal birth experience. Similarly, two women who had a positive experience of a CS selected RCS

> *16-03: I had a vaginal birth for my first baby and a caesarean section for my second baby. The experience of vaginal birth was excellent, so I have been thinking about having a vaginal birth for my third baby. I prefer to have a vaginal birth.* (Vaginal birth)

> *18-09: I feel that caesarean section was not really painful. I feel OK and I can endure it. Since I had the experience of a caesarean section for my first child, I will have my second child through the same method of caesarean section.* (RCS)

Negative experiences

A total of eight women had experienced a previous CS due to an unsuccessful induction of labour and in these instances cervical dilatation was limited to less than 2 cm during latent stage or 7-8 cm during active stage. These women lacked confidence with VBAC for this birth because of the previously unsuccessful experience of induction of labour.

> *05-01: Initially, I decided to have vaginal birth for the first birth but the doctor said it was less than two centimetres. So, I had induction of labour. However, the labour course was prolonged and I couldn't give birth for a long time.. So in the end, I still had a caesarean section. I am afraid to experience the same situation as before. So I have decided to have a caesarean section this time.*

Two women who had a negative experience with a CS were willing to attempt a VBAC. These two women reported that they were reluctant to have RCS because of the severe back pain and fear of anaesthesia from their last birth experience.

> *06-02: I felt that my caesarean section was terrible because it required anaesthesia and I felt terrible.*

Concern about the risks of vaginal birth

Concern about vaginal birth contributed to women selecting RCS. Two sub-categories were identified, uterine rupture and labour pain.

Uterine rupture

Some women were concerned about the issue of uterine rupture. They were fearful of uterine rupture associated with vaginal birth. Concern about the risk of uterine rupture in relation to the interval between previous CS and this pregnancy and caesarean wound healing was reported by women who had a strong intention to attempt VBAC. These women reported they had at least over a three-year interval between this birth and the previous birth and they were more willing to attempt VBAC.

> *11-02: Because I felt that [a caesarean section] was much safer, I was afraid that if the interval since the wound was too short, it might have caused problems at that time.*

Labour pain

Women were also fearful of not having the ability to cope with labour and birth because of fear of pain. A total of five women were reluctant to attempt VBAC because they were concerned about failure of VBAC leading to experiences of pain. Of the five women, one woman did not attempt a VBAC and four women underwent VBAC for their previous birth that resulted in a RCS. Women were concerned they would experience the pain of a labour and, in the event a CS was required, wound pain from the operation would result.

> *05-02: I am afraid that the result would be the same; that is, I will experience the pain twice!*

Evaluation of modes of birth

Women evaluated the different modes of birth and compared the advantages and disadvantages between CS and vaginal birth before deciding to have a RCS or a VBAC.

Positive evaluation

The majority of women stated that a vaginal birth is better than CS for mothers' and babies' health. In this study, three women had experienced births involving both a CS and vaginal birth; they were all determined to attempt a VBAC for the forthcoming birth.

> *07-01: It is for a quick recovery. My first baby was delivered by caesarean section, and my second baby was by vaginal birth. Comparing the two methods, I think the recovery was faster for the vaginal birth.*

Some women had a CS based on the consideration of safety and convenience. CS from their reports was viewed as much safer and more convenient than the uncertainty of a vaginal birth.

> *15-18: I felt that this method was more convenient. You do not need to worry when there is sudden and unexpected pain in the abdomen. I love things that can be done in accordance with a plan.*

Negative evaluation

Women compared the difference in pain and complications to evaluate the relative disadvantages between vaginal birth and CS. Pain was the most frequently cited negative influence on decision-making offered by women. They stated that vaginal birth was associated with pain before birth while there was pain after birth with CS.

> *16-04: I approve of vaginal birth more, and because I had a caesarean section before, I want to have a vaginal birth even more [for my next birth]. Because a caesarean section means that you feel the pain afterwards, but for a vaginal birth, you feel the pain on the day of the birth, and it's okay afterwards. For me, I am afraid of pain so I approve more of having a natural birth.*

When women compared the potential complications of the two modes of birth, they were concerned with the complication of adhesions if they had RCS, while incontinence was noted as the biggest concern by women if they selected VBAC.

> *07-17:For my previous birth, it was for almost two years, and I still have that kind of incontinence problem. I think it had a very far reaching impact!*

Current pregnancy situation

The situation of the current pregnancy affected women's decisions. In particular, if women wanted to have a VBAC, they were concerned about foetal presentation and foetal size.

Foetal presentation

Women who intended to attempt a VBAC continued to accept ultrasound examination before 38 weeks' gestation to confirm foetal presentation. Three women had foetal mal-presentation detected before 35 weeks' gestation but they all turned to a cephalic presentation between 35 and 38 weeks' gestation. All three women continued to plan for a RCS because they reported that they had already made this decision.

> *15-25: It was about the thirty-second week. The prenatal examination revealed an abnormal foetal position. In the later period (35weeks), I thought that I should make an appointment to have a caesarean section at that time, even though the foetal position was normal.*

Foetal size.

Women were also concerned about foetal size. They were concerned that they may not have VBAC if the foetus was too big.

> *17-19: Actually, my fear was more or less in my mind, and then based on the size of my baby, I was more worried. But I just wanted to see the baby's condition because my baby was not big, and then I thought, okay! Let's give it a try.*

Information resources

Women did not receive formal written information regarding VBAC from obstetricians and nurses. Instead, they received information from several sources, including obstetricians' recommendations, the experience of significant others, and impact of internet.

Obstetrician's recommendations

Of the information sources, obstetricians' recommendations were a critical factor influencing women's decisions. Eight women who decided to have a RCS were influenced by their obstetricians' recommendations that once a caesarean has been performed then the next birth should also be a caesarean. Four women reported that they did not receive any explanation from obstetricians but they complied with their obstetrician's choice.

> *13-01: Caesarean delivery! Doctor Z decided! It was not my decision. The doctor did not tell me the reason; he just took a look. Because my first baby was born with his assistance, he directly said caesarean delivery this time.*

The experience of significant others

Some women made birth choices based on their significant others' experience. Women's family members, in particular their mothers, mothers-in-law, sisters and sisters-in-law who had birth experiences were reported by women to have more influence on their decisions than other female friends or colleagues. The majority of significant others judged mode of birth based on their previous birth choices. For instance, they recommended RCS because they had a VBAC resulting in a RCS.

> *05-15: Because my older sister had the same results for her first baby, she suffered bad pain twice, exactly the same situation. She wanted to have a vaginal birth the first time, thinking that it is better for both the baby and the pregnant woman. But she tried to have a vaginal birth and got the same result. I made the decision because I asked my older sister.*

Impact of internet

Platforms such as Yahoo, Facebook, and Google were a common source of information for woman and some obstetricians also recommended women search for relevant information on the internet. On the internet, some women who had a previous CS shared their experiences regarding birth choices. These women stated that if you had the first baby by CS, you should have a CS for your second baby because the obstetrician made this recommendation. In addition, pregnant women were afraid to have a VBAC because of the dramatic descriptions of uterine rupture prevalent on the internet.

> *03-06: Many Internet rumours have been spread that the wound may rupture before the birth, and that the amniotic fluid will come out or the baby's hair will come out. Many opinions like that saying that vaginal birth after caesarean section also puts the baby and the mother at a high risk.*

Health insurance

Two sub-subcategories were identified, including National Health Insurance and private insurance. In Taiwan, the National Health Insurance System is a social insurance program administered by the government [39]. National Health Insurance is compulsory social insurance, providing all citizens with equal access to medical services. Insured people need to pay premiums regularly and they receive full medical care. Notably, National Health Insurance offers financial coverage for a subsequent pregnancy as long as women have had a previous CS.

National Health Insurance

National Health Insurance reimburses health care providers on a fee-for-service basis. For some women, the financial factor did not affect their decision for RCS because of the overriding considerations for safety.

> *14-13: The doctor said that the National Health Insurance program would cover it. If it did not provide cover, it would be very expensive. However, even in that situation, I would still choose a caesarean delivery because of the consideration of safety.*

Private insurance

In contrast to National Health Insurance, private insurance has strict criteria of financial coverage for RCS in Taiwan. Most private insurance does not cover RCS if women do not undergo a VBAC. Although a few women agreed to have a RCS based on their obstetricians' recommendations for consideration of safety, they were still upset their private insurance could not cover the cost.

> *19-30: I have private insurance! The doctor said that if you have an operation this time because of the previous caesarean delivery, it is not covered by insurance according to our insurance company.*

Decision-making processes of women

The decision-making process for women involved searching for information, listening to obstetricians' professional judgment, evaluating alternatives, and making a decision regarding mode of birth.

Searching for information Women sought relevant information regarding mode of birth from obstetricians, significant others or the internet and then discussed the options with obstetricians to confirm the mode of birth. Some (4/21) women did not receive information regarding VBAC from obstetricians and they complied with a RCS arrangement because their obstetrician had scheduled a RCS for them, without inquiring about the women's intention. These women accepted a decision for RCS in the first trimester of pregnancy.

Listening to obstetricians' professional judgment Although most women in this study wished for as natural a birth as possible, a total of 13 women on hearing their obstetrician's explanation and recommendation regarding mode of birth, selected RCS. The explanation of risks about uterine rupture from some obstetricians influenced women's decisions. Some more experienced obstetricians explained the monitoring systems, such as cardiotocography, used during labour to detect complications in women with risk factors, while the potential for urine rupture was described by less experienced obstetricians. Women were reluctant to have VBAC if the potential for uterine rupture was described.

Evaluating alternatives Women who had a preference for vaginal birth evaluated the advantages and disadvantages of alternatives, the condition of their health and that of their unborn baby, and obstetricians' professional recommendations to decide whether they would have a VBAC. In particular, women considered the interval between their pregnancies, current pregnancy status (such as foetal presentation and the estimated foetal size). In contrast, women who were willing to have VBAC reported equivalent proportions of risks between VBAC and vaginal birth, over a five-year birth interval between the current and the previous birth, and/or a well-equipped medical centre to manage emergency situations. These women were confident with vaginal birth and viewed vaginal birth positively.

Making a decision regarding mode of birth Some women made a decision for RCS/VBAC following evaluation of alternatives. A total of nine women who intended to have VBAC decided on this mode before 35-37 weeks gestation. Twelve women decided to have a RCS after considering their own condition and that of the foetus or once the risks were explained by obstetricians.

Postnatal women's interviews

Of the nine women who attempted a VBAC, six women were in their second pregnancy and three women were pregnant for the third time. All women who were in their third pregnancy achieved a VBAC; another two women achieved a vaginal birth; two women planned a VBAC but then scheduled a RCS because labour did not commence spontaneously by 38 weeks' gestation; and two women attempted a VBAC that resulted in a RCS as their labour course progressed slowly. Of the twelve women planning to give birth by RCS, all women delivered their second baby with RCS (Table 3). Half of the 21 postnatal women reported that they were satisfied with their decisions regarding preferred mode of birth, while a third of women accepted the outcome because of its perceived safety. Postnatal women evaluated their decisions regarding mode of birth in three areas, reflection on birth choices, reflection on factors influencing decisions, and reflection on outcomes of decisions.

Reflection on birth choice

Postnatal women who planned a VBAC reflected on the process of labour to form a view about the reason for their mode of birth. Women described being carefully monitored for signs of labour to evaluate whether the labour had started, such as a bloody show, water breaking, and labour pains.

> *17-22: I had labour induction for eight hours. After nine hours, [the contractions] were getting faster. I was three centimetres in nearly nine hours, but afterwards, [they became] faster, and I was fully dilated in half an hour.* (VBAC.)

Postnatal women who had RCS reflected on the process of RCS to evaluate their operative birth. These women reflected on their experience of an operation for their primary caesarean delivery compared with the RCS.

> *14-23: The doctor scheduled the operation for me and then performed a caesarean section directly. Last time, I did not feel anything; I was entirely asleep. But this time, I could feel pain and it felt quite terrible.* (RCS.)

Reflections on factors influencing decisions

After birth, postnatal women reflected on factors influencing their birth decisions. Obstetrician's advice was the main factor influencing a woman's decision. Some women in the study stated their obstetricians did not

Table 3 Women's intentions and their actual mode of birth

Birth mode	Intended mode of birth	Actual mode of birth	
		RCS	VBAC
VBAC	9 (42.9%)	4 (19.1%)	5 (23.8%)
RCS	12 (57.1%)	12 (57.1%)	0 (00.0%)
Total	21(100.0%)	16 (76.2%)	5 (23.8%)

provide them with any information to help them make birth choices but they complied with obstetricians' recommendation to have RCS. They also expressed their fear about asking questions of their obstetrician because the obstetrician had many patients waiting for consultation.

19-47 The doctor! I was that kind of person! What the doctor told me, that method, I just followed what he said. (RCS.)

10-47 The doctor was too busy. When you asked him questions, he just briefly understated it, telling you in just a few words. He could not answer all your doubts. (RCS.)

The study hospital offered information regarding general antenatal and postnatal care only. One woman, who attempted a VBAC that resulted in a RCS, attributed her failure to poor information provision.

08-58: I felt that the information was insufficient! (Woman attempted a VBAC that resulted in a RCS.)

Refection on outcomes of decisions

Postnatal women reflected on the outcomes of their decisions regarding mode of birth. All postnatal women were happy with their baby's health and wellbeing after birth except for one woman who attempted a VBAC that resulted in a RCS. These women reflected on their decisions from the perspectives of their recovery and their baby's health at birth.

02-39: I still felt weak but it was much better [than after the previous birth]. This birth was much better than the previous birth. (*Women had a* RCS.)

17-03: My physical strength was really different! Body recovery was pretty good. One month after birth, I felt good. My physical strength and vigour were good. (*Women had* a VBAC.).

Discussion

A qualitative approach was used to elicit Taiwanese women's decision-making processes and the influences on their mode of birth following a previous CS. Women's decision-making was identified using multiple data collection methods, including in-depth interviews, observations and field notes. In particular, this study used in-depth interviews to capture individual participants' viewpoints.

The Theory of Planned Behaviour (TPB) was used to assist in the interpretation of the findings. Specifically, the TPB framework assisted in discerning the reasons underpinning women's decisions and also assisted to understand women's actions regarding mode of birth. The TPB includes three psychometric determinants influencing human behavioural intentions [40]. These determinants are attitudes towards a behaviour, subjective norms and perceived behavioural control [41]. Taiwanese women's decisions were influenced by internal and external factors. Internal or personal factors related to an evaluation of mode of birth were reflected in the 'attitudes toward behaviour' construct of the TPB (Fig. 2). In this study, women who evaluated vaginal birth in a positive light were more willing to attempt VBAC. Conversely, women who had a negative attitude towards VBAC selected RCS. This finding is consistent with previous studies [14, 42].

Subjective norms include external factors influencing women's decision making such as obstetricians' recommendations, the experiences of significant others and health insurance. In this study, obstetricians' recommendations and the experiences of significant others (female families or friends) played an important role in women's decision-making. Obstetricians have been described as a major factor in driving the CS rate upward [10]. Research has shown that hospital physicians were the most frequent information providers; however, they provided women with information about procedural issues rather than possible health risks and benefits [43, 44]. In the present study, unbalanced explanations regarding the risk of uterine rupture potentially affected women in making decisions in favour of RCS. This finding corroborates findings of a recent Australian study [45]. Australian women who chose RCS reported that VBAC was the most risky option, based on the information they received from hospital obstetricians [45]. In addition, some pregnant women in the study complied with obstetricians' recommendation to opt for RCS because they found it difficult to oppose obstetricians' opinions. Medical recommendations, especially during the birth, were experienced as powerful and difficult for women to oppose [45]. Power and a knowledge imbalance, as well as trusting relationships with obstetricians continue to reinforce this momentum. Positive benefits of midwife led care indicate the recommencement of midwifery practice in Taiwan to optimise maternal care [46–49].

Perceived behavioural control is related to women's intention to participate in decision-making. Self-efficacy is a key concept of perceived behavioural control [40]. Four constructs in our findings are related to women's self-efficacy, including previous birth experience, current

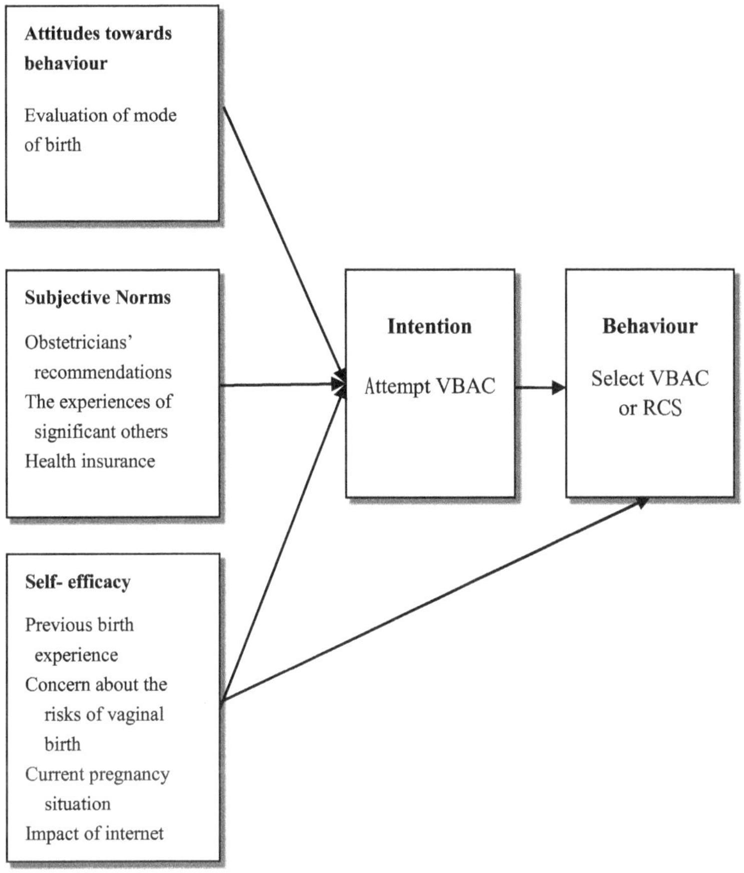

Fig. 2 Taiwanese women's decision-making regarding mode of birth as applied to TPB

pregnancy situation, concern about the risks of vaginal birth and impact of the internet. In this study, women who had a high sense of self-efficacy were more willing to attempt VBAC. Several studies have demonstrated that previous experiences influenced decision-making in women who had had a previous CS and these experiences have been found to affect women's subsequent birth choice [16, 50–53]. In the present study, Taiwanese women who had a positive experience selected the same mode of birth as their previous birth, while women who had a negative experience chose a different mode of birth. These findings are similar to those of a recent study, in which 85% of women who had an RCS stated they would make the same choice again, compared to 70.1% for the planned VBAC group [53]. In this study, most women lacked confidence to have VBAC because of their previous negative experience of induction. This finding is supported by findings of another Taiwanese study [54]. According to Kuan [54], Taiwanese women who were aiming to birth vaginally but had to have a CS were aware of medical intervention practices and they requested CS out of fear of "suffering twice". Kuan argued that Taiwanese women requested a CS for their first birth because hospitals enforce a significant amount of medical intervention [54]. Because of concern about the risks of vaginal birth, some women considered RCS as the safest method for mother and baby based on medical perspectives; they were therefore unwilling to attempt VBAC. However, this assumption has been based on a misunderstanding of the risks and benefits of VBAC [55]. In fact, several previous studies have shown that women who have had a previous CS lacked knowledge about the benefits and risks regarding the various birth options [12, 56, 57]. Internet has been found to play an important role for women in searching for information regarding mode of birth [44, 58]. Due to a lack of leaflets, booklets and newsletters regarding VBAC in organisations, Taiwanese women sought help from other women on the internet. However, a lack of comprehensive information and inaccurate information on the internet contributed to study participants' decision to avoid an attempt of VBAC. The findings of the present study in relation to use of the internet for information were consistent with those of a recent Swedish study [58]. This highlights the need for high quality information provision if the misconceptions are to be corrected.

Strengths and limitations

For geographical convenience, data were collected in a large private medical centre rather than in a public hospital or a clinic in Taiwan. Therefore, the findings may not be transferable to all pregnant women in Taiwan. Women were interviewed in a waiting room while awaiting their consultation, the location and time constraints may have limited their ability to fully share their stories. In spite of these limitations, the findings that emerged from participants' interviews were meaningful and offered greater depth than a survey would have produced. Additionally, this study comprised of interviews with prenatal and postnatal women which was helpful in capturing their actual thinking regarding mode of birth from different perspectives. Observation of women-obstetrician dyads during consultations enabled examination of the actual interactions between obstetricians and pregnant women, thereby providing a deeper understanding of the information sharing and decision-making process than would not have been obtained through the individual interviews alone.

Conclusions

The health and wellbeing of mother and baby were the major concern for women deciding on a mode of birth after a previous CS. Influenced by internal and external factors, women's interactions with obstetricians regarding mode of birth choices varied from complying with obstetricians' recommendations to shared communication styles. In the present study, if women participated passively in the decision-making process regarding their birth choices, their choices were primarily guided by risk reduction of uterine rupture. They were particularly influenced by obstetricians' recommendations in early pregnancy. By contrast, women who actively participated in decision-making regarding their birth choices were guided by a previous experience of vaginal birth. These women discussed with obstetricians their intention to attempt VBAC and were actively involved in the decision-making.

All women have the right to be informed of alternative options of birth. Internal factors, in particular, establishing a supportive birth environment such as Next Birth after Caesarean (NBAC) clinics is helpful in facilitating women's confidence in VBAC. Routine provision of explanations by obstetricians regarding risks associated with alternative birth options, in addition to financial coverage for RCS from National Health Insurance, would assist women's decision-making. Establishment of a website of decision aids to provide women with reliable information about birthing options may also assist women's decision-making. Finally, midwife-led models of care for information provision may hold promise for reducing risks of birth in Taiwan.

Abbreviations

CS: Caesarean Section; NBAC: Next Birth after Caesarean; RCS: Repeat Caesarean Section; VBAC: Vaginal Birth after Caesarean

Acknowledgments

We acknowledge that Deakin University offered a scholarship for principal investigator. We also sincerely thank the obstetricians and women who participated in the study and the secretary of the Department of Obstetrics and Gynaecology who assisted in recruitment.

Funding

No funding was received for the study.

Authors' contributions

SWC, TKB, AMH and CN contributed to the research design and methods development. SWC undertook recruitment, conducted the interviews, undertook data analysis, and led the preparation of the transcripts. All authors contributed to the analysis and interpretation of the data and the development of the manuscript. All authors have approved the final version of the manuscript.

Competing interests

The authors declare that they have no competing interest.

Author details

[1]Deakin University, Faculty of Health, School of Nursing and Midwifery, Geelong, Australia. [2]National Taipei University of Nursing and Health Science, School of Nursing, Taipei, Taiwan. [3]Centre for Quality and Patient Safety Research-Monash Health Partnership, Clayton, Australia. [4]James Cook University & Townsville Hospital and Health Service, School of Nursing and Midwifery, Townsville, Australia. [5]Centre for Quality and Patient Safety Research- Alfred Health Partnership, Melbourne, Australia.

References

1. Australian Institute of Health and Welfare. Australia's mothers and babies 2015—in brief Perinatal Stat Ser. 2017;33:18.
2. Curtin SC, Gregory KD, Korst LM, Uddin SF. Maternal Morbidity for Vaginal and Cesarean Deliveries, According to Previous Cesarean History: New Data From the Birth Certificate, 2013. Natl Vital Stat Rep. 2015;64(4):1–13.
3. Knight H, Gurol-Urganci I, Meulen J, Mahmood T, Richmond D, Dougall A, et al. Vaginal birth after caesarean section: a cohort study investigating factors associated with its uptake and success. BJOG. 2014;121(2):183–92.
4. Guise JM, Denman MA, Emeis C, Marshall N, Walker M, Fu R, et al. Vaginal birth after cesarean: new insights on maternal and neonatal outcomes. Obstet Gynecol. 2010;115(6):1267–78.
5. Al-Zirqi I, Stray-Pedersen B, Forsen L, Vangen S. Uterine rupture after previous caesarean section. BJOG. 2010;117(7):809–20.
6. Ma LK, Liu N, Bian XM, Teng LR, Qi H, Gong XM, et al. Pregnancy outcomes of repeat cesarean section in Peking union medical college hospital. Chin Med Sci J. 2009;24(3):147–50.
7. Fawsitt CG, Bourke J, Greene RA, Everard CM, Murphy A, Lutomski JE. At what price? A cost-effectiveness analysis comparing trial of labour after previous caesarean versus elective repeat caesarean delivery. PLoS One. 2013;8(3):e58577.
8. Cragin EB. Conservatism in obstetrics. N Y Med J. 1916;104:1–3. (Level III)
9. Mazzoni A, Althabe F, Liu NH, Bonotti AM, Gibbons L, Sánchez AJ, et al. Women's preference for cesarean section: a systematic review and meta-analysis of observational studies. Obstet Anesth Dig. 2012;32(1):23–4.

10. Weaver J, Statham H, Richards M. Are there "unnecessary" cesarean sections? Perceptions of women and obstetricians about cesarean sections for nonclinical indications. Birth. 2007;34(1):32–41.
11. Wang CK. Caesarean delivery on maternal request: systematic review on maternal and neonatal outcomes: the University of Hong Kong 2011.
12. Renner RM, Eden KB, Osterweil P, Chan BK, Guise JM. Informational factors influencing patient's childbirth preferences after prior cesarean. Am J Obstet Gynecol. 2007;196(5):e14–e6.
13. Farnsworth A, Pearson PH. Choosing mode of delivery after previous caesarean birth. British J Midwifery. 2007;15(4):188.
14. Godden B, Hauck Y, Hardwick T, Bayes S. Women's erceptions of contributory factors for successful vaginal birth after cesarean. Int J Childbirth. 2012;2(2):96–106.
15. Shoaib T, Memon S, Javed I, Pario S, Bhutta SZ. Decision-making and involvement of women with previous C-section in choosing their mode of delivery. J Pak Med Assoc. 2012;62(10):1038–41.
16. Fisher C, Hauck Y, Fenwick J. How social context impacts on women's fears of childbirth: a western Australian example. Soc Sci Med. 2006;63(1):64–75.
17. Roberts RG, Deutchman M, King VJ, Fryer GE, Miyoshi TJ. Changing policies on vaginal birth after cesarean: impact on access. Birth. 2007;34(4):316–22.
18. Cox KJ. Providers' perspectives on the vaginal birth after cesarean guidelines in Florida, United States: a qualitative study. BMC Pregnancy Childbirth. 2011;11(1):72.
19. Ministry of Health and Welfare. 2015 statistics of birth reporting system Taiwan: 2016.
20. Kuo S. Changes in nurse-midwifery practices in Taiwan. Hu li za zhi J Nurs. 2009;56(2):75–80.
21. Hatem M, Sandall J, Devane D, Soltani H, Gates S. Midwife-led versus other models of care for childbearing women (review). Database of Syst Rev. 2008;4
22. Chiou YL, Chou FH. History and prospect of the profession and education of midwifery in Taiwan Nurs J. 2006;5 (2):65-70.
23. Chu KH, Tai CJ, Hsu CS, Yeh MC, Chien LY. Women's preference for cesarean delivery and differences between Taiwanese women undergoing different modes of delivery. BMC Health Serv Res. 2010;10(1):138.
24. Liu CM, Lin Y Jr, Su YY, Chang SD, Cheng PJ. Impact of health policy based on the self-management program on cesarean section rate at a tertiary hospital in Taiwan. J Formos Med Assoc. 2013;112(2):93–8.
25. Guise JM, Berlin M, McDonagh M, Osterweil P, Chan B, Helfand M. Safety of vaginal birth after cesarean: a systematic review. Obstet Gynecol. 2004; 103(3):420–9.
26. Gamble J, Creedy DK, McCourt C, Weaver J, Beake S. A critique of the literature on women's request for cesarean section. Birth. 2007;34(4):331–40.
27. Tsai HT, Wu CH. Vaginal birth after cesarean section-The world trend and local experience in Taiwan. Taiwan J Obstet Gynecol. 2017;56(1):41–5.
28. Chu KH, editor Effect of Self-Efficacy Regarding a Smooth Labor on Cesarean Deliveries Among Primiparas in Taiwan. Sigma Theta Tau International's 25th International Nursing Research Congress. 2014. STTI.
29. Chu KH, Lee YH, Tai CJ, Lin YH, Huang CM, Chien LY. Caesarean delivery before 39 weeks associated with selecting an auspicious time for birth in Taiwan. Women Birth. 2015.
30. Chen CS, Liu TC, Chen B, Lin CL. The failure of financial incentive? The seemingly inexorable rise of cesarean section. Soc Sci Med. 2014;101:47–51.
31. Hastie P, Hay P. 7 qualitative approaches. Armour, K and Macdonald, D Research Methods in Physical Education and Youth Sport; 2012. p. 79–94.
32. Petty NJ, Thomson OP, Stew G. Ready for a paradigm shift? Part 2: introducing qualitative research methodologies and methods. Man Ther. 2012;17(5):378–84.
33. Kvale S. Interviews an introduction to qualitative research interviewing: sage publications. 1996.
34. McNamara C, editor. General guidelines for conducting interviews: Minnesota; 1999.
35. Corbin J, Strauss A. Basics of qualitative research: techniques and procedures for developing grounded theory. 3rd ed. Thousand Oaks, CA: Sage; 2008.
36. Speziale HS, Streubert HJ, Carpenter DR. Qualitative research in nursing: Advancing the humanistic imperative. Philadelphia: Lippincott Williams & Wilkins; 2011.
37. Flick U. An introduction to qualitative research. 5th ed. London: Sage; 2014.
38. Lincoln YS, Guba EG. Naturalistic inquiry. Newbury Park, CA: Sage Publications; 1985.
39. Administration NHI. National health insurance in Taiwan 2013-2014 annual report Taiwan: National Health Insurance Administration, 2014.
40. Ajzen I. Perceived behavioral control, self-efficacy, locus of control, and the theory of planned behavior. J Appl Soc Psychol. 2002;32(4):665–83.
41. Ajzen I. The theory of planned behavior. Organ Behav Hum Decis Process. 1991;50(2):179–211.
42. Mone F, Harrity C, Toner B, Mcnally A, Adams B, Currie A. Predicting why women have elective repeat cesarean deliveries and predictors of successful vaginal birth after cesarean. Int J Gynecol Obstet. 2014;126(1):67–9.
43. Emmett CL, Shaw ARG, Montgomery AA, Murphy DJ. Women's experience of decision making about mode of delivery after a previous caesarean section: the role of health professionals and information about health risks. BJOG. 2006;113(12):1438–45.
44. Lagan BM, Sinclair M, George KW. Internet use in pregnancy informs women's decision making: a web-based survey. Birth. 2010;37(2):106–15.
45. McGrath P, Phillips E, Vaughan G. Vaginal birth after caesarean risk decision-making: Australian findings on the mothers' perspective. Int J Nurs Pract. 2010;16(3):274–81.
46. White HK, le May A, Cluett ER. Evaluating a midwife-led model of antenatal Care for Women with a previous cesarean section: a retrospective. Comparative Cohort Study Birth. 2016;43(3):200–8.
47. Suzuki S. Trend analysis of primary midwife-led delivery care at a Japanese perinatal center. Int J Med Sci. 2014;11(5):466.
48. Ten Hoope-Bender P, de Bernis L, Campbell J, Downe S, Fauveau V, Fogstad H, et al. Improvement of maternal and newborn health through midwifery. The Lancet. 2014;384(9949):1226–35.
49. Renfrew MJ, McFadden A, Bastos MH, Campbell J, Channon AA, Cheung NF, et al. Midwifery and quality care: findings from a new evidence-informed framework for maternal and newborn care. Lancet. 2014;384(9948):1129–45.
50. Kringeland T, Daltveit AK, Moller A. How does preference for natural childbirth relate to the actual mode of delivery? A population-based cohort study from Norway. Birth. 2010;37(1):21–7.
51. Moffat MA, Bell JS, Porter MA, Lawton S, Hundley V, Danielian P, et al. Decision making about mode of delivery among pregnant women who have previously had a caesarean section: a qualitative study. BJOG. 2007; 114(1):86–93.
52. Nilsson C, Bondas T, Lundgren I. Previous birth experience in women with intense fear of childbirth. J Obstet Gynecol Neonatal Nurs. 2010;39(3):298–309.
53. Shorten A, Shorten B. The importance of mode of birth after previous cesarean: success, satisfaction, and postnatal health. J Midwifery Women's Health. 2012;57(2):126–32.
54. Kuan CI. A reinterpretation of maternal requests for cesarean sections in Taiwan. J Archaeology Anthropol 2010;72:97-136.
55. Ecker JL, Frigoletto FD. Cesarean delivery and the risk–benefit calculus. N Engl J Med. 2007;356(9):885–8.
56. Declercq E, Sakala C, Corry MP, Applebaum S. Listening to mothers II: report of the second national US survey of women's childbearing experiences. J Prinatal Educ. 2007;16(4):9.
57. Klein MC, Liston R, Fraser WD, Baradaran N, Hearps SJC, Tomkinson J, et al. Attitudes of the new generation of Canadian obstetricians: how do they differ from their predecessors? Birth. 2011;38(2):129–39.
58. Larsson M. A descriptive study of the use of the internet by women seeking pregnancy-related information. Midwifery. 2009;25(1):14–20.

4

Patterns of caesarean section in HIV infected and non-infected women in Malawi: is caesarean section used for PMTCT?

Lyson Tenthani[1,2,3*], Joep J. van Oosterhout[4,5], Andreas D. Haas[2], Malango Msukwa[6,8], Nozgechi Phiri[6,8], Frank Chimbwandira[1], Kali Tal[2], Karoline Aebi-Popp[7], Janne Estill[2,8,9] and Olivia Keiser[2,8]

Abstract

Background: Caesarean section (CS) is not recommended for PMTCT in Malawi HIV Guidelines, contrary to most high-income countries where CS is indicated if viral suppression is sub-optimal pre-delivery. We describe patterns of CS in HIV-infected and uninfected women in Malawi and explored if insight into the use of Elective CS (ECS) for PMTCT could be obtained.

Methods: We used routinely collected data from individual medical records from 17 large health facilities in the central and southern regions of Malawi, from January 2010 to December 2013. We included data from maternity registers from all HIV-positive women, and randomly selected around every fourth woman with negative or unknown HIV status. We used multivariable logistic regressions and cluster-based robust standard errors to examine independent associations of patient- and facility characteristics with CS and ECS.

Results: We included 62,033 women in the analysis. The weighted percentage of women who had a spontaneous vaginal delivery was 80.0% (CI 95% 79.5–80.4%); 2.4% (95% CI 2.3–2.6%) had a vacuum extraction; 2.3% (95% CI 2.2–2.5%) had a vaginal breech delivery; 14.0% (95% CI 13.6–14.4%) had a CS while for 1.3% (95% CI 1.2–1.4%) the mode of delivery was not recorded. Prevalence of CS without recorded medical or obstetric indication (ECS) was 5.1%, ($n = 3152$). Presence of maternal and infant complications and older age were independently associated with CS delivery. HIV-positive women were less likely to have ECS than HIV negative women (aOR 0.65; 95%-CI 0.57–0.74). Among HIV-positive women, those on antiretrovirals (ARV's) for ≥4 weeks prior to delivery were less likely to have ECS than HIV-positive women who had not received ARVs during pregnancy (aOR 0.81; 95% CI 0.68–0.96).

Conclusions: The pattern of CS's in Malawi is largely determined by maternal and infant complications. Positive HIV status was negatively associated with CS delivery, possibly because health care workers were concerned about the risk of occupational HIV transmission and the known increased risk of post-operative complications. Our results leave open the possibility that CS is practiced to prevent MTCT given that ECS was more common among women at high risk of MTCT due to no or short exposure to ARV's.

* Correspondence: ltenthani@gmail.com
[1]Department of HIV and AIDS, Ministry of Health, Lilongwe, Malawi
[2]Institute of Social and Preventive Medicine, University of Bern, Bern, Switzerland
Full list of author information is available at the end of the article

Background

In 2014, an estimated 1.1 million people were living with HIV in Malawi, including 130,000 children under fifteen [1]. Mother-to-child transmission (MTCT) is the most common cause of infection in children. Without intervention, risk of MTCT is estimated to be 5–10% over the course of pregnancy, 10–20% during labour, and 10–20% during breastfeeding; overall 30–45% of infants born to mothers with HIV will contract the virus [2]. With effective antiretroviral therapy (ART), the risk of MTCT can be reduced to less than 5% [3].

In Malawi the total fertility rate is estimated to be between 4.4 and 5.7 children per woman. High ratios of maternal mortality (460–680 per 100,000 live births) and neonatal mortality (27 per 1000 live births) have been recorded. The contraceptive prevalence rate varies between 44.4% (sexually active unmarried women) and 59. 2% (married women) [4]. Maternal mortality is believed to be strongly impacted on by the HIV epidemic, with a steep increase between 1992 and 2000 and a sharp decline since the start of free ART provision in 2004 [4].

In this context, Malawi implemented a test and treat policy ("Option B+") to facilitate access to ART for all HIV-infected pregnant and breastfeeding women [4]. The policy was adopted by other low-income countries and is now recommended by the World Health Organization [5]. Under Option B+, women are diagnosed with HIV during routine testing in antenatal care and they initiate ART within one week of diagnosis [4]. In 2011, Option B+ was implemented as Malawi's National PMTCT policy and the ART coverage among pregnant women increased strongly [6]. However, even with Option B+, a substantial proportion of women are likely not to be fully virologically suppressed when around 20% of pregnant women are not tested for HIV [7]; almost 20% discontinue treatment within the first months [8, 9]; and about 30% adhere to ART inadequately during pregnancy, with young age and Option B+ indication for ART as risk factors [10]. Overall, 9% of women who are on ART during pregnancy do not achieve adequate virological suppression at delivery [11].

Caesarean section (CS) can be used to reduce the risk of intrapartum HIV transmission [12–14]. In high-income countries CS is recommended for women with > 400 HIV RNA copies/ml at the time of delivery [15, 16]. In resource constrained settings like Malawi, elective caesarean section (ECS; defined here as a CS without documented obstetric or medical indication) is not a recommended PMTCT strategy [17] as the increased risk of morbidity and mortality that is associated with ECS is expected to outweigh its HIV prevention benefits [18, 19]. In addition, resources and capacity to perform CS are limited in low-income countries like Malawi [19, 20]. Despite this, it is possible that health care workers and pregnant women in Malawi opt for an ECS in circumstances where MTCT risk is known or believed to be high.

We describe the prevalence and pattern of indications of CS among deliveries of HIV positive and HIV negative women in Malawi. We also explore our data for the potential practice of using ECS for PMTCT.

Methods

Data sources

We entered routinely collected data from individual medical records in 17 large health facilities in the central and southern regions of Malawi, from January 2010 to December 2013. The selected facilities were among 20 study facilities that participate in the Umoyo+ study (http://aidsinfo.unaids.org/). Two of the 20 facilities were excluded because no CS's were done, another one because of missing data. In the Malawi government health care system, observations from labour and delivery are recorded on labour charts and summarized in a maternity register. These standard monitoring and evaluation tools capture demographic characteristics, obstetrical history, and observations on the delivery and infant. Theatre registers document detailed information about CS (i.e. indication, duration, observations and outcome of the procedure). At each health facility, we included data from maternity registers from all HIV positive women and from a randomly selected approximately one quarter of women with negative or unknown HIV status. We describe the sampling strategy in more detail in the Additional file 1: Appendix 1. In case the indication for CS could not be determined from the maternity register, we extracted relevant information from labour charts and theatre registers.

Definitions

Health care workers classified the mode of delivery either as CS or as vaginal delivery (including assisted vaginal deliveries that use vacuum and forceps extraction). The main outcomes of the study were CS and ECS. The delivery was defined as CS when it was conducted through CS irrespective of the reason for the procedure. A CS was classified as ECS if it was conducted electively without documentation of an obstetric or medical indication. In women with a previous CS, the current CS was counted as ECS only if there was no trial of vaginal delivery for the current delivery with no previous history of CS (if a previous CS was the indication for the current CS, this will be reported according to local guidelines). HIV status was positive if a woman was admitted for labour and delivery with documentation of a positive HIV test result or if she was on ART, or if she had a positive test result obtained between the onset of labour and the period immediately after delivery. A woman was classified as HIV negative if she had a negative test result in that same period or if she had a documented negative test result during the current pregnancy. HIV unknown status was assigned if testing was not documented, if it was documented as not done, or if test results were inconclusive or missing.

Statistical analysis

We provide patterns of indications for CS among HIV positive, unknown and negative women using descriptive statistics. To examine independent associations between CS or ECS and patient and facility characteristics, we used multivariable logistic regression analyses, with cluster-based robust standard errors adjusting for clustering of patients within facilities. We considered the following explanatory variables: year of admission, maternal complications (hemorrhage, obstructed/prolonged labour, pre-eclampsia, maternal sepsis, ruptured uterus, others when unspecified, unknown if nothing was recorded), infant complications (prematurity, low birth weight, asphyxia, other if unspecified, unknown if nothing was recorded), HIV status (negative, positive, unknown), and ARV use during pregnancy (no ARVs, ARVs for < 4 weeks, ARVs for≥4 weeks), number of deliveries (0, 1, 2–3, > 3), singleton (yes/no), age category (< 20, 20–24, 25–29, 30–34, > 34 years), facility ownership (government or Christian Health Association (CHAM)) and location (urban or rural). We ran 4 models each to examine predictors of CS and predictors of ECS. We included all women in the first CS model; women with unknown HIV status in the second, HIV negative women in the third model and HIV positive women in the fourth. In the four ECS models, we excluded women who had a previous CS and failed trial of vaginal delivery and women with a recorded maternal or infant complication (as these women were not at risk of ECS) (Fig. 1). In all analyses HIV negative women were weighted by the inverse of the probability that the observation was included because of the sampling design. HIV positive women were assigned a weight of 1 as data from all HIV positive women was analyzed (see sampling strategy description in Additional file 1: Appendix 1). We therefore report weighted prevalence rates throughout. All data were analyzed with STATA software (Version 13.1, Stata Corporation, Texas USA.

Results

Characteristics of study participants

Out of 62,033 women included in the analysis 56,292 (90.7%) had a known HIV status and 5741 (9.3%) had an unknown HIV status. Among women with known HIV status 23,193 were HIV positive and 33,099 were HIV negative, resulting in a weighted HIV prevalence of 9.7%. (95% CI 9.3–10.1%). Characteristics of study participants stratified

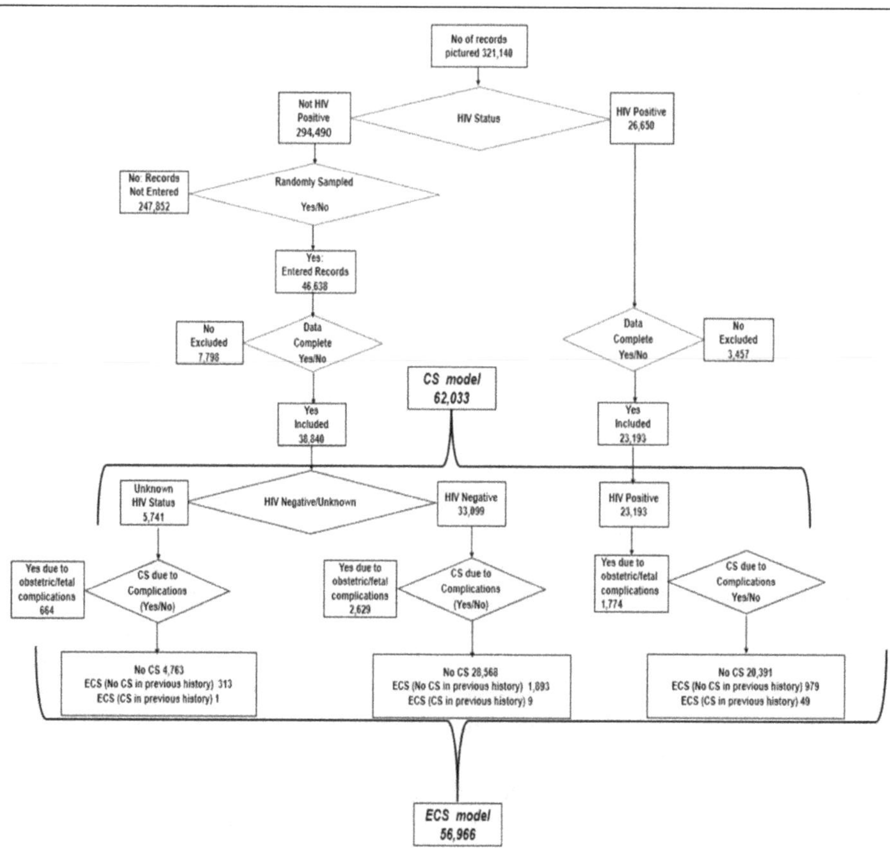

CS=Cesarean Section ECS=Elective Cesarean Section

Fig. 1 Flow chart showing the patients' records included in the study and the specific model according to their HIV status and mode of delivery

by HIV status are shown in Table 1. Their median age was 25 years (interquartile range [IQR] 20–30). Women had a median of one delivery (IQR 1–3). The majority of women (89.6%, 55,583) received care at government owned facilities and 10.4% (6450) were managed in faith-based clinics. About 76% of the women (47,215) attended clinics in rural settings and 24% (14,818) were seen at urban clinics.

Maternal and infant complications

The proportion of women with maternal complications was 12.5%(95% CI 12.1–12.9%). Maternal complications occurred more frequently among HIV positive (15.2%; 95% CI 14.8–15.7%) than among HIV negative women (11.5%; 95% CI 11.1–11.9%). Among women with unknown HIV status the corresponding percentage was 16.2% (95% CI 15. 2–17.3%). The percentage of infants who had complications was 14.5% (95% CI 14.1–14.8%). Infant complications were more common among HIV exposed infants (25.1%, CI 24. 5–25.7%) than among infants born to mothers with negative (12.7%, CI 12.3–13.1%) or unknown HIV status (18.3%, CI 17.2–19.5%). The distribution of specific maternal and infant complications by HIV status is shown in Table 1.

Mode of delivery

The percentage of women who had a spontaneous vaginal delivery was 80.0% (CI 95% 79.5–80.4%); 2.4% (95% CI 2.3–2.6%) had vacuum extraction; 2.3% (95% CI 2.2–2.5%) had a vaginal breech delivery; 14.0% (95% CI 13.6–14.4%) had CS while for 1.3% (95% CI 1.2–1.4%) of the women mode of delivery was not recorded.

Overall, prevalence of CS among women with unknown HIV status was significantly higher than among deliveries of HIV negative women, which in turn was significantly higher than among deliveries in HIV positive women (HIV unknown 16.2%, 95% CI 15.1–17.3%; HIV negative 13.8%, 95% CI 13.3–14.2%; HIV positive 12.1%, 95% CI 11.7–12.5%). The distribution of CS according to individual and facility-level characteristics stratified by HIV status is shown in Table 2. Among women with a recorded complication 64.4% (95% CI 63.9–64.9%) had a CS delivery compared to 6.8% (95% CI 6.7–6.9%) in women without a recorded complication. The prevalence of elective CS without recorded medical or obstetric indication (ECS) was 5.1% (95% CI 4.9–5.3%).

Associations of individual and facility level characteristics with CS

HIV positive women were less likely to have CS compared to HIV negative women (aOR 0.60; 95%-CI 0.51–0.71) while those with unknown HIV status had similar odds of CS as HIV negative women (aOR 1.01; 96% CI 0.84–1.20). Table 3 shows the results from the multivariable logistic regression analyses of variables associated with CS. Presence of maternal complications, infant complications and older age were independently associated with CS delivery in each of the three groups. Twin delivery and delivering for the first time were associated with a higher probability of CS in all groups. Year of admission was independently associated with a lower odds of CS after 2010 only in HIV negative women.

Associations of individual and facility level characteristics with ECS

Results from the multivariable logistic regression analyses of variables associated with ECS delivery among all women, HIV positive women, those with unknown HIV status and HIV negative women are presented in Table 4. HIV positive women were less likely to have ECS compared to HIV negative women (aOR 0.65; 95%-CI 0.57–0.74). Among HIV positive women, those who were on ARV's for ≥4 weeks prior to delivery were less likely to have ECS than HIV positive women who had not received ARVs during pregnancy. Older age and delivery in an urban facility were associated with higher odds of ECS in all groups. First deliveries and non-singleton deliveries were independently associated with an increased odds of ECS in all groups except in women with HIV unknown status. Delivery in 2010, was independently associated with ECS, except in HIV positive women.

Discussion

We found that the prevalence of CS in deliveries in 17 large health facilities in Malawi was 14.0% and was higher among deliveries of HIV negative women compared to HIV positive women. The 14% CS prevalence found in our study is almost three times higher than the 5% last reported in the 2010 nationally representative study [21, 22] and the 6.2% reported in a multinational study in sub-Saharan Africa [23]. However this can be explained by our exclusion of deliveries taking place in primary health facilities where CS services are not offered.

CS delivery was strongly associated with presence of maternal or infant complications. As expected, maternal and infant complications were more common among HIV positive women than HIV negative women, while those with unknown HIV status had similar frequency of complications to HIV positive women (possibly due to undiagnosed HIV among those with unknown status). We also found that among HIV positive women the chance of ECS was higher in those who had received less than 4 weeks or no exposure to ARVs during pregnancy. As in other studies the adjusted odds of a CS delivery increased with age and almost doubled among HIV positive women aged above 29 years compared to those below 20 years [24–27].

Our data suggest that patterns of CS in Malawi are also influenced by other factors than maternal and fetal obstetric conditions. The lower frequency of CS among HIV positive women in spite of their higher maternal and infant complication rates could be explained by

Table 1 Characteristics of study participants by HIV status

Item		All women ($n = 62,033$)		Women with unknown HIV status ($n = 5741$)		HIV negative women ($n = 33,099$)		HIV positive women ($n = 23,193$)	
		Total	Weighted %	Total	Weighted %	Total	Weighted %	Total	Weighted %
Year of admission	2010	10,526	20.8	675	18.4	4272	20.9	5579	24.1
	2011	16,216	30.9	1647	38.2	7056	29.4	7513	32.4
	`2012	16,749	22.6	1888	23.6	9889	22.5	4972	21.4
	2013	18,542	25.8	1531	19.9	11,882	27.2	5129	22.1
Maternal complication	None	52,992	86.8	4674	82.4	28,932	88.0	19,386	83.6
	Hemorrhage	1566	2.0	173	2.9	621	1.7	772	3.3
	OPL	2899	4.3	312	5.0	1413	4.7	1175	5.1
	Preeclampsia	511	0.8	78	1.2	260	0.7	173	0.7
	Sepsis	101	0.1	13	0.3	21	0.1	67	0.3
	RU	161	0.2	28	0.5	68	0.2	65	0.3
	Unspecified	3275	5.0	386	6.4	1610	4.7	1278	5.5
	Unknown	528	0.7	77	1.4	174	0.5	277	1.2
Infant complication	None	51,017	85.8	4691	82.1	28,892	87.6	17,435	75.2
	Prematurity	2609	3.6	281	4.7	1163	3.3	1156	5.0
	LBW	2166	3.0	261	4.8	844	2.5	1073	4.6
	Asphyxia	2140	3.4	246	3.9	1158	3.3	732	3.2
	Unspecified	1683	2.6	197	3.3	811	2.4	675	2.9
	Unknown	2418	1.6	65	1.2	231	0.8	2122	9.1
No of previous deliveries	0	14,446	29.1	1738	30.6	10,125	30.8	2583	11.1
	1	12,554	21.2	1138	19.9	7314	21.8	4102	17.7
	2–3	19,780	28.0	1505	26.2	8856	26.9	9419	40.6
	> 3	14,554	20.5	1180	20.4	6523	19.6	6851	29.5
	Unknown	699	1.2	180	2.9	281	0.9	238	1.0
Age in years	< 20	11,191	23.0	1428	26.3	8217	24.4	1546	6.7
	20–24	17,485	31.0	1738	30.5	10,491	32.0	5256	22.7
	25–29	14,003	20.0	1035	17.1	6374	19.5	6595	28.4
	30–34	10,960	13.9	740	12.5	4389	12.9	58,31	25.1
	> 34	7288	10.2	583	9.8	3094	9.6	3610	15.6
	Unknown	1106	1.9	217	4.0	534	1.6	355	1.5
Singleton	Yes	59,862	96.6	5519	96.1	32,068	96.7	22,274	96.0
	No	2171	3.4	222	3.9	1031	3.3	919	4.0
ARVs during pregnancy	None, HIV+	11,938	4.3	N/A				11,938	51.5
	<4wks	2716	1.0					2716	11.7
	≥4wks	8539	3.1					8539	36.8
	None, HIV-	38,840	91.6					N/A	
Facility ownership	Government	55,583	89.6	5476	95.3	29,447	88.1	20,660	89.1
	CHAM	6450	10.4	265	4.7	3652	11.9	2533	10.9
Facility location	Rural	47,215	80.4	4936	86.2	26,660	80.8	15,619	67.3
	Urban	14,818	19.6	805	13.8	6439	19.2	7574	32.7

aOR adjusted odds ratio, *OPL* obstructed/prolonged labor, *RU* Ruptured Uterus, *LBW* Low Birth Weight, *ARVs* antiretrovirals, *CHAM* Christian Health Association of Malawi

Table 2 Proportion of women who delivered through C-section according to baseline characteristics

Item		All Women (n = 62,033)	Women with unknown HIV status (n = 5741)	HIV negative women n = 33,099)	HIV positive women n = 23,193
Year of admission	2010	15.2 (14.2–16.3)	17.2 (14.3–20.7)	15.1 (13.9–16.4)	13.7 (12.8–14.6)
	2011	13.7 (12.9–14.5)	13.4 (11.7–15.4)	13.8 (12.9–14.9)	13.3 (12.5–14.1)
	2012	13.4 (12.8–13.9)	18.2 (16.6–20.1)	12.8 (12.2–13.5)	9.6 (8.8–10.5)
	2013	13.8 (13.3–14.4)	18.1 (16.2–20.1)	13.5 (12.9–14.1)	11.0 (10.2–11.9)
Maternal complication	None	6.6 (6.3–6.9)	6.3 (6.1–6.6)	6.8 (6.6–6.9)	5.1 (4.8–5.4)
	Hemorrhage	29.5 (26.5–32.8)	34.7 (32.0–37.6)	30.2 (28.7–31.7)	19.0 (16.4–22.0)
	OPL	68.2 (65.8–70.4)	68.0 (65.9–70.0)	69.2 (68.2–70.1)	60.9 (58.0–63.6)
	Preeclampsia	60.2 (55.0–65.2)	64.8 (60.4–69.1)	61.2 (58.7–63.6)	39.3 (32.3–46.8)
	Sepsis	16.5 (7.3–33.3)	5.1 (2.1–11.5)	30.7 (23.4–39.2)	6.0 (2.2–14.9)
	RU	87.4 (78.5–93.0)	84.7 (78.6–89.4)	90.7 (87.6–93.1)	72.3 (60.2–81.9)
	Unspecified	75.7 (73.5–77.8)	77.0 (75.3–78.6)	77.2 (76.3–78.0)	61.4 (58.7–64.1)
	Unknown	33.0 (27.6–38.8)	31.9 (28.1–36.1)	36.6 (33.8–39.4)	20.6 (16.2–25.8)
Infant complication	None	12.4 (12.0–12.8)	13.9 (13.5–14.3)	12.3 (12.1–12.4)	11.2 (10.7–11.7)
	Prematurity	17.0 (15.1–19.1)	21.7 (19.9–23.7)	16.1 (15.3–17.0)	15.2 (13.3–17.4)
	LBW	20.8 (18.4–23.4)	16.1 (14.5–17.8)	23.0 (21.9–24.1)	18.0 (15.8–20.4)
	Asphyxia	29.2 (26.7–31.8)	40.0 (37.5–42.5)	26.8 (25.8–27.8)	30.2 (27.0–33.6)
	Unspecified	32.4 (29.5–35.5)	36.8 (34.2–39.5)	31.8 (30.6–33.1)	29.2 (25.9–32.7)
	Unknown	15.7 (12.9–19.1)	15.5 (12.5–19.0)	31.2 (29.1–33.4)	2.7 (2.1–3.5)
No of previous deliveries	0	16.3 (15.5–17.1)	16.2 (15.5–16.9)	16.2 (16.0–16.5)	18.7 (17.3–20.3)
	1	14.2 (13.3–15.0)	15.9 (15.1–16.8)	14.0 (13.7–14.3)	12.6 (11.6–13.6)
	2–3	13.3 (12.6–14.0)	17.8 (17.0–18.5)	12.7 (12.5–13.0)	11.6 (11.0–12.3)
	> 3	11.2 (10.5–12.1)	13.8 (13.0–14.6)	11.0 (10.7–11.3)	9.9 (9.2–10.6)
	Unknown	17.4 (14.1–21.3)	20.2 (18.0–22.7)	16.2 (14.6–17.9)	14.3 (10.4–19.3)
Age in years	< 20	14.3 (13.5–15.1)	13.3 (12.6–14.0)	14.5 (14.2–14.8)	13.6 (12.0–15.5)
	20–24	14.6 (13.9–15.4)	18.5 (17.8–19.3)	14.2 (13.9–14.4)	12.3 (11.4–13.2)
	25–29	14.6 (13.8–15.5)	18.7 (17.8–19.6)	14.4 (14.1–14.7)	11.8 (11.1–12.6)
	30–34	12.1 (11.2–13.0)	13.7 (12.8–14.7)	11.8 (11.4–12.2)	11.9 (11.1–12.8)
	> 34	12.6 (11.5–13.8)	15.3 (14.2–16.5)	12.2 (11.8–12.7)	11.9 (10.9–13.0)
	Unknown	13.6 (11.1–16.4)	15.3 (13.6–17.3)	13.0 (11.9–14.1)	12.4 (9.3–16.3)
Singleton	Yes	13.7 (13.4–14.1)	16.0 (15.7–16.4)	13.6 (13.4–13.7)	11.7 (11.3–12.2)
	No	20.4 (17.9–23.0)	19.7 (17.8–21.8)	20.4 (19.5–21.4)	20.8 (18.2–23.4)
ARVs during pregnancy	None	11.7 (11.1–12.3)	N/A		11.7 (11.1–12.3)
	<4wks	12.4 (11.3–13.7)			12.4 (11.3–13.7)
	≥4wks	12.5 (11.9–13.2)			12.5 (11.9–13.3)
	HIV- & Unknown	14.1 (13.7–14.6)			N/A
Facility ownership	Government	13.8 (13.4–14.2)	16.2 (15.8–16.5)	13.5 (13.4–13.7)	12.2 (11.8–12.7)
	CHAM	15.3 (14.1–16.7)	16.6 (15.0–18.4)	15.7 (15.2–16.1)	11.3 (10.1–12.5)
Facility location	Rural	13.6 (13.4–13.7)	16.0 (15.6–16.4)	13.3 (13.1–13.4)	11.4 (10.9–11.9)
	Urban	15.7 (15.4–16.0)	17.3 (16.3–18.3)	15.9 (15.5–16.2)	13.6 (12.9–14.4)
Totals		14.0 (13.6–14.4)	16.2 (15.1–17.3)	13.8 (13.3–14.2)	12.1 (9.1–15.1)

OPL obstructed/prolonged labor, *RU* Ruptured Uterus, *CHAM* Christian Health Association of Malawi, *LBW* Low Birth Weight, *aOR* adjusted odds ratio, *ARVs* antiretrovirals

Table 3 Individual and facility-level factors associated with C-Section among women delivering in 17 large health facilities in Malawi

Item		aOR (95% CI) All Women (55,443)	*p*	aOR (95% CI) Women with Unknown HIV status (*n* = 5302)	*P*	aOR (95% CI) HIV- Women (n = 31,978)	*p*	aOR (95% CI) HIV+ Women (*n* = 20,436)	*P*
Year of admission	2010	1	0.07	1	0.09	1	0.02	1	0.06
	2011	0.71 (0.50–1.01)		0.58 (0.37–0.91)		0.71 (0.50–1.00)		1.00 (0.73–1.38)	
	2012	0.65 (0.45–0.93)		0.71 (0.42–1.19)		0.61 (0.43–0.88)		0.83 (0.56–1.22)	
	2013	0.67 (0.49–0.92)		0.67 (0.43–1.07)		0.65 (0.48–0.87)		1.04 (0.73–1.49)	
Maternal Obstetric Complication	None	1	< 0.01	1	< 0.01	1	< 0.01	1	< 0.01
	Hemorrhage	5.85 (3.12–10.97)		7.02 (4.26–11.58)		5.80 (3.03–11.12)		4.25 (1.72–10.47)	
	OPL	32.23 (17.15–60.57)		29.43 (17.75–48.80)		33.61 (16.99–66.47)		29.88 (11.89–75.13)	
	Preeclampsia	21.76 (10.32–45.86)		27.18 (14.18–52.09)		22.14 (9.83–49.88)		11.23 (4.56–27.68)	
	Sepsis	4.25 (1.30–13.85)		1.35 (0.14–13.18)		8.13 (1.57–42.16)		1.20 (0.36–4.02)	
	RU	160.25 (75.41–340.51)		141.95 (34.98–576.08)		186.48 (66.45–523.27)		94.91 (43.33–207.89)	
	Others	52.85 (31.25–89.39)		51.75 (35.26–75.97)		55.-81 (33.24–93.69)		38.01 (15.13–95.52)	
Infant Complication	None	1	0.01	1	< 0.01	1	< 0.01	1	< 0.01
	Prematurity	0.99 (0.77–1.29)		1.12 (0.61–2.05)		0.95 (0.61–1.46)		1.11 (0.87–1.42)	
	LBW	1.40 (1.07–1.83)		0.77 (0.38–1.58)		1.75 (1.28–2.39)		1.09 (0.77–1.53)	
	Asphyxia	1.86 (1.29–2.67)		3.02 (1.83–4.96)		1.65 (1.08–2.53)		1.92 (1.33–2.76)	
	Others	1.59 (1.15–2.19)		2.20 (1.07–4.52)		1.53 (1.10–2.11)		1.14 (0.73–1.78)	
No of previous deliveries	0	1	< 0.01	1	0.31	1	< 0.01	1	< 0.01
	1	0.83 (0.74–0.93)		0.84 (0.63–1.12)		0.84 (0.74–0.95)		0.61 (0.49–0.76)	
	2–3	0.68 (0.56–0.83)		0.79 (0.55–1.13)		0.68 (0.55–0.84)		0.50 (0.40–0.62)	
	> 3	0.52 (0.41–0.66)		0.72 (0.50–1.05)		0.51 (0.39–0.67)		0.35 (0.26–0.45)	
Age (years)	< 20	1	< 0.01	1	0.02	1	0.01	1	< 0.01
	20–24	1.28 (1.12–1.47)		1.75 (1.25–2.44)		1.20 (1.04–1.39)		1.37 (1.12–1.67)	
	25–29	1.56 (1.27–1.93)		1.96 (1.23–3.11)		1.49 (1.16–1.92)		1.72 (1.34–2.21)	
	30–34	1.44 (1.15–1.81)		1.66 (0.99–2.78)		1.35 (1.03–1.78)		1.98 (1.50–2.61)	
	> 34	1.63 (1.34–1.99)		1.62 (1.00–2.64)		1.57 (1.21–2.03)		2.24 (1.75–2.85)	
Singletons	Yes	1	< 0.01	1	0.35	1	0.03	1	0.04
	No	1.49 (1.10–2.03)		1.31 (0.74–2.33)		1.51 (1.05–2.16)		1.58 (1.03–2.43)	
ARVs during Pregnancy	None	N/A		N/A		N/A		1	0.83
	<4wks	N/A		N/A		N/A		0.98 (0.72–1.32)	
	≥4wks	N/A		N/A		N/A		0.96 (0.81–1.12)	
Facility Ownership	Govt.	1	0.90	1	0.57	1	0.36	1	0.77
	CHAM	1.42 (0.65–3.13)		1.27 (0.55–2.94)		1.48 (0.64–3.41)		1.09 (0.62–1.90)	
Facility Location	Rural	1	0.27	1	0.26	1	0.13	1	0.23
	Urban	1.39 (0.91–2.12)		1.19 (0.88–1.62)		1.47 (0.89–2.41)		1.16 (0.91–1.46)	

OPL obstructed/prolonged labor, *RU* Ruptured Uterus, *CHAM* Christian Health Association of Malawi, *LBW* Low Birth Weight, *aOR* adjusted odds ratio, *ARVs* antiretrovirals

strict CS indication setting by health care workers in recognition of the increased post-operative morbidity and mortality [28–30]. Clinicians may also be reluctant to perform ECS in HIV infected women due to a perceived risk of occupational HIV transmission [31]. Stigma and discrimination related to HIV infection may also play a role on health care workers' decision making [32]. On the other hand, we observed that among HIV positive women the prevalence of CS and ECS was higher in those who had no or less than 4 weeks of exposure to ARVs (i.e. were at high MTCT risk) than in women with longer ARV drug usage in pregnancy. This suggests that high MTCT risk is being considered as an indication for CS in Malawian clinical practice.

Table 4 Individual and facility-level factors associated with Elective Caesarean Section

Item		aOR (95% CI) All Women (55,443)	p	aOR (95% CI) Women with Unknown HIV status (n = 4764)	p	aOR (95% CI) HIV- Women (n = 29,747)	p	aOR (95% CI) HIV+ Women (n = 20,932)	p
Year of Admission	2010	1	0.03	1	0.01	1	0.02	1	< 0.09
	2011	0.63 (0.42–0.94)		0.47 (0.29–0.76)		0.64 (0.43–0.96)		0.84 (0.55–1.30)	
	2012	0.55 (0.34–0.88)		0.61 (0.31–1.22)		0.53 (0.33–0.86)		0.55 (0.28–1.06)	
	2013	0.53 (0.35–0.83)		0.40 (0.21–0.78)		0.54 (0.36–0.82)		0.68 (0.39–1.19)	
No of deliveries	0	1	< 0.01	1	0.11	1	< 0.01	1	< 0.01
	1	0.76 (0.66–0.87)		0.74 (0.57–0.96)		0.77 (0.66–0.90)		0.59 (0.46–0.75)	
	2–3	0.65 (0.51–0.82)		0.68 (0.42–1.11)		0.65 (0.51–0.83)		0.49 (0.38–0.63)	
	> 3	0.46 (0.34–0.63)		0.68 (0.40–1.16)		0.45 (0.31–0.65)		0.31 (0.22–0.43)	
Age (years)	< 20	1	< 0.01	1	< 0.01	1	< 0.01	1	< 0.01
	20–24	1.38 (1.18–1.61)		2.07 (1.42–3.03)		1.29 (1.09–1.53)		1.46 (1.12–1.91)	
	25–29	1.68 (1.35–2.09)		2.11 (1.21–3.67)		1.60 (1.25–2.06)		1.86 (1.33–2.60)	
	30–34	1.46 (1.10–1.92)		1.44 (0.81–2.54)		1.37 (1.00–1.88)		2.19 (1.40–3.43)	
	> 34	1.68 (1.24–2.27)		1.93 (1.07–3.50)		1.58 (1.08–2.32)		2.26 (1.57–3.27)	
Singletons	Yes	1	< 0.01	1	0.13	1	< 0.01	1	< 0.01
	No	1.98 (1.55–2.54)		1.48 (0.90–2.46)		2.06 (1.54–2.77)		2.27 (1.51–3.41)	
ARVs during Pregnancy	None	N/A		N/A		N/A		1	0.04
	<4wks	N/A		N/A		N/A		0.96 (0.73–1.27)	
	≥4wks	N/A		N/A		N/A		0.81 (0.68–0.96)	
Facility Ownership	Government	1	0.69	1	0.47	1	0.72	1	0.80
	CHAM	1.63 (0.69–3.83		1.19 (0.74–1.91)		1.75 (0.72–4.27)		1.08 (0.59–1.99)	
Facility Location	Rural	1	0.03	1	0.01	1	0.03	1	< 0.01
	Urban	1.95 (1.06–3.56)		1.52 (1.17–1.98)		2.02 (1.05–3.86)		2.15 (1.27–3.64)	

CHAM Christian Health Association of Malawi, *aOR* adjusted odds ratio, *ARVs* antiretrovirals

We are not aware of other publications that assessed why women or health care workers opt for an ECS in sub-Saharan Africa. Most of the recent publications focused on the effect of early ART and Option B+ on PMTCT [33, 34]. A recent systematic review [35] assessed the risks and benefits of ECS in women with HIV. Of 36 studies included, only 3 were done in sub-Saharan Africa. Two of these studies described risk factors for MTCT [36, 37]. Unger et al. analyzed the use of CS over time, and assessed postpartum morbidity and mortality; but they did not discuss why the use of CS increased over time [38].

Our data showed that ECS was more frequent among women who delivered in urban than rural facilities. Several studies observed a higher prevalence of CS in urban settings and this was mostly driven by demands from mothers or by provider preferences [20, 32, 39] although it is also possible that the difference reflects the larger availability of surgery facilities in urban areas. The reason why this difference was only observed in analyses of ECS and not of all CS, may be due to the fact that demands from mothers and provider preferences are not formally accepted indications for CS in guidelines, thus are not reported in registers and delivery charts or due to the fact that knowledge about the potential use of CS for MTCT is higher in urban areas.

Some studies have shown a declining trend in CS upon wider availability of ARVs [40]. We also saw a reduction in CS and ECS deliveries after 2010, but remarkably not in HIV positive women, suggesting that other factors than increased ART coverage determined this [6].

The study has several strengths and limitations. It is based on a large dataset and includes health facilities in different regions in Malawi. Generalization of the results of this study needs to be considered with care because the data were from large health facilities only. Another limitation is that we used routinely collected medical records which may have affected data quality. The proportion of missing data from explanatory variables was below 5%, except for infant complications (Table 1) and we believe it is unlikely that data were systematically missing for particular groups. In our study, the HIV status variable could be determined by HIV test results that became available before the onset of labour and immediately after delivery. In the latter case HIV status could not have impacted on a CS/ ECS decision. Because all HIV testing in Malawi is with rapid point-of-care tests that provide a result within

30 min, most results would have been obtained before delivery, but we do not have data to document this. Further, we assumed that CS was elective when no obstetric indication was recorded, while there could simply be missing obstetric data. We limited this as much as possible by complimenting maternity register data with information from labour charts and theatre registers.

We did not have data on ART adherence or treatment interruptions. Health care workers may have considered CS more frequently in patients with poorer adherence because they know that suboptimal adherence impairs the preventive effect of PMTCT.

Conclusions

We have shown that patterns of CS in Malawi are largely determined by maternal and infant complications. Positive HIV status was inversely associated with CS delivery, possibly related to health care workers' perceived risk of occupational HIV transmission and the recognition of the known higher rate of post-operative complications. Our results leave open the possibility that CS is practiced as a means of PMTCT in Malawi as we found that ECS was significantly more common among women with a high risk of MTCT due to no or short exposure to ARVs in pregnancy in a setting with limited access to viral load testing. Further studies are needed to confirm our findings, including surveys among providers of CS services and qualitative research involving patients and practitioners about factors related ECS decisions including stigma and wealth.

Abbreviations

aOR: adjusted odds ratio; ART: Antiretroviral therapy; ARVs: Antiretrovirals; CHAM: Christian Health Association of Malawi; CI: Confidence interval; CS: Caesarean section; ECS: Elective caesarean section; IQR: Interquartile range; I-TECH: International Training and Education Center for Health; LBW: Low Birth Weight; MOH: Ministry of Health; MTCT: Mother to child transmission; OPL: Obstructed/prolonged labour; PEER: Partnerships for Enhanced Engagement in Research; PMTCT: Prevention of mother to child transmission

Acknowledgements

We would like to acknowledge all the health facility staff and MOH and CHAM management who supported the data collection. Further we would like to thank all the data entry team who diligently entered the data management and staff of Baobab Health Trust and I-TECH Malawi for the support provided during this study.

Funding

This work was supported by the Bill and Melinda Gates Foundation (Global Health Grant OPP1090200), The United States Agency for International Development- National Institute of Health Initiative Partnerships for Enhanced Engagement in Research Health (PEER Health) grant AID OAA-A-11-0012. OK was supported by PROSPER Fellowship Grant (Grant 3233 B-150 934) and by a professorship grant from the Swiss National Science Foundation (#PP00P3_163878). The funding agencies played no role in the design of the study, the collection, analysis, and interpretation of data, and in writing the manuscript.

Authors' contributions

LT developed the study protocol, conducted the initial analysis and interpretation of data. OK, JJO, ADH and JE contributed in the data analysis and helped with the interpretation of the results. NP, MM, FC, KAP and KT contributed to the interpretation of the results. LT drafted the manuscript which was critically revised by OK, JJO, ADH, NP, MM, JE, FC, KAP and KT. FC, MM, ADH and NP actively participated in data collection and management. All authors have read the final version of the manuscript and have given final approval of this version to be published.

Competing interests

The authors declare that they have no competing interests.

Author details

Department of HIV and AIDS, Ministry of Health, Lilongwe, Malawi. [2]Institute of Social and Preventive Medicine, University of Bern, Bern, Switzerland. International Training and Education Center for Health, P.O Box 30369, Lilongwe 3, Malawi. [4]Dignitas International, Zomba, Malawi. [5]Department of Medicine, College of Medicine, Blantyre, Malawi. [6]The Baobab Health Trust, Lilongwe, Malawi. [7]Department of Infectious Diseases, University Hospital Bern, Bern, Switzerland. [8]Institute of Global Health, University of Geneva, Geneva, Switzerland. [9]Institute of Mathematical Statistics and Actuarial Science, University of Bern, Bern, Switzerland.

References

1. UNAIDS. AIDSinfo 2014 [Available from: http://aidsinfo.unaids.org/. Accessed 18 June 2016.
2. De Cock KM, Fowler MG, Mercier E, de Vincenzi I, Saba J, Hoff E, et al. Prevention of mother-to-child HIV transmission in resource-poor countries: translating research into policy and practice. JAMA. 2000;283(9):1175–82.
3. WHO. Global Update on HIV Treatment 2013.
4. Schouten EJ, Jahn A, Midiani D, Makombe SD, Mnthambala A, Chirwa Z, et al. Prevention of mother-to-child transmission of HIV and the health-related millennium development goals: time for a public health approach. Lancet. 2011;378(9787):282–4.
5. WHO. Consolidated guidelines on the use of antiretroviral drugs for treating and preventing HIV infection: what's new. 2015.
6 CDC. Impact of an innovative approach to prevent mother-to-child transmission of HIV–Malawi, July 2011-September 2012. MMWR Morb Mortal Wkly Rep. 2013;1(62):148–51.
7 Tenthani L, Haas AD, Egger M, Van Oosterhout JJ, Jahn A, Chimbwandira F, et al. Brief report: HIV testing among pregnant women who attend antenatal Care in Malawi. J Acquir Immune Defic Syndr. 2015;69(5):610–4.
8 Haas AD, Tenthani L, Msukwa MT, Tal K, Jahn A, Gadabu OJ, et al. Retention in care during the first 3 years of antiretroviral therapy for women in Malawi's option B+ programme: an observational cohort study. Lancet HIV. 2016;3(4):e175–82.
9 Tenthani L, Haas AD, Tweya H, Jahn A, van Oosterhout JJ, Chimbwandira F, et al. Retention in care under universal antiretroviral therapy for HIV-infected pregnant and breastfeeding women ('Option B+') in Malawi. J Acquir Immune Defic Syndr. 2015;69(5):610–4.
10 Haas AD, Msukwa MT, Egger M, Tenthani L, Tweya H, Jahn A, et al. Adherence to antiretroviral therapy during and after pregnancy: cohort study on women receiving Care in Malawi's "option B+" programme. Clin. Infect Dis. 2016;63(9):1227–35.
11 Ministry of Health Malawi. Integrated HIV Program Report January–March 2016.
12 Brocklehurst P. Interventions for reducing the risk of mother-to-child transmission of HIV infection. Cochrane Database Syst Rev. 2002;(1). Art. No.: CD000102. https://doi.org/10.1002/14651858.CD000102.
13 European Mode of Delivery C. Elective caesarean-section versus vaginal delivery in prevention of vertical HIV-1 transmission: a randomised clinical trial. Lancet. 1999;353(9158):1035–9
14 Read JS, Newell MK. Efficacy and safety of cesarean delivery for prevention of mother-to-child transmission of HIV-1. Cochrane Database Syst Rev. 2005;(4). Art. No 4:CD005479. https://doi.org/10.1002/14651858.CD005479.

15 de Ruiter A, Taylor GP, Clayden P, Dhar J, Gandhi K, Gilleece Y, et al. British HIV association guidelines for the management of HIV infection in pregnant women 2012 (2014 interim review). HIV Med. 2014;15(Suppl 4):1–77.
16 Panel on Treatment of HIV-Infected Pregnant Women and Prevention of Perinatal Transmission. Recommendations for Use of Antiretroviral Drugs in Pregnant HIV-1-Infected Women for Maternal Health and Interventions to Reduce Perinatal HIV Transmission in the United States. Available at http://aidsinfo.nih.gov/contentfiles/lvguidelines/PerinatalGL.pdf. Accessed 12 June 2016.
17 WHO. Consolidated guidelines on the use of antiretroviral drugs for treating and preventing HIV infection: recommendations for a public health approach June 2013.` Available from: http://apps.who.int/iris/bitstream/10665/85321/1/9789241505727_eng.pdf?ua=1. Accessed 12 June 2016.
18 Fenton PM, Whitty CJ, Reynolds F. Caesarean section in Malawi: prospective study of early maternal and perinatal mortality. BMJ. 2003;327(7415):587.
19 WHO. Caesarean sections should only be performed when medically necessary. Switzerland: Geneva; 2015.
20 Buekens P, Curtis S, Alayon S. Demographic and health surveys: caesarean section rates in sub-Saharan Africa. BMJ. 2003;326(7381):136.
21 Macro. National Statistical Office. Calverton, Maryland: Malawi Demographic and Health Survey 2004; 2005.
22 Macro National Stastical Office. Malawi demographic and health survey 2010. Malawi, and Calverton, Maryland, USA: Zomba; 2011.
23 Chu K, Cortier H, Maldonado F, Mashant T, Ford N, Trelles M. Cesarean section rates and indications in sub-Saharan Africa: a multi-country study from Medecins sans Frontieres. PLoS One. 2012;7(9):e44484.
24 Carolan M. Maternal age >/=45 years and maternal and perinatal outcomes: a review of the evidence. Midwifery. 2013;29(5):479–89.
25 Carolan M, Frankowska D. Advanced maternal age and adverse perinatal outcome: a review of the evidence. Midwifery. 2011;27(6):793–801.
26 Cavazos-Rehg PA, Krauss MJ, Spitznagel EL, Bommarito K, Madden T, Olsen MA, et al. Maternal age and risk of labor and delivery complications. Matern Child Health J. 2015;19(6):1202–11.
27 Aebi-Popp K, Mulcahy F, Glass TR, Rudin C, Martinez de Tejada B, Bertisch B, et al. Missed opportunities among HIV-positive women to control viral replication during pregnancy and to have a vaginal delivery. J Acquir Immune Defic Syndr. 2013;64(1):58–65.
28 Ferrero S, Bentivoglio G. Post-operative complications after caesarean section in HIV-infected women. Arch Gynecol Obstet. 2003;268(4):268–73.
29 Kourtis AP, Ellington S, Pazol K, Flowers L, Haddad L, Jamieson DJ. Complications of cesarean deliveries among HIV-infected women in the United States. AIDS. 2014;28(17):2609–18.
30 Read JS, Tuomala R, Kpamegan E, Zorrilla C, Landesman S, Brown G, et al. Mode of delivery and postpartum morbidity among HIV-infected women: the women and infants transmission study. J Acquir Immune Defic Syndr. 2001;26(3):236–45.
31 Gounden YP, Moodley J. Exposure to human immunodeficiency virus among healthcare workers in South Africa. International journal of gynaecology and obstetrics: the official organ of the. Int J Gynaecol Obstet. 2000;69(3):265–70.
32 Neuman M, Alcock G, Azad K, Kuddus A, Osrin D, More NS, et al. Prevalence and determinants of caesarean section in private and public health facilities in underserved south Asian communities: cross-sectional analysis of data from Bangladesh, India and Nepal. BMJ Open. 2014;4(12):e005982.
33 Haas AD, van Oosterhout JJ, Tenthani L, Jahn A, Zwahlen M, Msukwa MT, et al. HIV transmission and retention in care among HIV-exposed children enrolled in Malawi's prevention of mother-to-child transmission programme. J Int AIDS Soc. 2017;20(1):21947.
34 Gourlay A, Birdthistle I, Mburu G, Iorpenda K, Wringe A. Barriers and facilitating factors to the uptake of antiretroviral drugs for prevention of mother-to-child transmission of HIV in sub-Saharan Africa: a systematic review. J Int AIDS Soc. 2013;16:18588.
35 Kennedy CE, Yeh PT, Pandey S, Betran AP, Narasimhan M. Elective cesarean section for women living with HIV: a systematic review of risks and benefits. AIDS. 2017;31(11):1579–91.
36 Bobat R, Coovadia H, Coutsoudis A, Moodley D. Determinants of mother-to-child transmission of human immunodeficiency virus type 1 infection in a cohort from Durban, South Africa. Pediatr Infect Dis J. 1996;15(7):604–10.
37 Ilohl KK, Ilohl ON, Ikefunal AN, Ibeziakol NS, Ubesiell AC, Emodi IJ. Determinants of mother-to-child transmission of HIV despite PMTCT interventions in Enugu, Nigeria. S Afr J Child Health. 2015;9(2):49–52.
38 Unger JA, Richardson BA, Otieno PA, Farquhar C, Wamalwa D, John-Stewart GC. Mode of delivery and postpartum HIV-1 disease progression and mortality in a Kenyan cohort. BMC Pregnancy Childbirth. 2014;14:257.
39 Khanal V, Karkee R, Lee AH, Binns CW. Adverse obstetric symptoms and rural-urban difference in cesarean delivery in Rupandehi district, western Nepal: a cohort study. Reprod Health. 2016;13:17.
40 European Collaborative S, Boer K, England K, Godfried MH, Thorne C. Mode of delivery in HIV-infected pregnant women and prevention of mother-to-child transmission: changing practices in Western Europe. HIV Med. 2010;11(6):368–78.

5

Factors associated with caesarean deliveries among child-bearing women in Pakistan: secondary analysis of data from the Demographic and Health Survey, 2012–13

Aisha Amjad[1], Uzair Amjad[1], Rubeena Zakar[1], Ahmed Usman[1], Muhammad Zakria Zakar[1] and Florian Fischer[2*]

Abstract

Background: The increasing rate of caesarean deliveries has become a serious concern for public health experts globally. Various medical and non-medical factors, such as maternal socio-demographics, are found to be responsible for this upsurge. Like in other countries, the rate of caesarean sections has increased in Pakistan as well. Therefore, there is a need to investigate the factors behind this increase. This study aims to assess the determinants associated with caesarean deliveries among child-bearing women aged 15–49 years in Pakistan.

Methods: Secondary data analysis was conducted on nationally representative cross-sectional survey data from the Pakistan Demographic and Health Survey, 2012–2013. The analysis was limited to mothers aged 15–49 years, who had given birth to at least one child during the 5 years immediately preceding the survey ($n = 7461$). Maternal socio-demographic characteristics and pregnancy-related variables, including antenatal care utilisation, place of delivery and pregnancy complications were considered as independent variables. The association between caesarean section deliveries (outcome variable) and its determinants was assessed by calculating unadjusted and adjusted odds ratios with 95% confidence intervals using a multivariable binary logistic regression.

Results: Of the women who had given birth to at least one child during the previous 5 years, the percentage of mothers who delivered their babies through caesarean section was found to be 13.6%. The likelihood of caesarean deliveries was associated with mothers aged more than 24 years, women residing in Punjab province, women belonging to the richest class, women with higher education, women employed at professional/managerial/technical level, and women residing in an urban setting. Additionally, the women who had pregnancy complications, a high utilisation of antenatal care and delivered their babies in private hospitals were found to have higher chances of caesarean deliveries.

Conclusions: The study revealed that there are a high percentage of women delivering babies through caesarean section in Pakistan. Therefore, strict measures need to be taken to deal with this concern. For example, detailed medical justifications by doctors for performing caesarean sections and awareness among women regarding the reduction of pregnancy complications can help to reduce the chances of malpractice related to caesarean deliveries.

Keywords: Caesarean delivery, Vaginal delivery, Pregnancy complication, Antenatal visit

* Correspondence: f.fischer@uni-bielefeld.de
[2]Department of Public Health Medicine, School of Public Health, Bielefeld University, Bielefeld, Germany
Full list of author information is available at the end of the article

Background

The role of caesarean section deliveries is acknowledged worldwide for dealing with complications related to childbirth and reducing the mortality rates of mother and foetus [1]. However, during the last decade, the increase in caesarean section deliveries has become a matter of serious concern for public health experts globally [2]. In most countries, the caesarean section rate (CSR) has exceeded the level of 10–15% recommended by the World Health Organization (WHO) [1]. Among high-income countries, CSR is 30.3% in the USA, 22% in the United Kingdom, 26% in Canada, 19% in France, 28% in Germany and 30% in Australia [2]. Similarly, in low-income countries, CSR is increasing on a yearly basis. For example, in Bangladesh, caesarean deliveries increased from 2% (2000) to 17% (2011); in India from 3% (1992) to 11% (2006) and in Nepal from 1% (2000) to 5% (2011) [3]. Similarly, an increasing rate of caesarean deliveries has been documented in Pakistan. The findings of studies conducted in different areas of Pakistan report a current CSR of 16–20%, approximately [4, 5].

Increasing CSR worldwide has prompted public-health professionals to discuss the medical and non-medical determinants responsible for this increase [6]. Certain obstetric risks such as dystocia, previous caesarean section, foetal distress, breach births, post-term pregnancy, multiple pregnancy and hypertensive disorder are considered to be justifiable medical reasons for caesarean deliveries [7, 8]. Furthermore, socio-demographic, cultural and psychological factors may also influence the increase in CSR [6]. Maternal socio-demographics such as age, social class, education, occupation and type of residence have been found to be strongly correlated with the type of delivery [9]. In terms of cultural aspects, studies have shown that the cultural context plays a pivotal role in constructing the patterns of women's behaviour towards pregnancy-related issues and mode of delivery [10–12]. Additionally, psychological factors which may be due to fear related to prolonged labour and vaginal delivery pain reinforce women's preferences for caesarean delivery [13].

Furthermore, doctors' decisions and patient demand are contributing factors affecting the escalation of CSR across the globe [14]. In developed countries, where patients are given the option to choose between vaginal and caesarean delivery, women's preference for caesarean delivery has appeared as an important determinant [15]. In developing countries, doctors' referrals to perform caesarean surgery appear to be a more significant determinant than the woman's preference [16].

The high rate of caesarean deliveries in both developed and developing countries also underlines the growing medicalisation of the childbirth process [6]. Over the past few years, a greater reliance on medical technology to deal with childbirth complications has resulted in increasing rates of caesarean deliveries [17, 18]. This medicalisation of childbirth has also increased concerns regarding malpractice associated with the use of medical technology by doctors, who may perform unnecessary caesareans for their own convenience, quick handling to save time or economic incentives [19]. Moreover, expectant mothers' inadequate knowledge about childbirth complications is likely to increase the chances of their exploitation for economic gain. In such cases, doctors and hospital authorities might easily persuade patients to opt for caesarean deliveries by associating the method with the security of mother and child health, even when the baby could be delivered normally [20].

The discussion mentioned above underlines several medical and non-medical factors that lie behind high CSR in different countries across the world. However, despite an alarming increase in CSR, there is a paucity of literature systematically investigating the determinants associated with the increase in caesarean deliveries in Pakistan. Given this background, this paper aims to assess the maternal socio-demographic characteristics and pregnancy-related variables associated with caesarean deliveries among child-bearing women aged 15–49 years in Pakistan.

Methods

Sample of participants

Secondary data analysis was used to analyse data obtained from the Pakistan Demographic and Health Survey (PDHS) 2012–13 [21]. This was the third time the global programme of Demographic and Health Surveys had conducted the survey in Pakistan. The main aim was to provide updated and reliable data on fertility and family planning, childhood mortality, maternal and child health, women's and children's nutritional status, women's empowerment, domestic violence and knowledge about HIV/AIDS. The PDHS dataset comprises a nationally representative household-based sample of 12,943 households, selected by using a two-stage, stratified, random sample design. However, owing to security and political reasons, the Federally Administered Tribal Areas, the Federally Administered National Areas, Azad Jammu and Kashmir, and restricted military areas were excluded from the survey.

During the first stage, the whole area, comprising of urban and rural regions of four provinces in Pakistan and Gilgit Baltistan, was divided into mutually exclusive smaller areas known as enumeration blocks. About 200–250 households were situated in each enumeration block, and these were further classified into low, middle and high income categories. In the second stage, households situated in both urban and rural areas were selected by using a systematic random sampling technique. Out of 12,943 households interviewed, a total of 14,569 ever-married women aged 15–49 years were identified, of whom 13,558 were successfully interviewed by using individual women's questionnaires, a response rate of 93%. Depending upon the preferences of household members, trained interviewers conducted a verbally administered survey in their national or regional language. Detailed methodology, with complete information on survey design and data collection, has been published elsewhere [21]. For this study, the data was limited to mothers aged 15–49 years who had given birth during the previous 5 years ($n = 7461$).

Survey instrument and data management

Maternal socio-demographic characteristics and pregnancy-related variables, including antenatal care utilisation, place of delivery and pregnancy complications, were considered as independent variables. Maternal socio-demographic variables were assessed through questions related to the mother's age when she gave birth (< 18, 18–20, 21–24, > 24 years), level of education (no education, primary, middle, secondary, or higher education), area of residence (urban, rural), national region of residence (Punjab, Sindh, Balochistan, Khyber Pukhtunkhwa, Gilgit Baltistan, or Islamabad Capital Territory). Depending upon the possession of consumer items and residential characteristics, the wealth index was measured in quintiles (poorest, poorer, middle, richer, richest). Mothers' employment status was assessed through a question asking whether they were working at the time of interview. The working mothers were subdivided into categories (unskilled, skilled, or professional/managerial/technical), whereas non-employed mothers were placed in the category of "not working". The birth order of children born to the women during the previous 5 years was recoded as "1", "2–3", "4–5", "6 or more". The birth order refers to the order of a child born in his/her family. Considering the recommendations of the WHO [22], a woman without pregnancy complications should have at least four antenatal visits to reduce the probability of adverse pregnancy outcomes. Keeping this aspect in mind, the number of antenatal visits of the mothers during pregnancy was categorised as "None", "1–3" or "4 and more". Pregnancy complications were assessed with the help of a question investigating whether the mothers were informed about any pregnancy complications during their antenatal visits or not. The response category for pregnancy complications was termed "Yes" for those women who had a medical history of health problems such as anaemia, hypertension, diabetes and/or haemorrhage during pregnancy. Similarly, the mothers were asked where they had delivered their babies. The place of delivery was recoded as "private" or "public" sectors, excluding those cases of deliveries which took place at home, because caesarean section deliveries cannot be performed at home. In the Pakistani context, the public sector includes government hospitals and rural health centres while the private sector includes private hospitals and clinics.

Caesarean section was used as the outcome variable. It was assessed by asking mothers whether their last-born baby during the previous 5 years was delivered by caesarean section or not. In the PDHS, the birth of children by caesarean section was defined as "delivery by caesarean section", and the response categories were termed "Yes" and "No". However, data were not available to differentiate between medically indicated and non-medically indicated cases of caesarean deliveries.

Statistical analysis

All the data were weighted and SPSS version 21 was used to analyse the secondary data obtained from the PDHS to account for women who delivered by caesarean section versus women who did not. Weighting was performed to account for the complex sampling design and allows us to generalise our findings to all women in Pakistan. Descriptive statistics for both groups and maternal socio-demographic variables were presented as frequency distributions and percentages. We calculated weighted percentages of the national population from the original sample. We assessed the association between caesarean section deliveries and its determinants by calculating unadjusted odds ratios (OR) and adjusted odds ratios (AOR) with 95% confidence intervals (CI). A simple binary logistic regression analysis was carried out to assess the relationship between deliveries by caesarean section and the independent variables. In the multivariate logistic regression analysis, the inclusion of independent variables was based on a significance level of $p < 0.05$. The AOR was obtained by simultaneously entering all the independent variables that were found to be significant at less than 0.05 level in the bivariate analyses.

Results

Maternal socio-demographic characteristics

Of the women who had given birth during the previous 5 years ($n = 7461$), 32.1% were in the age range of 21–24 years. In terms of education, 55.8% never attended school. 72.2% were non-working mothers and 22.8% belonged to the poorest quintile of wealth. As far as the region and place of residence was concerned, it was found that more than half of the mothers (69.9%) resided in rural areas, while 56.1% were inhabitants of Punjab province (Table 1).

Of the women who had given birth to at least one child during the previous 5 years, the percentage of mothers who delivered their babies through caesarean section was found to be 13.6% ($n = 1014$).

Table 1 Socio-demographic characteristics of child-bearing women aged 15–49 years

Variables	Number of participants n = 7461	Weighted percentage
Mother's age at birth (in years)		
Less than 18	2025	27.2
18–20	1661	22.3
21–24	2394	32.1
More than 24	1367	18.4
Mother's education		
No education	4155	55.8
Primary	1230	16.5
Middle	587	7.9
Secondary	792	10.6
Higher	682	9.2
Mother's occupation		
Not working	5378	72.2
Unskilled	938	12.6
Skilled	990	13.3
Professional/Technical/Managerial	140	1.9
Wealth index		
Poorest	1698	22.8
Poorer	1544	20.7
Middle	1464	19.7
Richer	1469	19.4
Richest	1272	17.1
Type of residence		
Urban	2244	30.1
Rural	5202	69.9
Region		
Punjab	4180	56.1
Sindh	1714	23.0
Khyber Pakhtunkhwa	1117	15.0
Balochistan	348	4.7
Gilgit Baltistan	56	0.7
Islamabad Capital Territory	31	0.4

Determinants of caesarean deliveries

Simple binary logistic regression

The data shows that women aged more than 24 years (OR = 5.001; 95% CI: 4.041–6.187) and with a child at first birth order (OR = 5.059; 95% CI: 3.953–6.475) have a higher chance of delivering babies by caesarean section. As far as the maternal socio-economic status was concerned, the probability of caesarean deliveries was higher among mothers belonging to the richest class (OR = 11.421; 95% CI: 8.681–15.027), having higher education (OR = 7.860; 95% CI: 6.509–9.492) and employed at professional/technical/managerial levels (OR = 2.147; 95% CI: 1.527–3.020). Similarly, the odds of caesarean deliveries were higher among the mothers residing in urban areas (OR = 2.425; 95% CI: 2.115–2.780). Additionally, women who had high a high risk of pregnancy complication (OR = 1.677; 95% CI: 1.453–1.936) and received antenatal care more than four times (OR = 25.4; 95% CI: 17.219–37.471) had greater chances of delivering babies through caesarean section. Moreover, the women who delivered babies in private hospitals (OR: 1.326; 95% CI: 1.140–1.53) were found to have higher probability of undergoing caesarean delivery (Table 2).

Multivariable logistic regression

Using multivariable logistic regression analysis, the data showed that women with pregnancy complications (AOR = 1.307; 95% CI: 1.107–1.545), and who utilised antenatal care more than four times (AOR = 2.811; 95% CI: 1.823–4.33) had higher chances of delivering babies by caesarean. Similarly, women age at first birth more than 24 years (AOR = 1.883; 95% CI: 1.452–2.438) were found to have a greater chance of giving birth by caesarean section than younger women. Women who lived in Punjab province (AOR = 1.911; 95% CI: 1.457–2.506) were more likely to deliver children by caesarean section. Contrarily, women living in Baluchistan (AOR = 0.376; 95% CI: 0.228–0.622) had lower risk of caesarean deliveries as compared to Islamabad. Women belonged to the richest class (AOR = 1.588; CI: 1.036–2.435) were found to have a higher probability of delivering through caesarean section. Additionally, the women who delivered babies in private hospitals (AOR = 1.052 CI: 0.883–1.254) had a greater chance of caesarean deliveries (Table 3).

Discussion

The prevalence of caesarean deliveries among women in Pakistan rose from 7.3% in 2008 to 14% in 2013 [21, 23]. Various studies conducted at local hospitals in Pakistan have highlighted obstetric risks such as foetal distress, failed induction, wound sepsis, repeated caesarean and massive haemorrhage as the medical causes of increasing CSR [24–26]. The cultural belief that caesarean is a symbol of better socio-economic status [11] could also be a possible reason for the increasing rate of caesarean deliveries. However, in developing countries like Pakistan, caesareans are not performed on the demand of the patient; rather, the doctor generally determines the choice of a caesarean delivery [6]. Therefore, another factor influencing the caesarean rate in the Pakistani context could be the referrals of doctors [27].

Among the socio-demographic characteristics of mothers, the association between maternal age and

Table 2 Simple binary logistic regression for the predictors associated with cesarean section among women aged 15–49 years

Socio-demographic characteristics	Delivery by caesarean (weighted percentage)		OR	95% CI	p-value[1]
	No	Yes			
Mother's age at birth (in years)					
Less than 18	92.8	7.2	1		
18–20	88.1	11.9	1.658	1.307–2.103	< 0.001
21–24	81.1	18.9	2.743	2.231–3.372	< 0.001
More than 24	72.4	27.6	5.001	4.041–6.187	< 0.001
Children birth order					
More than 6	93.9	6.1	1		
1	74.5	25.5	5.059	3.953–6.475	< 0.001
2–3	80.4	19.6	3.425	2.706–4.334	< 0.001
4–5	89.5	10.5	1.558	1.189–2.042	< 0.001
Mother's education					
No education	92.5	7.5	1		
Primary	82.9	17.1	2.661	2.150–3.294	< 0.001
Middle	78.7	21.3	3.519	2.737–4.523	< 0.001
Secondary	68.5	31.5	5.221	4.262–6.397	< 0.001
Higher	59.8	40.2	7.860	6.509–9.492	< 0.001
Mother's occupation					
Not working	81.9	18.1	1		
Unskilled	88.6	11.4	0.759	0.599–0.962	0.023
Skilled	94.7	5.3	0.355	0.248–0.507	< 0.001
Professional/Technical/Managerial	70.0	30.0	2.147	1.527–3.020	< 0.001
Wealth index					
Poorest	94.5	5.5	1		
Poorer	93.0	7.0	1.622	1.167–2.255	< 0.001
Middle	88.1	11.9	2.456	1.801–3.348	< 0.001
Richer	76.4	23.6	5.487	4.123–7.303	< 0.001
Richest	64.7	35.3	11.421	8.681–15.03	< 0.001
Type of residence					
Rural	88.5	11.5	1		
Urban	74.4	25.6	2.425	2.115–2.780	< 0.001
Region					
Islamabad Capital Territory	71.9	28.1	1		
Punjab	80.9	19.1	0.709	0.563–0.894	< 0.001
Sindh	82.6	17.4	0.655	0.516–0.832	< 0.001
Khyber Pakhtunkhwa	94.8	5.2	0.203	0.153–0.269	< 0.001
Baluchistan	98.3	1.7	0.061	0.039–0.095	< 0.001
Gilgit Baltistan	96.4	3.6	0.156	0.106–0.229	< 0.001
Pregnancy complication					
No	85.1	14.9	1		
Yes	74.8	25.2	1.677	1.453–1.936	< 0.001
Antenatal care utilization					
None	97.9	22.1	1		
1–3	89.3	10.7	6.212	4.147–9.307	< 0.001

Table 2 Simple binary logistic regression for the predictors associated with cesarean section among women aged 15–49 years *(Continued)*

Socio-demographic characteristics	Delivery by caesarean (weighted percentage)		OR	95% CI	p-value[1]
	No	Yes			
More than 4	69.9	30.1	25.401	17.219–37.471	< 0.001
Place of delivery					
Public	71.1	28.9	1		
Private	68.8	31.2	1.326	1.140–1.543	< 0.001

Abbreviations: *1* reference category, *OR* odds ratio, *CI* confidence interval
[1]By using X^2 test

mode of delivery is found to be an important factor [28]. Several pieces of research have demonstrated that the chance of caesarean delivery is higher among older mothers [29]. Similarly, our data found that the probability of delivery by caesarean increases with rising age of the mother. While the reasons for the increased number of caesarean deliveries among older women are still uncertain, it is believed that older mothers are more prone to pregnancy complications that may lead to caesarean deliveries [30]. In Pakistan, the rising trend among women of getting married or conceiving at a later age due to their orientation towards career, educational, financial and other goals tends to increase their chances of undergoing caesarean delivery [31]. Thus, this may possibly be a factor in the upsurge in the rate of caesarean sections in Pakistan.

The literature has shown that women who report chronic health problems (including chronic hypertension, cardiac disease, lung disease or other medical risk factors) are more likely to undergo caesarean section [3]. Supporting the results of these studies, our data also shows that women who were reported to have pregnancy complications such as anaemia, hypertension, haemorrhage, or diabetes during pregnancy had a greater likelihood of caesarean delivery.

Clinical studies have shown that antenatal care utilisation, pregnancy complications and mode of delivery are interlinked [32]. Keeping in view the significance of antenatal care utilisation in determining the mode of delivery, the WHO recommends every pregnant woman to have at least four antenatal care visits during her pregnancy [22]. Similarly, the literature elucidates that antenatal care serves as a precautionary measure to prevent complications which may lead to caesarean sections [7]. In contrast, our data shows that mothers who received antenatal care more than four times delivered babies by caesarean section. Although the reason for this is still unclear, the risk-avoiding behaviour of gynaecologists towards women who reported having pregnancy complications could be one of the reasons for this preference for caesarean delivery.

In terms of regional demographics, the findings of this study indicate that mothers living in Punjab province have a higher probability of undergoing caesarean section; the reason could be the easy access, availability and utilisation of maternal healthcare facilities at private and public hospitals in the province [4]. On the other hand, limited access to health facilities, poor maternal socio-economic status and lower educational level can be identified as important factors associated with a lesser likelihood of caesarean section in other provinces.

Studies conducted in different South Asian countries, including Bangladesh, India and Nepal, suggest that women with a higher socio-economic background are more likely to undergo caesarean section [3]. Likewise, literature from other countries indicates that the rate of caesareans was higher among mothers with higher socio-economic status [33]. Correspondingly, the findings of our study also show that mothers with better socio-economic status are more likely to opt for caesarean deliveries than their poorer counterparts. Arguably, mothers belonging to a higher socio-economic class have adequate financial resources to afford the expense of a caesarean section.

Although the role of caesarean delivery in reducing maternal and neonatal deaths has been widely acknowledged, the possibility of malpractice associated with this surgical procedure is also on the increase [6]. When discussing its misuse, several studies argue that in developing countries the rate of caesarean deliveries is higher in private hospitals than public hospitals because of the financial benefits [3, 33]. Conversely, our study has found that the rate of caesarean deliveries is increasing in both private and public-sector hospitals in Pakistan without significant variation. Arguably, the malpractice associated with caesarean deliveries may exist in both settings for different reasons. For instance, the high operating expenses of performing a caesarean procedure may be identified as one of the reasons that has led to an increase in the caesarean delivery rate in private hospitals. Whereas, in the case of public hospitals, the desire of doctors to improve their surgical experience, a shortage of paramedical staff, a need for quick handling and convenience may be considered as other possible reasons for the increase in caesarean deliveries [34]. However, the PDHS (2012–2013) does not provide any data to distinguish between medically indicated

Table 3 Adjusted odd ratios for multivariable logistic regression of factors independently associated with among women aged 15–49 years[a]

Variables	AOR	95% CI	p-value[3]
Mother's age at birth (years)			
Less than 18	1		
18–20	1.134	0.866–1.485	0.360
21–24	1.479	1.161–1.884	0.002
More than 24	1.883	1.452–2.438	< 0.001
Children birth order			
More than 6	1		
1	1.208	0.909–1.606	0.193
2–3	1.282	0.959–1.713	0.093
4–5	0.901	0.656–1.239	0.523
Mother's education			
No education	1		
Primary	1.047	0.808–1.358	0.727
Middle	1.018	0.749–1.385	0.908
Secondary	1.164	0.889–1.524	0.270
Higher	1.268	0.966–1.666	0.088
Mother's occupation			
Not working	1		
Unskilled	1.003	0.753–1.337	0.983
Skilled	0.786	0.506–1.222	0.285
Professional/Technical/Managerial	1.018	0.686–1.511	0.930
Wealth index			
Poorest	1		
Poorer	0.974	0.652–1.455	0.896
Middle	1.026	0.692–1.520	0.898
Richer	1.330	0.894–1.979	0.159
Richest	1.588	1.036–2.435	0.034
Type of residence			
Rural	1		
Urban	1.043	0.789–1.166	0.675
Region			
Islamabad Capital Territory	1		
Punjab	1.911	1.457–2.506	< 0.001
Sindh	1.428	1.072–1.903	0.009
KPK	0.647	0.468–0.896	< 0.001
Baluchistan	0.376	0.228–0.622	< 0.001
Gilgit Baltistan	0.432	0.278–0.670	< 0.001
Pregnancy complication			
No	1		
Yes	1.307	1.107–1.545	0.002
Antenatal care utilization			
None	1		
1–3	1.522	0.985–2.354	0.059

Table 3 Adjusted odd ratios for multivariable logistic regression of factors independently associated with among women aged 15–49 years[a] *(Continued)*

Variables	AOR	95% CI	p-value[3]
More than 4	2.811	1.823–4.333	< 0.001
Place of delivery			
Public	1		
Private	1.052	0.883–1.254	0.570

Abbreviations: *1* reference category, *AOR* adjusted odds ratio, *CI* confidence interval
[3]By using X^2 test
[a]Multivariate logistic regression analysis was carried out to obtain AOR after entering all the independent variables simultaneously that were significant at level 0.05 in binary analysis

and non-medically indicated caesarean section deliveries in private and public hospital settings.

Limitations

The results of this study need to be considered in the light of several limitations. Firstly, the PDHS 2012–2013 does not provide data on the type of pregnancy complications a mother might experience during pregnancy. Owing to the scarcity of relevant information, this study could not identify any specific type of pregnancy complication that resulted in caesarean delivery. Secondly, the PDHS 2012–2013 data does not provide details of medical or non-medical reasons for performing caesarean sections. Therefore, the given data does not provide adequate information to relate the increase in the caesarean section rate with malpractice involving surgical procedures. Thirdly, owing to the cross-sectional design, the study could not assess the causal relationship between any of the independent variables and caesarean section deliveries. Moreover, the mothers' questionnaire does not provide information on the type of delivery (caesarean or vaginal) for each childbirth; so it could not be established whether a previous caesarean section emerged as one of reasons for a caesarean for the following deliveries or not.

Conclusions

Our study shows that the current CSR in Pakistan is approximately 14%. Using data from the Pakistan Demographic and Health Survey 2012–13, our study revealed strong associations between maternal age, mother's education, region, pregnancy complications, utilisation of antenatal care, place of birth of a child, area of residence and the wealth profiles of mothers and the probability of caesarean section deliveries. It was found that women aged more than 24 years, having pregnancy complications, and utilising antenatal care more than four times during pregnancy were more likely to have a caesarean delivery. Furthermore, the results revealed that women living in an urban setting, residing in Punjab province, who were highly educated and had a better socioeconomic background were independently associated with caesarean delivery. The study has argued that there is an increasing misuse of caesarean interventions in both private and public hospitals in Pakistan. The present study recommends that, in order to reduce the escalating caesarean rate, a detailed medical justification for performing caesareans by doctors should be provided. Adequate awareness regarding the reduction of pregnancy complications can also help to reduce the chances of malpractice involving caesareans. Additionally, qualitative research needs to be conducted to understand the cultural beliefs, psychological factors and perceptions of Pakistani women that may be contributing to the upsurge in the CSR in Pakistan.

Abbreviations

AOR: adjusted odds ratio; CI: confidence interval; CSR: caesarean section rate; OR: odds ratio; PDHS: Pakistan Demographic and Health Survey; WHO: World Health Organization

Acknowledgements

We acknowledge support of the publication fee by Deutsche Forschungsgemeinschaft and the Open Access Publication Funds of Bielefeld University.

Authors' contributions

AA and UA drafted the initial manuscript. RZ supervised and reviewed manuscript writing and data analysis. AU, MZ and FF contributed in reviewing the final manuscript. All authors have read the manuscript. All authors read and approved the final manuscript.

Competing interests

The authors declare that they have no competing interests.

Author details

[1]Institute of Social and Cultural Studies, University of the Punjab, Lahore, Pakistan. [2]Department of Public Health Medicine, School of Public Health, Bielefeld University, Bielefeld, Germany.

References

1. Betran AP, Torloni MR, Zhang JJ, Gülmezoglu AM, for the WHO Working Group on Caesarean Section. WHO statement on caesarean section rates: a commentary. BJOG. 2015; https://doi.org/10.1111/1471-0528.13526.

2. Gibbons L, Belizán JM, Lauer JA, Betrán AP, Merialdi M, Althabe F. The global numbers and costs of additionally needed and unnecessary caesarean sections performed per year: overuse as a barrier to universal coverage. World Health Report 2010, Background Paper 30. Geneva, World Health Organization; 2010.
3. Neuman M, Alcock G, Azad K, et al. Prevalence and determinants of caesarean section in private and public health facilities in underserved South Asian communities: cross-sectional analysis of data from Bangladesh, India and Nepal. BMJ Open. 2014;4:e005982.
4. Nazir S. Determinants of cesarean deliveries in Pakistan, Pide working papers; 2015.
5. Qazi Q, Akhtar Z, Khan K, Khan AH. Pregnant women view regarding cesarean section in Northwest Pakistan. Tropical Medicine & Surgery. 2013;1:105.
6. Ghosh S. Increasing trend in cesarean section delivery in India: role of medicalisation of maternal health, Working paper. Bangalore: Institute for Social and Economic Change; 2010.
7. Mishra US, Ramanathan M. Delivery-related complications and determinants of caesarean section rates in India. Health Policy Plan. 2002;17:90–8.
8. El-Ardat MA, Izetbegovic S, Mehmedbasic E, Duric M. Frequency of vaginal birth after cesarean section at clinic of gynecology and obstetrics in Sarajevo. Med Arh. 2013;67(6):435–7.
9. Nilsen C, Østbye T, Daltveit AK, Mmbaga BT, Sandøy IF. Trends in and socio-demographic factors associated with caesarean section at a Tanzanian referral hospital, 2000 to 2013. Int J Equity Health. 2014;13:87.
10. Karlström A, Nystedt A, Johansson M, Hildingsson I. Behind the myth–few women prefer caesarean section in the absence of medical or obstetrical factors. Midwifery. 2011;27:620–7.
11. Latifnejad RR, Zakerihamidi M, Merghati KE, Kazemnejad A. Cultural perceptions and preferences of Iranian women regarding cesarean delivery. Iranian J Nurs Midwifery Res. 2014;19:S28–36.
12. Lori JR, Boyle JS. Cultural childbirth practices, beliefs, and traditions in post-conflict Liberia. Health Care Women Int. 2011;32(6):454–73.
13. Béhague DP, Victora CG, Barros FC. Consumer demand for caesarean sections in Brazil: informed decision making, patient choice, or social inequality? A population based birth cohort study linking ethnographic and epidemiological methods. BMJ. 2002;324:942.
14. Mazzoni A, Althabe F, Liu NH, Bonotti AM, Gibbons L, Sanchez AJ. Women's preference for caesarean section: a systematic review and meta-analysis of observational studies. BJOG. 2011;118(4):391–9.
15. Ash A, Okah D. What is the right number of caesarean sections? Lancet. 1997;349:1557.
16. Lauer JA, Betrán AP, Merialdi M, Wojdyla D. Determinants of caesarean section rates in developed countries: supply, demand and opportunities for control. Geneva: World Health Organization; 2010.
17. Buekens P. Over-medicalisation of maternal care in developing countries. In: De Brouwere V, Van Lerberghe W, editors. Safe, motherhood strategies: a review of the evidence. Antwerp: ITG Press; 2001. p. 195–206.
18. Johanson R, Newburn M, Macfarlane A. Has the medicalisation of childbirth gone too far? BMJ. 2002;324:892–5.
19. Pai M. Unnecessary medical interventions: caesarean sections as a case study. Econ Polit Wkly. 2000;35:2755–61.
20. Johnson EM, Rehavi MM. Physicians treating physicians: information and incentives in childbirth, NBER working paper; 2013.
21. NIPS. Pakistan demographic and health survey 2012–13. Islamabad: National Institute of Population Studies and Macro International Inc; 2008.
22. World Health Organization. Provision of effective antenatal care: integrated management of pregnancy and childbirth. Geneva: World Health Organization; 2006.
23. NIPS. Pakistan demographic and health survey 2006–2007. Islamabad: National Institute of Population Studies and Macro International Inc; 2008.
24. Hafeez M, Yasin A, Badar N, Pasha MI, Akram N, Gulzar B. Prevalence and indications of caesarean section in a teaching hospital. JIMSA. 2014;27:15–6.
25. Iftikhar T, Rizvi U, Ejaz L. Evaluation of causes of increasing cesarean section rate in tertiary care hospital. J Sheikh Zayed Medical College. 2010;1:1.
26. Jabeen J, Mansoor MH, Mansoor A. Analysis of indications of cesarean sections. J Rawalpindi Medical College. 2013;17(1):101–3.
27. Martinez PA. C-section boom: all about the $?. 2013. http://www.parents.com/blogs/everythingpregnancy/2013/09/04/must-read/cesarean-section-birth-monetary-incentive/. Accessed 19 Apr 2018.
28. Carolan M, Davey M-A, Biro MA, Kealy M. Older maternal age and intervention in labor: a population-based study comparing older and younger first-time mothers in Victoria, Australia. Birth. 2011;38(1):24–9.
29. Bayrambour H, Heaman M. Advanced maternal age and the risk of cesarean birth: a systematic review. Birth. 2010;37(3):219–26.
30. Lin HC, Sheen TC, Tang CH, Kao S. Association between maternal age and the likelihood of a cesarean section: a population-based multivariate logistic regression analysis. Acta Obstet Gynecol Scand. 2004;83:1178–83.
31. Hanif HM. Association between maternal age and pregnancy outcome: implications for the Pakistani society. J Pak Med Assoc. 2011;61:313–9.
32. Ashraf-Ganjoei T, Mirzaei F, Anari-Dokht F. Relationship between prenatal care and the outcome of pregnancy in low-risk pregnancies. Open J Obstet Gynecol. 2011;1:109–12.
33. Padmadas SS, Suresh KS, Nair SB, Anitha Kumari KR. Cesarean section delivery in Kerala, India: Evidence from National Family Health Survey. Soc Sci Med Sci. 2000;519(4):511–21.
34. Sial MA. Increasing number of C-sections crosses all danger thresholds. https://www.pakistantoday.com.pk/2012/01/08/increasing-number-of-c-sections-crosses-all-dangerthresholds/. Accessed 19 Apr 2018.

6

Caesarean section audit to improve quality of care in a rural referral hospital in Tanzania

Luuk Dekker[1,2], Tessa Houtzager[1,2], Omary Kilume[1,3], John Horogo[1], Jos van Roosmalen[2] and Angelo Sadock Nyamtema[1,3*]

Abstract

Background: Caesarean section (CS) is often a life-saving procedure, but can also lead to serious complications, even more so in low-resource settings. Therefore unnecessary CS should be avoided and optimal circumstances for vaginal delivery should be created. In this study, we aim to audit indications for Caesarean sections and improve decision-making and obstetric management.

Methods: Audit of all cases of CS performed from January to August 2013 was performed in a rural referral hospital in Tanzania. The study period was divided in three audit blocks; retrospective (before auditing), prospective 1 and prospective 2. A local audit panel (LP) and an external auditor (EA) judged if obstetric management was adequate and indications were appropriate or if CS could have been prevented and yet retain good pregnancy outcome. Furthermore, changes in modes of deliveries, overall pregnancy outcome and decision-to-delivery interval were monitored.

Results: During the study period there were 1868 deliveries. Of these, 403 (21.6%) were Caesarean sections. The proportions of unjustified CS prior to introduction of audit were as high as 34 and 75%, according to the respective judgments of LP and EA. Following introduction of audit, the proportions of unjustified CS decreased to 23% ($p = 0.29$) and 52% ($p = 0.01$) according to LP and EA respectively. However, CS rate did not change (20.2 to 21.7%), assisted vacuum delivery rate did not increase (3.9 to 1.8%) and median decision-to-delivery interval was 83 min (range 10 - 390 min).

Conclusions: Although this is a single center study, these findings suggest that unnecessary Caesarean sections exist at an alarming rate even in referral hospitals and suggest that a vast number can be averted by introducing a focused CS audit system. Our findings indicate that CS audit is a useful tool and, if well implemented, can enhance rational use of resources, improve decision-making and harmonise practice among care providers.

Keywords: Caesarean section, Assisted vaginal delivery, Vacuum delivery, Audit, Tanzania, Decision-to-delivery interval

Background

Caesarean section (CS) is a lifesaving procedure when spontaneous or assisted vaginal delivery is not possible. The World Health Organization (WHO) recommends a rate of 5 – 15% for any community and above that is considered unnecessary overuse of the procedure. In Tanzania, the population-based CS-rate in 2010 was 4.5% and in rural areas only 3.2%, indicating general underuse [1, 2]. However, in some health facilities CS-rates are much higher and probably overused.

Although CS in general is a safe operation, the procedure can lead to serious complications. These include endometritis, wound haematoma and infection, venous thromboembolism, anaesthetic complications, infertility and abdominal adhesions which can lead to chronic abdominal and pelvic pain as well as a risk of injury to adjacent organs in future surgeries [3–8]. Furthermore, CS bears consequences for subsequent pregnancies, with higher risks of excessive blood loss, uterine scar rupture,

* Correspondence: nyamtema_angelo@yahoo.co.uk; anyamtema@ttcih.ac.tz
[1]Department of Obstetrics and Gynaecology, St. Francis Referral Hospital, Ifakara, Tanzania
[3]St. Francis University College of Health and Allied Sciences, P.O Box 175, Ifakara, Tanzania
Full list of author information is available at the end of the article

placenta accreta, placenta praevia and abruptio placentae [9–12]. Most of these complications are more serious in resource-limited settings, reinforcing the restraint which should be used in deciding to perform CS.

In addition to these medical complications, CS is associated with considerable costs for patients and hospitals, resulting in a longer hospital stay, whilst the number of available beds in most centres is limited. Therefore, to avoid unnecessary CS, management of women in labour should be appropriate and the decision for CS be made only in situations where no better alternatives are available [13].

Few audits measuring adequacy of decision-making for CS have formally been evaluated in countries such as Tanzania [14–17]. In an attempt to improve health care and reduce maternal and perinatal mortality and morbidity, audit was introduced in St. Francis Referral Hospital (SFRH) in Ifakara, Tanzania [18]. The research questions in this study were: 'What is the current magnitude of unnecessary CS at SFRH?' 'Can CS audit be used to reduce unnecessary CS?' 'Can CS audit lead to harmonisation of decision-making, enhance alternative delivery modalities and improve maternal care?' To answer these questions, we established a CS audit system at SFRH, hoping that if successful the initiative may provide an appropriate template for the future use of an audit-based system to reduce unnecessary CS and enhance alternative modes of deliveries in resource-poor settings.

Methods

The study was conducted in St. Francis Referral Hospital, a referral hospital located in Ifakara, headquarters of Kilombero district in Morogoro region in south-western Tanzania. The district covers an area of 14,918 km^2 with a population of 407,880 as per 2012 population census. Seventy-two percent of inhabitants live in rural areas, 81% of the population being farmers [19]. SFRH has 372 beds and an average annual delivery rate of 5200 [18]. Although prenatal services are provided at all levels of health care including dispensaries, patients requiring higher level of care may have to walk up to 75 km to get to SFRH. In view of this, SFRH also provides care to patients from the neighbouring districts (Ulanga, Kilosa and Morogoro rural districts).

Cases of CS were collected retrospectively up to 7 weeks from January until February and prospectively in two blocks from February until August, 2013. For data-collection, the same sources were used for the retro- and prospective periods, being case files, partographs, antenatal-care cards and delivery records books. Data items collected included gravidity, parity, modes of previous deliveries including the number of previous Caesarean sections, gestational age, time at decision for CS and time at start of surgery.

The local investigators summarised all cases of CS and presented them anonymously to a local audit panel (LP) using powerpoint-presentations. This local panel included all obstetricians, intern doctors, assistant medical officers, medical students and midwives present at the time of clinical morning discussions. Involvement of all doctors was encouraged in order to improve knowledge and harmonise obstetric practices in the department. They critically discussed the cases and reached consensus if obstetric management was appropriate and indications were conform the hospital standards or if CS could have been prevented. The investigators were present during presentations and the LP was able to ask them for extra information if needed before making its final judgment. Furthermore, an external auditor (EA) evaluated the cases as well, since it is known that external and internal analysis can differ significantly [20]. The EA was a senior obstetrician who was familiar with the resources available and the circumstances in which obstetric care is provided in SFRH. The same presentations, complemented with additional information if requested, were sent to the EA for second judgment. These judgments were based on, among others, the National CEmOC management guidelines, WHO recommendations and other nationally recommended reference books [21, 22]. Unjustified indications for an emergency CS were for example: 'prolonged/obstructed labour' with intact membranes, 'prolonged/obstructed labour' in primigravidae without oxytocin augmentation, 'prolonged/obstructed labour' with descent ≤3/5 (level of the Ischial Spine, station 0) without a trial of vacuum extraction or 'prolonged/obstructed labour' before crossing of the action line. If CS was judged to be unjustified, this did not mean CS could have definitely been prevented, but it implies that optimal circumstances for vaginal delivery were not created and that CS might have been avoided.

Main outcome measures were: Modes of deliveries, indications for CS, judgment on obstetric management and justification of CS by local audit panel and external auditor, maternal morbidity and mortality and decision-to-delivery interval.

In order to further enhance analysis, indications for CS were classified into groups based on their similarities and agreed management approaches. CS performed in women with ≥2 previous uterine scars were excluded from the analyses, since this indication is always considered to be justified based upon the national guidelines for emergency obstetric care. Asides from these, a classification system of indications was developed because there usually was more than one indication contributing to the decision to perform CS such as 'Foetal Distress + Prolonged Labour', 'Obstructed Labour + inadequate contractions' or 'Cephalopelvic Disproportion + Foetal Heart Rate <100 bpm'. In these combinations of indications, no consistency in primary indication could be identified. Moreover, often indications such as prolonged labour and obstructed labour were not distinguished consistently. Lastly, classification in these groups was also done in order to retain enough statistical power to demonstrate clinically important differences.

The three groups of indications were:

- Group 1: failed trial of scar;
- Group 2: cephalopelvic disproportion/prolonged or obstructed labour/arrested descent/foetal distress (without previous scars);
- Group 3: other than group 1 & 2.

Group 3 included indications such as malpresentation, (pre)eclampsia, multiple pregnancy, bad obstetric history, cord prolapse, placenta praevia or abruptio placenta.

Judgments of local audit panel and external auditor were documented and analysed. Furthermore, to determine the impact of the audit, proportions of unjustified CS and trends of CS and vacuum delivery rate were compared between the three study blocks. For exploring the quality of health care, maternal outcome was assessed. Morbidity was evaluated using the Haydom-variant of the internationally established Maternal-Near-Miss criteria of the WHO, since these criteria are better suited in low-resource settings like SFRH [23].

All statistical analyses were computed using SPSS version 20 (SPSS, Inc., USA). Differences in modes of deliveries and judgments over the audit periods were analysed using chi-square tests with two-sided p-values. Outcomes were considered significant if $p < 0.05$. Case by case correlation was calculated using Cohen's kappa for agreement between local panel and external auditor. Permission to conduct the study was obtained from the hospital management and ethical clearance as part of the larger audit project in the hospital [17]. After having evaluated all cases locally, a final presentation was held in SFRH with tentative results. These were discussed and recommendations were made for improving future obstetric care.

Results

The study period covered 179 days which were divided into three audit blocks, one retrospective block followed by two prospective blocks. Over this period, 1868 deliveries took place in SFRH. Mean maternal age was 27 years, mean parity 1.6 and mean gestational age 39 weeks (Table 1).

Out of all deliveries, 403 (21.6%) were by Caesarean section and 44 (2.4%) were assisted by vacuum (Table 2). Of all cases of CS, 334 (82.9%) were summarised and discussed. Cases were not analysed either because files from the retrospective block could not be retrieved or due to other logistical reasons in the prospective blocks, most often being the investigator temporarily not being present at SFRH for a limited period of time. Out of these 334 cases, 99 (30%) were primigravidae and 156 (47%) had at least one previous uterine scar. There were 26 maternal-near-misses, almost all of them due to eclampsia, ≥2 units of blood, uterine rupture or a combination of these. Furthermore, five (1.5%) maternal deaths occurred. Two of these were due to complications of abruptio placentae, one was due to eclampsia, one due to uterine rupture and one due to postpartum haemorrhage. In four of five maternal deaths (80%) CS was found unjustified. All CS in six cases of uterine rupture were justified, however one CS was found to be performed too late. Over the three audit blocks there were no significant changes in modes of deliveries.

Table 1 Characteristics of women who delivered by Caesarean section during the study period

Basic indicators	Number	Mean (SD)
Maternal age in years		26.6 (6.5)
Gravidity		2.7 (1.6)
1	99	
2	75	
3+	160	
Parity		1.6 (1.6)
0	101	
1	80	
2+	153	
Number of living children		1.3 (1.4)
0	120	
1	87	
2+	120	
(unknown)	(7)	
Gestational age in weeks		38.8 (2.8)
HIV-positive status	20 (10.2%)	
Maternal-near-miss	26 (7.8%)	
Maternal deaths	5 (1.5%)	

The table provides a statistical description of the population of women who were included in this study and an overview of the maternal morbidity (defined as maternal-near-misses) and mortality

Mean APGAR at 1 min was 8.0 and after 5 min was 9.5, two neonates having an APGAR < 4 after 5 min. Of 190 neonates of which outcome is known, 21 (11.1%) were admitted to the neonatal ward. Asides, six neonates (3.2%) , of which one pair were twins, died after CS. Of these five cases of CS, two were judged as unjustified. There were seven cases of intra-uterine fetal death (3.7%), of which in five CS was unjustified. None of the adverse pregnancy outcomes was directly attributed to the CS procedure.

Of the 334 analysed cases, 64 CS (19%) were performed due to a history of two or more previous uterine scars and these were excluded from further analysis. Of the remaining 270 cases over all three blocks in total, LP judged 70 (26%) and EA judged 157 (58%) CS to be unjustified. Cohen's

Table 2 Overtime trends of proportions of modes of deliveries and decision-to-delivery interval

Delivery indicators	Retrospective block *n* (%)	Prospective block 1 *n* (%)	Prospective block 2 *n* (%)	Total *n* (%)	Chi-square test for differences in mode of delivery across the blocks
Audit period in days	51	39	89	179	
Total deliveries	415 (100)	429 (100)	1024 (100)	1868 (100)	
Vaginal deliveries	315 (75.9)	322 (75.1)	784 (76.6)	1421 (76.1)	$p = 0.83$ (χ^2=0.4)
Caesarean sections	84 (20.2)	97 (22.6)	222 (21.7)	403 (21.6)	$p = 0.70$ (χ^2=0.7)
Vacuum deliveries	16 (3.9)	10 (2.3)	18 (1.8)	44 (2.4)	$p = 0.06$ (χ^2=5.7)
Caesarean sections analysed	70 (83.3)	96 (99.0)	168 (75.7)	334 (82.9)	
Decision-to-delivery interval for emergency CS in minutes; median (range)	75 (15-340)	60 (15-390)	95 (10-365)	83 (10-390)	

The table shows a numerical overview of the blocks, including the number of cases collected, modes of deliveries (with chi-square tests for differences in modes of deliveries over the blocks) and decision-to-delivery intervals per block

kappa for case by case correlation was 0.27, suggesting fair agreement between LP and EA.

Of retrospectively analysed cases, proportions of unjustified CS were 34% according to the local audit panel and 75% according to the external auditor. Following introduction of audit, this dropped to 23% for LP ($p = 0.29$) and 52% for EA ($p = 0.01$) (Fig. 1). In view of the different groups of indications, the most notable declines of unjustified CS, especially according to the local panel, were seen in group 1 [trial of scar] and 2 [cephalopelvic disproportion/prolonged or obstructed labour/arrested descent/foetal distress] (Table 3). The major reasons for persistent unjustified CS in these groups were failure to adhere to the principles of trial of labour or trial of scar. These included the presence of intact membranes at time of decision for emergency CS, absence of oxytocin augmentation in case of inadequate contractions or not attempting to perform vacuum delivery prior to emergency CS when the cervix was fully dilated and descent ≤3/5. Almost a quarter (24%) of 152 women who had emergency CS after a failed trial of labour or scar (group 1 or 2) still had intact membranes when CS was performed and 28 (18%) reached full dilatation and a descent of ≤3/5, indicating that they could have had a trial of assisted vacuum delivery. Of all 152 cases of emergency CS, two women had a failed trial of vacuum prior to CS.

After introduction of audit, Caesarean section rate did not change (20.2 to 21.7%) and assisted vacuum delivery rate did not increase (3.9 to 1.8%). However, it was noted that assisted vacuum delivery was registered by midwives in the delivery book as spontaneous vaginal delivery quite often. Because of incomplete documentation only 215 emergency CS cases could be assessed for the time interval from decision for emergency CS to the start of surgery.

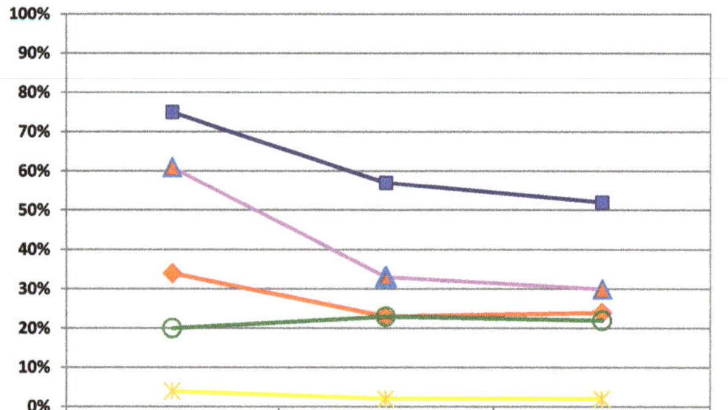

	Retrospective Block (n=70)	Prospective Block 1 (n=96)	Prospective Block 2 (n=168)
Unjustified by LP	34%	23%	24%
Unjustified by EA	75%	57%	52%
Unjustified by LP & EA*	61%	33%	30%
CS rate	20%	23%	22%
Vacuum delivery rate	4%	2%	2%

Fig. 1 Overtime trends of the proportions of unjustified Caesarean sections and modes of deliveries. Content: A multiple line graph with concomitant table displaying the trends of the percentages of unjustified CS over the blocks as judged by the local audit panel and the external auditor, as well as the trends of modes of deliveries (CS-rate and vacuum delivery rate). *Abbreviations: SFRH = St. Francis Referral Hospital; LP = local audit panel; EA = external auditor; CS = Caesarean section*

Table 3 Overtime trends of proportions of unjustified Caesarean sections per group of indications

Groups of indications for CS	Retrospective Block		Prospective Block 1		Prospective Block 2		Chi-square test for differences across the blocks
	Total *n*	Unjustified *n* (%)	Total *n*	Unjustified *n* (%)	Total *n*	Unjustified *n* (%)	
Group 1 [Failure of trial of scar]							
Judgment by LP	10	3 (30%)	15	3 (20%)	20	4 (20%)	$p = 0.80$ (χ^2=0.5)
Judgment by EA	10	8 (80%)	15	7 (47%)	20	12 (60%)	$p = 0.25$ (χ^2=2.8)
Group 2 [Cephalopelvic disproportion/obstructed or prolonged labour/arrested descent/foetal distress]							
Judgment by LP	27	14 (52%)	24	6 (25%)	56	13 (23%)	$p = 0.24$ (χ^2=7.5)
Judgment by EA	27	23 (85%)	24	14 (58%)	56	34 (61%)	p = *0.06* (χ^2=5.8)
Group 3 [other than group 1&2]							
Judgment by LP	22	3 (14%)	38	9 (24%)	58	15 (26%)	$p = 0.50$ (χ^2=1.4)
Judgment by EA	22	13 (59%)	38	23 (61%)	58	23 (40%)	$p = 0.09$ (χ^2=4.9)

The table shows a numerical overview of the subgroups by indications per block, including the number of unjustified CS within those, with chi-square tests for differences in justification over the blocks
Abbreviations: *LP* local audit panel, *EA* external auditor, *CS* Caesarean section

The median interval was 83 min (range 10 – 390). Only one third (33%) got an emergency CS within an hour after decision and in 28 cases (13%) CS was performed three hours or more after the decision was made.

Discussion

Introduction of audit was associated with a reduction of unjustified CS of 11% (from 34 to 23%) and 23% (from 75 to 52%) according to the LP and EA, suggesting audit is a promising tool. This reduction of unjustified CS suggests enhancement of knowledge and harmonisation of decision-making among care providers, indicating improved quality of management of labour.

However, this study also has limitations. Firstly, this was a single center study, although SFRH is quite representative for rural hospitals in Tanzania. It would be interesting to see whether similar results could be acquired in other hospitals. Secondly, the drop of unjustified CS could be explained by the presence of high proportions of unjustified CS from the start. Thirdly, one fifth of CS could not be analysed due to poor documentation or logistical reasons. However, we found no reason to assume these CS are different from the analysed CS and may have led to bias. Finally, in order to maintain these results CS audit should be regularly done so that knowledge and harmony of the decision-making process is continuously transmitted to new care providers joining the obstetric department.

Globally, there is increasing concern about the rising trends of CS rates. General agreement is that, although Caesarean sections have become a much safer procedure over the years, it cannot replace vaginal delivery in terms of low maternal and neonatal morbidity and less expense [24]. In accordance with other reports, almost half (47%) of women who delivered by CS at SFRH had at least one previous uterine scar [25]. It is known that repeat CS rates are high in Western countries as well, numbers up to 76% having been reported [26]. These findings suggest that primary Caesarean section usually determines the future obstetric course of women and therefore should be avoided if possible. This is probably even more important in the more rural areas with limited access to health care. Again similar to other reports, our study shows that failure to progress and foetal distress were the leading indications for emergency CS, while two or more previous uterine scars was the most common indication for elective CS [27, 28].

The fact that a vast number of CS performed before introduction of audit at SFRH was unjustified suggests an alarming rate of unnecessary CS in this hospital and probably also in other Tanzanian hospitals. This needs urgent attention. Like many other studies from resource-limited countries, unjustified CS are mainly attributed to poor decision-making. Decisions for CS are often made by junior care providers who are less trained and get little supervision [29]. The LP acknowledged the difficulty not to rely too much on intern doctors, since senior doctors are not always present. They agreed that decision-making for CS requires more experience and knowledge and should be discussed more extensively with midwives and senior doctors. There was long-existing peer review by the obstetric department team of the Caesarean sections performed in the preceding 24 h during clinical morning discussions. This practice, however, did not seem to improve decision-making or harmonise practice on CS. This suggests a need to restructure clinical morning discussions to enhance decision-making and improve quality of care.

The difference in judgements between local audit panel and external auditor was notable. Although cases were submitted anonymously and the majority of staff would not have been involved in the management of most patients, the LP was judging their own actions, perhaps causing a less critical approach of the cases than the EA. Since the EA analysed all patients on his own and was not present during the panel meetings, he might have interpreted available information differently. Furthermore, since the EA is particularly involved in reducing unnecessary interventions he could be biased against actual appropriate indications.

Although no significant changes in trends of proportions of unjustified CS per group were found, probably due to the small number of cases per group per block, a decrease of unjustified CS was seen in all different groups of indications after introduction of the audit. The LP itself also thought the audit to be very useful and was positive about its effects, especially regarding its function as a "learning platform". Considering the impact found in this study, introduction of CS audit is recommended in all hospitals in Tanzania and other resource-limited countries.

Unexpectedly, despite the decrease in unjustified CS, Caesarean section rate nor assisted vacuum delivery rate changed significantly (20.2 to 21.7% and 3.9 to 1.8% respectively). A possible explanation could be that a group of women existed who needed CS, but did not receive it before the start of this audit. During the course of the audit, this group may have been acknowledged as suitable candidates for CS, while a group of women in whom CS was not indicated did not get the operation. This is subject for further study. Part of the low rate of assisted vacuum deliveries could be attributed to incorrect documentation, as investigators noticed that deliveries by vacuum were sometimes recorded by midwives as spontaneous vaginal deliveries. However, considering that assisted vacuum delivery could have been attempted in 18% of women from group 1 and 2 and was attempted in only two cases prior to emergency CS, it is likely that it is currently not used to its full potential. Operative vaginal delivery is known to be safe and contributes to more than 10% of deliveries in most European and Northern American countries [30]. All together, these findings prompt a need to promote the use of vacuum delivery, as it may also contribute to further reduction of unnecessary CS. During the final discussion, the LP recognised this issue and explained that vacuum extractions fell from grace because of a possibly increased risk of HIV-infection for the foetus. However, they agreed that no convincing scientific data was available to support this and that too few vacuum deliveries were performed in HIV-negative women as well, although they make up almost 90% of population.

Considering the generally accepted period of time between decision for and start of emergency CS is 60 min at most, the median decision-to-delivery interval of 83 min was striking. Furthermore, 13% were performed more than three hours after decision for emergency CS, while it is known that a decision-to-delivery interval of more than 75 min is already associated with poorer maternal and neonatal outcome [31]. This delay may be caused by the amount of time that elapses for haemoglobin and blood group analysis and preparation of the operating theatre, although there are two other operating theatres that could also be used in case of emergencies. Also, the limited number of available staff may contribute to this delay. However, the LP realised that a necessity for a reduction of the decision-to-delivery interval was obvious and stated that another study was needed to investigate the causes of this delay and to assess methods for improvement of the current situation.

Conclusions

Even though this was a relatively small study performed in one center, our findings suggest that unjustified Caesarean sections exist at alarming rates, even in referral hospitals, and suggest that a vast part can be averted by introducing a focused CS audit system. Our study findings suggest that CS audit is a very useful tool and, if well implemented, can improve decision-making and harmonise practice among care providers. Furthermore, decision-to-delivery interval should be reduced and monitored and the use of vacuum delivery should be emphasised. In view of these results CS audit is strongly recommended in all hospitals in resource-limited countries.

Abbreviations

CS: Caesarean section; EA: External auditor; LP: Local (audit) panel; SFRH: St. Francis Referral Hospital; WHO: World Health Organization

Acknowledgments

The authors would like to thank SFRH staff and hospital administration for allowing us to conduct this research. Furthermore, we wish to thank all doctors, AMO's, interns, students and midwives who took part in the local audit panel.

Authors' contributions

This study was designed by LD, TH, JvR and ASN. Data collection and presentation of cases was performed by LD and TH. OK, JH and ASN took place in the audit panel. JvR functioned as EA. LD carried out the statistical analyses and drafted the manuscript. All authors provided important input in interpretation of results and revision of the manuscript. All authors read and approved the final manuscript.

Competing interests

The authors declare that they have no competing interests.

Author details

[1]Department of Obstetrics and Gynaecology, St. Francis Referral Hospital, Ifakara, Tanzania. [2]Department of Obstetrics, Leiden University Medical Centre, Leiden, The Netherlands. [3]St. Francis University College of Health and Allied Sciences, P.O Box 175, Ifakara, Tanzania.

References

1. Cavallaro FL, Cresswell JA, Franca GV, Victora CG, Barros AJ, Ronsmans C. Trends in caesarean delivery by country and wealth quintile: cross-sectional surveys in southern Asia and sub-Saharan Africa. Bull World Health Organ. 2013;91:914–922D.
2. National Bureau of Statistics. United Republic of Tanzania demographic and health survey 2010. Tanzania: Dar-Es-Salaam; 2011.
3. Burrows LJ, Meyn LA, Weber AM. Maternal morbidity associated with vaginal versus cesarean delivery. Obstet Gynecol. 2004;103:907–12.
4. Liu S, Liston RM, Joseph KS, Heaman M, Sauve R, Kramer MS, et al. Maternal mortality and severe morbidity associated with low-risk planned cesarean delivery versus planned vaginal delivery at term. CMAJ. 2007;176:455–60.
5. Jacobsen AF, Skjeldestad FE, Sandset PM. Incidence and risk patterns of venous thromboembolism in pregnancy and puerperium–a register-based case-control study. Am J Obstet Gynecol. 2008;198:233. e1-7
6. Murphy DJ, Stirrat GM, Heron J, Team AS. The relationship between caesarean section and subfertility in a population-based sample of 14.541 pregnancies. Hum Reprod. 2002;17:1914–7.
7. Nikolajsen L, Sorensen HC, Jensen TS, Kehlet H. Chronic pain following caesarean section. Acta Anaesthesiol Scand. 2004;48:111–6.
8. Nisenblat V, Barak S, Griness OB, Degani S, Ohel G, Gonen R. Maternal complications associated with multiple cesarean deliveries. Obstet Gynecol. 2006;108:21–6.
9. Daltveit AK, Tollanes MC, Pihlstrom H, Irgens LM. Cesarean delivery and subsequent pregnancies. Obstet Gynecol. 2008;111:1327–34.
10. Usta IM, Hobeika EM, Musa AA, Gabriel GE, Nassar AH. Placenta previa-accreta: risk factors and complications. Am J Obstet Gynecol. 2005;193:1045–9.
11. Yang Q, Wen S, Oppenheimer L, Chen X, Black D, Gao J, et al. Association of caesarean delivery for first birth with placenta praevia and placental abruption in second pregnancy. BJOG. 2007;114:609–13.
12. Gurol-Urganci I, Cromwell DA, Edozien LC, Smith GC, Onwere C, Mahmood TA, et al. Risk of placenta previa in second birth after first birth cesarean section: a population-based study and meta-analysis. BMC Pregnancy Childbirth. 2011;11:95.
13. Souza JP, Gulmezoglu A, Lumbiganon P, Laopaiboon M, Carroli G, Fawole B, et al. Caesarean section without medical indications is associated with an increased risk of adverse short-term maternal outcomes: the 2004-2008 WHO global survey on maternal and perinatal health. BMC Med. 2010;8:71.
14. Maaløe N, Bygbjerg IC, Onesmo R, Secher NJ, Sorensen BL. Disclosing doubtful indications for emergency cesarean sections in rural hospitals in Tanzania: a retrospective criterion-based audit. Acta Obstet Gynecol Scand. 2012;91:1069–76.
15. Maaløe N, Sorensen BL, Onesmo R, Secher NJ, Bygbjerg IC. Prolonged labour as indication for emergency caesarean section: a quality assurance analysis by criterion-based audit at two Tanzanian rural hospitals. BJOG. 2012;119:605–13.
16. Heemelaar S, Nelissen E, Mdoe P, Kidanto H, van Roosmalen J, Stekelenburg J. Criteria-based audit of caesarean section in a referral hospital in rural Tanzania. Tropical Med Int Health. 2016;21:525–34.
17. Nyamtema AS, de Jong AB, Urassa DP, van Roosmalen J. Using audit to enhance quality of maternity care in resource limited countries: lessons learnt from rural Tanzania. BMC Pregnancy Childbirth. 2011;11:94.
18. St. Francis Referral Hospital website. Available online at: http://www.ifakara.org/en/st-francis-hospital/hospital.php (accessed August 10th, 2015).
19. National Bureau of Statistics. United Republic of Tanzania population and housing census 2012. Tanzania: Dar-Es-Salaam; 2013.
20. Sorensen BL, Elsass P, Nielsen BB, Massawe S, Nyakina J, Rasch V. Substandard emergency obstetric care - a confidential enquiry into maternal deaths at a regional hospital in Tanzania. Tropical Med Int Health. 2010;15:894–900.
21. WHO, UNFPA, UNCEF, World Bank. Integrated Management of Pregnancy and Childbirth. Managing Complications in Pregnancy and Childbirth: a guide for doctors and midwives. WHO; 2000.
22. Cunningham F, Leveno K, Bloom S, Hauth J, Gilstrap L, Wenstrom K. Williams obstetrics. 22nd ed. USA: The McGraw Hill Companies, Inc.; 2005.
23. Nelissen E, Mduma E, Broerse J, Ersdal H, Evjen-Olsen B, van Roosmalen J, et al. Applicability of the WHO maternal near miss criteria in a low-resource setting. PLoS One. 2013;8:e61248.
24. Sachs BP, Kobelin C, Castro MA, Frigoletto F. The risks of lowering the cesarean-delivery rate. N Engl J Med. 1999;340:54–7.
25. Wareham V, Bain C, Cruickshank D. Caesarean section audit by peer review. Eur J Obstet Gynecol Reprod Biol. 1993;48:9–14.
26. Wray J. Review of the National Sentinel Caesarean Section Audit Report. Pract Midwife. 2001;4:24–5.
27. CPY R. A clinical audit on caesarean section: indications and outcomes [PhD thesis]. Hong Kong: University of Hong Kong; 2003.
28. Naidoo N, Moodley J. Rising rates of caesarean sections: an audit of caesarean sections in a specialist private practice. SA Fam Pract. 2009;51:254–8.
29. Ion R, Alatt H. Reducing the caesarean section rate in a rural hospital in south-West Uganda. Arch Dis Child Fetal Neonatal Ed. 2013;98:A68.
30. Thomas J, Paranjothy S. Royal College of Obstetricians and Gynaecologists clinical effectiveness support unit: National Sentinel Caesarean Section Audit Report. London: RCOG Press; 2001.
31. Thomas J, Paranjothy S, James D. National cross sectional survey to determine whether the decision to delivery interval is critical in emergency caesarean section. BMJ. 2004;328:665.

7

Reintroducing vacuum extraction in primary health care facilities

Sunday Dominico[1*], Patricia E. Bailey[2], Nguke Mwakatundu[1], Mkambu Kasanga[1] and Jos van Roosmalen[3]

Abstract

Background: In rural Tanzania access to emergency obstetric and newborn care is threatened by poor roads and understaffed facilities among other challenges. Districts in Kigoma, Pwani and Morogoro regions were targeted by a local non-governmental organization to assist local government to build capacity and improve access to clinical management of severe obstetric and newborn complications. The program upgraded ten primary health care centres to provide comprehensive emergency obstetric and newborn care. This paper describes the process of reintroducing vacuum extraction into ten health centres and five hospitals, highlighting patterns in uptake, mode of delivery and lessons learned.

Methods: This observational study uses facility-based trend data collected between 2011 and 2016.Descriptive outcomes include institutional caesarean delivery rates, vacuum extraction rates, and the ratio of caesareans to vacuum-assisted deliveries.

Results: Institutional caesarean delivery rates remained stable at about 10–11% and the vacuum extraction rate rose from virtually no procedures in 2011 to about 2% in 2016. The increase was more visible in upgraded health centres than in hospitals. In 2016 vacuum extraction rates in newly upgraded health centres ranged from 0.5 to 7. 8%. Between 2011 and 2016, the ratio of caesareans to vacuum extractions in hospitals changed from 304 caesareans to 1 vacuum extraction to 10:1, while in health centres the ratio changed from 22: 1 to 3: 1.

Conclusions: Reintroduction of vacuum extraction into clinical practice in primary health care facilities with task-shifting is feasible. Reintroduction of this procedure was more successful when part of an integrated upgrading of health centres to provide comprehensive emergency obstetric care than when reintroduced into busy hospital environments. Turnover of trained staff in hospitals contributed to the uneven uptake of vacuum extraction. Lessons learned are applicable to further national scale up and to other countries.

Keywords: Vacuum extraction, Caesarean delivery, Task-shifting

Background

Timely delivery of a newborn in the second stage of labour can mean the difference between life and death in childbirth for some women and their babies. Prolonged labour, a frequent complication, especially among nulliparous women [1], or suspicion of foetal distress, often leads to the need for rapid intervention. When labour is well monitored and indications align, assisting delivery with vacuum extraction (VE) can be successful in a short time. Taking the woman to an operating theatre for caesarean delivery, however, is the more frequent path of action, but one that takes longer, is costlier, and leaves the woman at high risk of serious complications in the index and future pregnancies.

Assisted vaginal delivery has slipped out of favour in many countries over the last few decades [2], but it has never been widely used in most low- and middle-income countries despite high rates of use in Western Europe, Canada and Australia. As caesarean rates rise, instrumental delivery is seen as one strategy to temper that rise, especially by preventing first caesareans among

* Correspondence: sdominico@thaminiuhai.or.tz
[1]Thamini Uhai, Kigoma, Tanzania
Full list of author information is available at the end of the article

singleton term nulliparous women with spontaneous or induced labour [3]. In fact, VE is safer than surgery for the woman and her baby experiencing prolonged second stage of labour (unless signs of cephalopelvic disproportion are clear) [4]. Nevertheless, caesarean deliveries save thousands of lives each year and must be available when medically indicated, but a non-surgical option for women should also be encouraged when appropriate.

The socio-economic context for women with prolonged labour or foetal distress helps to determine what actions are taken. In Tanzania, a country with high levels of maternal and neonatal mortality (398 maternal deaths per 100,000 births, and 34 neonatal deaths/1000 live births, respectively) [5], the option of either procedure is undermined by lack of medical infrastructure, limited human resources, lack of training and equipment, and a fragmented referral system. Poor roads and limited transport options contribute to the difficulties labouring women face. According to the Tanzania Demographic Health Survey (DHS) 2015–16, the top two barriers to care-seeking were lack of money and distance to health facilities, two factors entwined [6]. Despite strong policy support from the government for institutional childbirth and a substantial investment in the primary health care system, for these and other reasons, over one-third of all births still occur at home without a skilled attendant at birth [6].

In 2008,[1] the government of Tanzania supported by the World Lung Foundation embarked on a project known as Thamini Uhai (Swahili for 'Value Life') to improve access to, availability, and quality of comprehensive emergency obstetric and newborn care (C-EmONC) in 15 facilities in three regions (Kigoma, Morogoro and Pwani). The C-EmONC project started with two innovative core strategies for achieving its goals: 1) decentralization of life-saving services from district or regional hospitals to primary health care centres, and 2) task-shifting obstetric procedures from doctors, who are in short supply, to advanced level associate clinicians or assistant medical officers (AMOs), and anaesthesia to associate clinicians or nurse anaesthetists and clinical officers. Nine remote rural primary health centres and one urban health centre were upgraded to provide C-EmONC, i.e. they were staffed and equipped to provide obstetric surgery, blood transfusion as well as the basic EmONC signal functions [7]. The strategy of expanding the role of selected health centres was strongly embraced by Tanzania's Ministry of Health that included decentralization and task-shifting as leading interventions in the nation's health policies and strategies to reduce maternal and perinatal mortality.

Five district or regional hospitals that received referrals from the ten health centres also benefitted from project quality improvement aspects (human resource support, training, clinical audit, on-going mentoring supervision). The project has demonstrated that traditional and innovative strategies were not only feasible but they also substantially increased institutional childbirth rates, access to life-saving services, and the quality of care. Furthermore, they decreased the need for referral [8, 9].

This paper describes a lesser recognized aspect of Thamini Uhai's implementation success, namely how they reintroduced VE into mainstream clinical practice. It also describes patterns in the uptake of VE, trends in mode of delivery, and lessons learned in the process.

Methods

The VE reintroduction process

Assisted vaginal delivery in Tanzania had been all but abandoned in 2008 when Thamini Uhai began implementation. Obstetric forceps was never popular and although national guidelines recognized VE as a sanctioned obstetric procedure, its utilization was often not considered [10, 11]. Quality improvement audits in two Tanzanian hospitals suggested that fear of HIV contributed to the reluctance to use VE [11, 12].[2] A guiding principle to capacity building was that all associate clinicians who were going to engage in surgery also needed the skills to use a vacuum extractor.

Before implementing VE training at project sites, advocacy efforts strategically began with clinical training at the two largest medical training centres in the country: Muhimbili Medical School and Bugando Teaching Hospital, where the country's leading obstetrician/gynaecologists worked. International experts teamed up with local champions to conduct these trainings. Some participants expressed reservations while paediatricians in some regions, at least, spoke against the practice. Nevertheless, the outcome of this early attempt to elicit the support of local leaders in the field was one of strong endorsement by the Ministry of Health and it fostered a favourable climate for including VE in the toolbox of obstetric skills.

The task-shifting strategy that Thamini Uhai embraced builds on a long history in Tanzania of working with AMOs for surgery [13] and nurse-midwives and clinical officers for anaesthesia. The 3 months of EmONC training for teams of surgeons and anaesthetists has been described elsewhere [14]. It also included skills-building in VE, removal of retained products, manual removal of placenta, cervical and perineal repairs, and adult and neonatal resuscitation.

This training was followed by weeklong Continuing Medical Education (CME) sessions that focused on specific topics that were identified as requiring further confidence- and skills-building such as VE. CMEs were conducted at the five hospitals in the three regions. Two rounds of VE CMEs have taken place, one in 2012 and the other in 2016. The CME focused on a review of the partograph and VE. Trainees used anatomical models for practice but had relatively few opportunities themselves to perform a vacuum-assisted delivery on a patient, but all observed the procedure being performed. Between nine and 14 individuals made up a batch for a CME session. The training used both soft and metal cups and the project distributed Malmström extractors and Kiwi equipment. The training was considered competency-based in the context of anatomical models and followed a protocol adapted from the American College of Obstetricians and Gynecologists. Training in VE also included how to treat complications such as postpartum haemorrhage and perineal lacerations, if they occurred. Because all sites had an operating theatre (OT), if vacuum-assisted delivery was not successful, a woman was transferred to the OT for caesarean delivery.

Multiple activities were put in place to support the newly trained AMOs, nurse-midwives and clinical officers, and to improve the quality of care. These included supportive supervision and clinical audits. Obstetrician/gynaecologists or experienced AMOs and an expert anaesthetist visited each site monthly, spending two to three-days at each site, providing on-the-job coaching and hands-on mentoring. The project established weekly teleconferences allowing staff to discuss specific cases with clinicians as well as closed user group networks enabling each facility to make calls for free within the network. The closed user groups facilitated specialists to be 'on call' so that emergency consultations were possible day and night; in Kigoma, they created a "WhatsApp" group.

The supportive supervision and clinical audit visits were helpful in identifying when a CME was warranted as staff rotated and others were transferred. In addition to the hands-on CMEs, eLearning sessions were developed. In the case of VE, the trainers adopted WHO's video on VE and translated it into Swahili.

The supervisory teams also reviewed the contents of a monthly monitoring form that tracked aggregated service statistics – births, maternal and neonatal deaths, intrapartum stillbirths, near misses, and audits of all caesareans, which were used for quality improvement purposes and immediate feedback [8]. The data extracted from these forms were used in the analyses below. When retrieving this information, staff had no contact with patients and no names were captured on the form. Given that the primary purpose of the data was for internal quality improvement and feedback for the staff and to document high level changes over time, neither patient consent nor Institutional Review Board approval was sought. However, the Ministry of Health and Social Welfare, the Regional and District health management teams and medical directors of participating facilities granted permission and approval of project activities.

In 2015 four additional health centres were selected for C-EmONC upgrading in Kigoma and began receiving a similar package of interventions that the other sites received, including training in VE for AMOs and nurse-midwives.

For this paper, the monitoring counts were used to calculate percentages, rates and ratios, for example, the ratio of the number of caesareans to VE procedures. No statistical tests were used.

Results

Anaesthesia and caesarean delivery skills-building was a central thrust of upgrading health centres between 2008 and 2011. Although VE was included, the first intensively focused CME on VE was conducted in 2012. Over the course of the project, at least four persons were trained in the use of VE at each hospital, and two at each health centre. At last count, more than 80 providers completed the three-months C-EmONC course and were trained to perform VE; 56 providers received CME training in 2016 alone. Initially, most VE trainees were AMOs, who were called only when midwives encountered a difficult delivery or complications. In the last Continuous Medical Education workshop, 75% of trainees were nurse-midwives purposefully.

As a backdrop to the uptake and performance of emergency obstetric procedures, the annual number of women giving birth in the project facilities increased by 26% at the five hospitals, from 10,950 deliveries to 13,810, between 2011 and 2016 (Table 1). The increase at the ten health centres was 22%, from 10,788 deliveries to 13,152, for an overall increase of 24% (Table 1). The increase was not evenly spread across project sites; it was highest (30%) in Pwani region (two project sites), next highest (28%) in Morogoro (four sites) and lowest (17%) in Kigoma (nine sites).

In Fig. 1, the total *assisted delivery rate*, defined as the proportion of women requiring an intervention for

Table 1 Deliveries in detail in the original 15 project supported facilities (2011–2016)

Years	2011	2012	2013	2014	2015	2016
Hospitals ($n = 5$)						
Total deliveries	10,950	12,056	12,376	13,729	13,910	13,810
Caesarean deliveries	1822	1858	1609	1901	1857	2163
Vacuum extractions	6	71	185	115	133	219
Health centres ($n = 10$)						
Total deliveries	10,788	11,436	10,861	12,299	12,279	13,152
Caesarean deliveries	624	692	580	670	709	852
Vacuum extractions	28	136	307	285	198	247
All facilities ($n = 15$)						
Total deliveries	21,738	23,492	23,237	26,028	26,189	26,962
Caesarean deliveries	2446	2550	2189	2571	2566	3015
Vacuum extractions	34	207	492	400	331	466

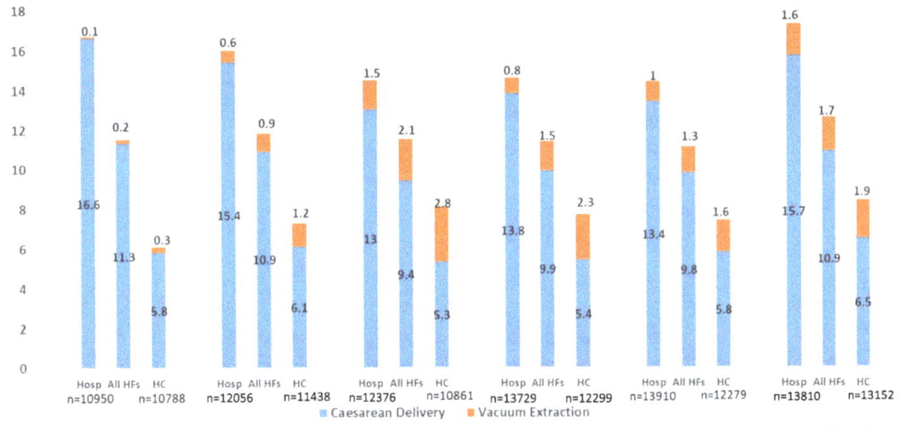

Fig. 1 Trends in caesarean delivery and vacuum extraction rates (per 100 deliveries) among the 15 original project facilities

delivery, either abdominal or vaginal [15], ranged from 11.5% in 2011 to 12.6% in 2016, not much change overall. The proportion of deliveries by caesarean ranged from 9.4 to 11.3% and of VE deliveries 0.2 to 2.8%. The year 2013, following the VE CME training in 2012, showed the lowest caesarean rate and the highest VE rate, suggesting that the uptake of VE marginally might have replaced a few caesarean deliveries. Mentoring and supervision might have played a role in building confidence and encouraging the use of VE.

The upgrading of health centres to C-EmONC centres was a departure from the conventional division of services within the national health system. Hospitals provided approximately twice the "assisted delivery" interventions to their patient mix than did health centres (Fig. 1). From an external source of data, the*2016 Pregnancy Outcomes Study in Kigoma Region*, the investigators observed that the Kigoma hospitals received proportionately about twice as many complications as did health centres [16]. The incorporation of VE into providers' daily practice was reportedly easier at health centres than hospitals and Fig. 1 supports this observation. Beginning in 2012, proportionately more deliveries were assisted with VE in health centres than in hospitals.

A more nuanced way of showing the variation in provider practice between hospitals and health centres is the ratio of caesarean deliveries to vacuum extractions (Table 2). In 2011 among hospitals, for every VE performed, clinicians and AMOs conducted 304 caesareans. In 2016 this ratio was 10 caesareans to 1 VE. In health centres, we see the same direction of change but at a different magnitude: from 22 caesareans to 1 VE in 2011 to a ratio of 3: 1 in 2016.

Table 2 Trends in the ratio of caesarean deliveries to vacuum extractions in hospitals and health centres

	2011	2012	2013	2014	2015	2016
Hospitals	303.7	26.2	8.7	16.5	14.0	9.9
Health centres	22.3	5.1	1.9	2.4	3.6	3.4

The aggregation of facilities shows overall trends but masks provider practice variation at health facility level. The disaggregation of facilities (Fig. 2) into health centres and hospitals reveals an uneven pattern in uptake and raises the question why uptake was greater in some facilities than in others. In these figures, the deliveries and VEs performed between 2011 and 2016 were reported. Four health centres had a VE rate of greater than 3% while three had a rate of less than 1%. The hospital of Utete was the only hospital with a VE rate of 3.1% while less than 1% of deliveries were delivered by VE in three of the five hospitals.

Based on data from the four health centres in Kigoma that were added to Thamini Uhai's scope of support in 2015, we see a similar uneven pattern of the uptake in VE in Fig. 3. At Kifura and Nyanzige health centres 7.8 and 5.1% of deliveries, respectively, were assisted with VE while less than 1% of deliveries at the other two health centres involved vacuum assistance. In fact, at Kifura, marginally more deliveries were assisted by VE than delivered by surgery.

Impact on intrapartum stillbirths

Improved emergency obstetric care should bring about improved perinatal outcomes, specifically fewer intrapartum stillbirths and early neonatal deaths. The *2016 Pregnancy Outcomes Study in Kigoma Region*, carried out by the USA Centers for Disease Control and Prevention, indicated a decline in the overall institutional stillbirth rate (from 28/1000 births to 22/1000 births) as well as the intrapartum stillbirth rate (from 16/1000 births to 12/1000 births) between 2011 and 2015, respectively. The highest rates were identified in project-supported hospitals but these facilities also showed the greatest declines

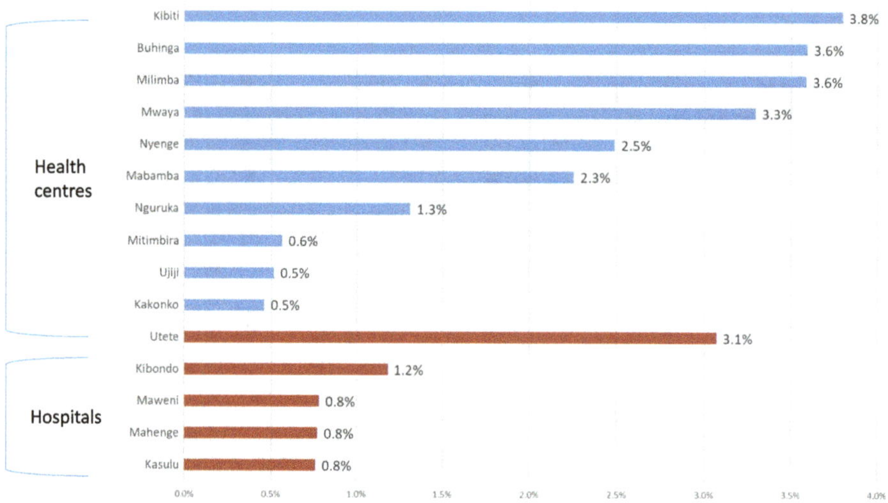

Fig. 2 Proportion of vacuum-assisted deliveries in supported sites 2011–2016

(from 37 to 20/1000 births). Project-supported health centres showed a small increase (from 12 to 16/1000 births) [16]. Unfortunately, no similar data exist for project sites in Morogoro or Pwani.

Discussion

This paper describes an experience reintroducing vacuum extraction into a context where it was rarely practiced. Vacuum extraction was reintroduced not as a reaction to rising costs due to soaring caesarean delivery rates as it has been in several Latin American hospitals [17, 18], but motivated by providing evidence-based care and preventing highly interventionist strategies that sometimes lose focus of a woman's well-being, the physical and mental hardships related to recovery from surgery, future pregnancy risks, and the financial costs to families and the health system.

In this case, VE has become part of an expanded skill set aimed at providing care to pregnant women who live in rural and often remote areas. Nyamtema and co-authors have described many successes of Thamini Uhai – the increase in institutional childbirth [8], effective task-shifting [14], and improved quality of care measured by a decrease in unjustified caesarean deliveries, and a lower risk of dying from complications of caesarean delivery [9]. VE has played a role in this changing environment since a non-surgical option now exists for selected cases of foetal distress and prolonged second stage of labour. Surely, some caesarean deliveries have been averted and intrapartum stillbirth rates are on the decline, although the introduction of VE is likely to be just one of several contributing factors.

Caesarean rates in the three regions that Thamini Uhai has supported are not excessive. According to the 2015–16 DHS and Multiple Indicator Survey, the population-based

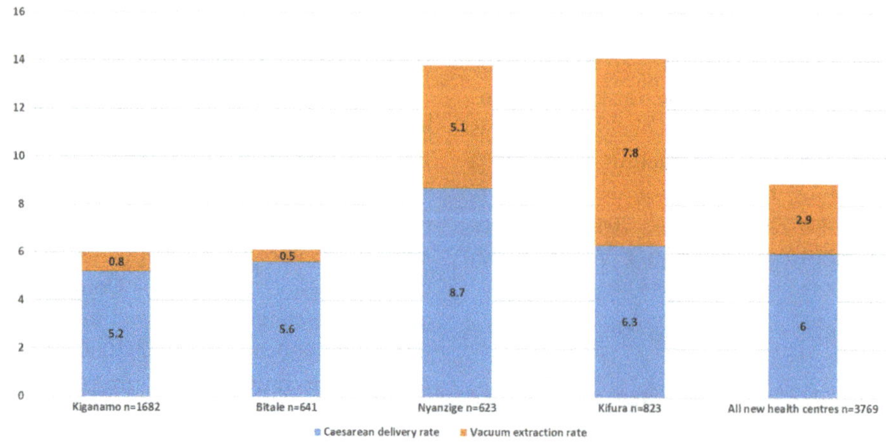

Fig. 3 Proportion of deliveries by caesarean and vacuum extraction in 2016 among health centres added in 2015

caesarean rates in Kigoma, Morogoro, and Pwani were 4.0, 6.2, and 3.0%, respectively [6]. In this paper, we saw rates of VE ranging from less than 1 to 7.8% among facility-based deliveries. The ratio of caesarean deliveries to VE, however, changed dramatically over the 6 years that Thamini Uhai collected mode of delivery data. By 2016 hospitals were intervening at a 10: 1 caesarean to VE ratio while upgraded health centres intervened at a 3: 1 ratio. To put these in a global context, the ratio in Scotland, Ireland, Canada, Australia and England (between 2004 and 2009) hovered around 2 to 1, and in the United States 7 to 1 [15]. In several sub-Saharan African countries, however, there is a tendency towards a higher dependency on caesarean surgery, for example, 27 caesareans to 1 VE in Congo Brazzaville in 2012 and 22: 1 in Ghana in 2010 [2].

This experience points to several lessons learned and challenges when reintroducing an underutilized clinical practice. It took the 2012 CME session dedicated to VE to jumpstart its integration into practice and another in 2016 to reinvigorate its use. Frequent staff turnover meant that training and coaching became an on-going need. This is not unique to VE but a universal complaint of training [19–21]; too often a person with a newly desirable skills-mix is transferred to a non-supportive or unequipped environment and skills are lost. Equipment is often cited as a barrier to performing VE [2], but it has not been a major issue in the context of the Thamini Uhai project environment. Yet maintenance and the acquisition of new equipment could become a challenge as the government takes greater responsibility of the project sites. To our knowledge, adverse outcomes related to VE have not produced a setback. Each hospital and health centre where VE is practiced has had caesarean surgery as a backup. That said, based on the monitoring of birth outcomes, the project has yet to show a definitive decrease in the intrapartum stillbirth rate at all levels, unlike a recent study in a well-known university hospital in Uganda that showed a strong association between VE reintroduction and fewer intrapartum stillbirths [22]. The lack of progress on this parameter has concerned staff; efforts to improve referral, audits of newborn deaths, training in neonatal resuscitation, and careful monitoring of newborn outcomes at health centres are underway.

The observation of the uneven uptake of VE across facilities is important for scaling up VE or for others attempting to reintroduce VE into an established practice. Major differences in training were ruled out as an explanation since the trainees from different facilities were brought together and trained by the same trainers using the same methodology. Several facilities – Utete, Buhingu, Nyenge, Mabamba and Mwaya – enjoyed more favourable ratios of health workers to delivery volume than other facilities, which might have helped explain their success of mainstreaming VE. The difficulty of monitoring labour that adheres to standards is not surprising where there is a shortage of staff. What the facilities with the highest VE rates seem to have had in common were AMOs and nurse-midwives that stood out for their commitment and activity level. Where the uptake of VE was particularly slow, additional staff members were trained, hoping that would provide a solution. Yet the procedure mix has not changed, suggesting that there may be pockets of resistance to the use of VE specifically, or resistance to changing practices more generally.

The low VE practice at supported hospitals could partially be explained by high staff-turnover as there have been staff rotations at least annually, and these have been replaced with others possibly without the skills or interest. The number of staff trained in VE does not seem to be the significant factor, since during the last phase of training between two and four providers were trained at each of the supported health centres and hospitals. High turnover of staff, however, is probably not the only explanation for low VE usage or for high reliance on caesarean delivery in hospitals. We also know that hospitals attended twice the number of obstetric complications than health centres did, and a large proportion of these were referrals of women with more serious conditions and with a wider range of indications for surgery.

The relatively rapid uptake of VE by the newly renovated health centres compared with hospitals where caesarean delivery was well entrenched may not come as a surprise for those who study the phenomenon of early adoption. The personal risk of using a new skill in a recently enhanced environment where the clinical staff was trained together may be lower than in facilities with more staff, not all of whom received the same training, and where clinical practices may be harder to change. It has been noted that the project stimulated and motivated staff, giving them a greater sense of satisfaction and confidence by enabling them to provide more services in improved conditions. Providing feedback to the facilities themselves on the wide variations in VE practice and adoption, much like an audit cycle, may also lead to internal discussion and reflection.

As Thamini Uhai's support shifts towards working less on the front line to more support to government structures to ensure the sustainability of what has been achieved, continued use of VE may be tested. Local policy support will be needed to keep unnecessary medical interventions at a minimum while championing the nurse-midwives, AMOs and specialists who currently mentor and train new staff arrivals.

Strengths of this case study include the project's ability 1) to monitor facility service statistics for at least 6 years by a stable implementation support team using the same methodology, 2) to observe not just long-term changes but short-term changes in sites that were added in 2015, and 3) to compare hospitals with health centres that have undergone substantial transition to fully functioning C-EmONC centres. A limitation, as implied above, is a lack of firm understanding of why staffs at some facilities perform VE more than others. Other gaps in information included indications for VE and caesarean delivery as well as any adverse outcomes related to each procedure, all of which would enrich the policy and program debate in Tanzania and elsewhere. Although not systematically recorded, serious complications resulting from vacuum extraction would have been revealed during project expert teams' monthly and quarterly supportive supervision and mentorship visits to the facilities. Finally, like many multi-faceted programmatic interventions, without a more rigorous evaluation design, attribution of cause and effect may be driven more by plausibility than definitive proof.

The maturity of the program should facilitate initiating an opportunity to qualitatively explore whether newly trained staff lack confidence, if physical or political environments are not supportive and how training and coaching might be modified. Simply listening and learning from both the slow and the early adopters, in both hospitals and health centres will provide much needed insight to support further efforts to reintroduce VE. Continuing to document this long term, multi-site experience to show safety of VE, cost savings and improvements in outcomes, will not only help local scale up but also influence national policy and provide guidance to others.

Conclusions

Although reintroduction of vacuum extraction is feasible, it requires a supportive environment that is sensitive and follow-up to when refresher training is needed. In this Tanzanian context, it seems to have been easier to reintroduce vacuum extraction as part of an integrated upgrading of health centres to provide C-EmONC than it has been to introduce it into a busy hospital environment.

Endnotes

[1]In 2006 groundwork for the project started but it was not formally supported by Bloomberg Philanthropies or the World Lung Foundation until 2008.

[2]The 2017 edition of *Managing complications in pregnancy and childbirth: a guide for midwives and doctors* recommends that artificial rupture of membranes not be the sole intervention for labour augmentation in areas of high HIV prevalence, but the authors do not caution against vacuum-assisted delivery in these same settings.

Abbreviations

AMO: Assistant medical officer; C-EmONC: Comprehensive emergency obstetric and newborn care; CME: Continuing medical education; DHS: Demographic and Health Survey; Ob/gyn: Obstetrician/gynaecologist; OT: Operating theatre; VE: Vacuum extraction

Acknowledgements

We would like to acknowledge Ms. Samantha Lobis for her long-standing support of Thamini Uhai and her helpful review. We also acknowledge Dr. Hamed Mohamed, Clinical Director during the early years of the project, for his role in pioneering the reintroduction of vacuum extraction, his clinical training, coaching, and setting up the monthly and quarterly monitoring system.

Funding

Thamini Uhai acknowledges the generous financial support of Bloomberg Philanthropies, Fondation H & B Agerup, the Swedish International Development Cooperation Agency, Svenska Postkod Stiftelsen, and Merck for Mothers. The funders played no role in the design of the study, the collection, analysis and interpretation of the data, or writing of the manuscript.

Authors' contributions

SD and PB conceived and planned the paper; SD and PB drafted the paper; MK oversaw the data collection and along with NM and JvR, contributed to the analysis, interpretation, and critically revised the content. All authors approved the final version for publication.

Competing interests

None declared for all authors except JvR who is a section editor of BMC Pregnancy and Childbirth.

Author details

[1]Thamini Uhai, Kigoma, Tanzania. [2]Pittsboro, USA. [3]Department of Obstetrics, Leiden University Medical Center and Athena Institute, VU University, de Boelelaan 1105, 1081 HV Amsterdam, The Netherlands.

References

1. Nystedt A, Hildingsson I. Diverse definitions of prolonged labour and its consequences with sometimes subsequent inappropriate treatment. BMC Pregnancy Childbirth. 2014;14:233.
2. Bailey PE, van Roosmalen J, Mola G, Evans C, de Bernis L, Dao B. Assisted vaginal delivery in low and middle income countries: an overview. BJOG. 2017;124(9):1335–44.
3. Zhang J, Geerts C, Hukkelhoven C, Offerhaus P, Zwart J, de Jonge A. Caesarean section rates in subgroups of women and perinatal outcomes. BJOG. 2016;123(5):754–61.
4. Murphy DJ, Liebling RE, Verity L, Swingler R, Patel R. Early maternal and neonatal morbidity associated with operative delivery in second stage of labour: a cohort study. Lancet. 2001;358(9289):1203–7.
5. World Health Organization (WHO), United Nations Children's Fund (UNICEF), United Nations Population Fund (UNFPA), World Bank, United Nations Population Division. Trends in maternal mortality: 1990 to 2015. Estimates by WHO, UNICEF, UNFPA, the World Bank and the United Nations Population Division. Geneva: WHO; 2015. http://apps.who.int/iris/bitstream/handle/10665/194254/9789241565141_eng.pdf;jsessionid=466CCBE1A9101C90B599087C83800C2B?sequence=1. Accessed 5 Nov 2017.
6. Ministry of Health, Community Development, Gender, Elderly, Children - MoHCDGEC/Tanzania Mainland, Ministry of Health - MoH/Zanzibar, National Bureau of Statistics - NBS/Tanzania, Office of Chief Government Statistician - OCGS/Zanzibar, ICF: Tanzania Demographic and Health Survey and Malaria Indicator Survey 2015–2016. Dar es Salaam, Tanzania: MoHCDGEC, MoH, NBS, OCGS, and ICF; 2016.

7. WHO, UNFPA, UNICEF, AMDD. Monitoring emergency obstetric care: a handbook. Geneva: World Health Organization; 2009. p. 152.
8. Nyamtema AS, Mwakatundu N, Dominico S, Mohamed H, Pemba S, Rumanyika R, Kairuki C, Kassiga I, Shayo A, Issa O, et al. Enhancing maternal and perinatal health in under-served remote areas in sub-Saharan Africa: a Tanzanian model. PLoS One. 2016;11(3):e0151419.
9. Nyamtema A, Mwakatundu N, Dominico S, Mohamed H, Shayo A, Rumanyika R, Kairuki C, Nzabuhakwa C, Issa O, Lyimo C, et al. Increasing the availability and quality of caesarean section in Tanzania. BJOG. 2016;123(10): 1676–82.
10. Ministry of Health: Advanced Life Saving Skills - Volume 2: Modules 1-10 Trainee's Manual. Dar-es-salaam, United Republic of Tanzania: Reproductive and Child Health Section, Ministry of Health; 2005.
11. Maaloe N, Bygbjerg IC, Onesmo R, Secher NJ, Sorensen BL. Disclosing doubtful indications for emergency cesarean sections in rural hospitals in Tanzania: a retrospective criterion-based audit. Acta Obstet Gynecol Scand. 2012;91(9):1069–76.
12. Maaloe N, Sorensen BL, Onesmo R, Secher NJ, Bygbjerg IC. Prolonged labour as indication for emergency caesarean section: a quality assurance analysis by criterion-based audit at two Tanzanian rural hospitals. BJOG. 2012;119(5):605–13.
13. McCord C, Mbaruku G, Pereira C, Nzabuhakwa C, Bergstrom S. The quality of emergency obstetrical surgery by assistant medical officers in Tanzanian district hospitals. Health Aff (Millwood). 2009;28(5):w876–85.
14. Nyamtema A, Pemba S, Mbaruka G, Rutasha F, van Roosmalen J. Tanzanian lessons in training non-physician clinicians to scale up comprehensive emergency obstetric care in remote and rural areas. Hum Resour Health. 2011;9:28.
15. Gei AF. Prevention of the first cesarean delivery: the role of operative vaginal delivery. Semin Perinatol. 2012;36(5):365–73.
16. Centers for Disease Control and Prevention: Reducing Maternal Mortality in Tanzania: Pregnancy Outcomes Findings from Kigoma Region, Tanzania. Atlanta: Reproductive Health division USA Centers for disease control and Prevention; 2016.
17. Ayala-Yanez R, Bayona-Soriano P, Hernandez-Jimenez A, Contreras-Rendon A, Chabat-Manzanera P, Nevarez-Bernal R. Forceps, actual use, and potential cesarean section prevention: study in a selected Mexican population. J Pregnancy. 2015;2015:489267.
18. Chang X, Chedraui P, Ross MG, Hidalgo L, Penafiel J. Vacuum assisted delivery in Ecuador for prolonged second stage of labor: maternal-neonatal outcome. J Matern Fetal Neonatal Med. 2007;20(5):381–4.
19. van Lonkhuijzen L, Dijkman A, van Roosmalen J, Zeeman G, Scherpbier A. A systematic review of the effectiveness of training in emergency obstetric care in low-resource environments. BJOG. 2010; 117(7):777–87.
20. Fixen D, Naoom S, Blase K, Friedman R, Wallace F: Implementation Research: A Synthesis of the Literature. *FMHI Publication #231*. Edited by Network TNIR. Tampa, FL: University of South FLorida, Louis de la Parte Florida Mental Health Institute; 2005.
21. Bluestone J, Johnson P, Fullerton J, Carr C, Alderman J, BonTempo J. Effective in-service training design and delivery: evidence from an integrative literature review. Hum Resour Health. 2013;11:51.
22. Nolens B, Lule J, Namiiro F, van Roosmalen J, Byamugisha J. Audit of a program to increase the use of vacuum extraction in Mulago hospital, Uganda. BMC Pregnancy Childbirth. 2016;16:258.

8

Management of Caesarean scar pregnancy with or without methotrexate before curettage: human chorionic gonadotropin trends and patient outcomes

Sheng Wang, Rajluxmee Beejadhursing, Xiangyi Ma and Ya Li*

Abstract

Background: To evaluate the effects of systemic methotrexate in cesarean scar pregnancy (CSP) patients treated with ultrasound-guided suction curettage.

Methods: A retrospective review of all women presenting with CSP treated with ultrasound-guided suction curettage at Tongji Hospital, Wuhan, China, between January 1, 2013 and December 31, 2015, was conducted. Patients were grouped into those not treated with methotrexate before curettage (group 1), treated with methotrexate by intramuscular injection (group 2) and treated with methotrexate by intravenous injection (group 3). The clinical characteristics and outcomes were analyzed.

Results: Among 107 patients, 47 patients were not treated with methotrexate before curettage, 46 patients had methotrexate administered by intramuscular injection and 14 patients had methotrexate injected intravenously. There were no significant differences among the groups in basic and clinical characteristics, such as age, gravity, parity, positive fetal heart beat and gestational age at diagnosis. Patients presented similar initial human chorionic gonadotropin (hCG) levels in all groups. After treatment with methotrexate or curettage, the percentage changes and varied ranges of the hCG levels were also similar in all groups. There were no significant differences in intraoperative blood loss and retained products of conception among the three groups. However group 1 had significantly shorter hospital stays than the two groups that were treated with methotrexate ($p<0.001$).

Conclusion: By grouping CSP patients who shared similar age, gravity, parity, fetal heart beat positive and gestational age at diagnosis, we found that the presence or absence of methotrexate treatment before curettage resulted in comparable outcomes and hCG levels, although patients who were not treated with methotrexate had significantly shorter stays in the hospital.

Keywords: Cesarean scar pregnancy, Human chorionic gonadotropin, Methotrexate, Suction curettage, Protocol comparisons

* Correspondence: yalitjh@163.com
Department of Obstetrics and Gynecology, Tongji Hospital, Tongji Medical College, Huazhong University of Science and Technology, Wuhan 430030, People's Republic of China

Background

Cesarean scar pregnancy (CSP) is defined as the implantation of a gestational sac within the scar of a previous cesarean surgery. If CSP is maintained, there are potentially higher risks that include uterine rupture, devastating hemorrhage, loss of subsequent fertility and even maternal mortality [1]. Therefore, the standard protocol for CSP management is to terminate the pregnancy. Nevertheless, while the optimal management of CSP remains unclear, there is a variety of therapeutic strategies are currently in use, such as medical treatment with systemic MTX, medical treatment with systemic and local MTX, uterine curettage, hysteroscopy, resection of CSP through a transvaginal approach, uterine artery embolization, laparoscopy, and high-intensity focused ultrasound [2]. Some complicated case may require combined application of several methods [3].

MTX is a folic acid antagonist that inhibits the enzyme dihydrofolate reductase, thereby interfering with DNA synthesis in rapidly dividing cells such as trophoblasts. The first usage of MTX in the treatment of ectopic pregnancy was reported by Tanaka et al. in an interstitial ectopic pregnancy in 1982 [4]. Recently, MTX has also used in treatment of cervical pregnancy, which is another form of ectopic pregnancy [5]. CSP is a special type ectopic pregnancy and as such, some researchers have investigated the use of MTX in conservative management or preliminary treatment of CSP prior to curettage [6, 7]. The application of the systemic administration of MTX in CSP is controversial. Semih Z. reported that systemic MTX manifested similar results compared to local MTX in terms of treatment success and reproductive outcomes [8]. Some researchers have further suggested that systemic MTX may be less effective in cases with higher serum hCG concentrations [9]. The effects of systemic MTX before curettage and whether it is recommended before curettage are still unknown. The aim of this study was to evaluate the hCG levels and outcomes in CSP patients treated with or without MTX before curettage to assess the efficacy of MTX.

Methods

This retrospective study analysed CSP patients treated at the Tongji Hospital, Wuhan, China, between 2013 and 2015. Data were collected through archived medical records. The study was approved by the hospital's ethics committee. Due to the retrospective nature of this study, informed consent from the patients was not deemed necessary at the time of data collection. However, the authors wish to disclose that, in accordance with hospital policy, patients were clearly informed of their treatment modalities and provided signed consent prior to their intervention. A diagnosis of CSP relied on routine sonographic criteria, including 1) empty uterine cavity and cervical canal; 2) a gestational sac located anteriorly at the level corresponding to the prior lower uterine segment of the cesarean section scar; 3) evidence of functional trophoblastic/placental circulation on Doppler scans; and 4) a negative sliding organs sign, which was defined as the inability to displace the gestational sac from its position at the level of the internal os [10]. Patients who were unsuccessfully treated and then transferred to our hospital were excluded from this study.

The protocol for treating CSP in our hospital included suction evacuation, chemotherapy with MTX, hysteroscopy, laparoscopy, transabdominal approach or a combination of two or more treatment options. In this study, our aim was to only assess the effects of MTX used before curettage. In the assessment of treatment outcome, we included patients who met the following criteria: (1) they were diagnosed with CSP and (2) either underwent medical treatment with MTX by intramuscular injection, by intravenous injection or were not treated with MTX before ultrasound-guided suction curettage. MTX was administered according to the protocol originally described by Stovall et al. [11] in 1991. In brief, MTX was administered intramuscularly two times (Day 0 and Day 4) or intravenously for 5 days (Day 0 to Day 5), with the same total dose of 50 mg/m^2. Suction curettage was performed the day following MTX treatment without awaiting a decline in serum hCG levels.

The clinical characteristics of the patients, such as age, gravity, parity, and number of previous cesarean sections, were reviewed. Retained products of conception, intraoperative blood loss and duration of hospital were analyzed. The volume of blood lost during surgery was determined by measuring contents of the suction container. In all patients, any material aspirated from the uterus was collected in suction container. After operation, the container was filtered with a screen filter, and the blood was measured in a graduated volume flask. Any other significant blood loss collected on surgical swabs and drapes and was subjectively assessed by the operating surgeon. Three days after operation, a transvaginal scan was performed to verify any retained products of conception, and serum hCG was also performed. If the scans were cleared and serum hCG had markedly declined by more than half of the pre-operation value, patients were subsequently discharged. Statistical analysis was performed using the IBM SPSS version 17.0 software (SPSS Inc., Chicago, IL). Quantitative data are presented as the mean ± SD, frequency and percentage; between-group differences were assessed by Student's t-test for continuous variables and the chi-squared test for categorical variables. P-values < 0.05 were considered indicative of a statistically significant difference.

Results

During the study period, our institution received a total of 317 patients with CSP; 107 patients underwent ultrasound-guided suction curettage, of which 47 patients were

Table 1 Comparison of the basic and clinical characteristics of patients not treated with MTX (Group 1), treated with MTX by intramuscular injection (Group 2) or treated with MTX by intravenous injection (Group 3)

	Mean ± SD/Rate			*P* value
	Group 1(*n* = 47)	Group 2(*n* = 46)	Group 3(*n* = 14)	
Age (years)	32.04 ± 6.283	31.15 ± 5.597	34.14 ± 4.865	0.206
Previous cesarean section (n)	1.17 ± 0.380	1.17 ± 0.383	1.57 ± 0.514	0.004
Gravidity (n)	4.13 ± 1.24	4.20 ± 1.470	5.0 ± 1.519	0.186
Parity (n)	1.21 ± 0.414	1.22 ± 0.513	1.50 ± 0.519	0.08
Gestational age at diagnosis (days)	52.68 ± 11.66	48.76 ± 8.945	52.15 ± 13.619	0.292
Fetal heart beat positive, n (%)	15(31.9%)	21(45.7%)	5(35.7%)	0.466

not treated with MTX before curettage, 46 patients were treated with MTX intramuscularly and 14 patients were treated with MTX by intravenous injection before curettage.

The baseline characteristics of the patients in the 3 groups are described in Table 1. The incidence of previous cesarean sections was significantly different among the 3 groups (1.17 ± 0.380, 1.17 ± 0.383, and 1.57 ± 0.514, respectively; $P = 0.004$). There were no significant differences between the 3 groups with respect to age, gravity, parity, fetal heart beat positive and gestational age at diagnosis.

Patients had similar initial hCG levels before MTX administration in group 2 and group 3 (Table 2). When we examined hCG trends, we found that the mean decline of hCG after MTX treatment was not significantly different between group 2 and group 3 ($p = 0.196$). In both surveys before and 3 days after curettage, the average hCG levels of the 3 groups were similar. We further examined the range of the changes in hCG levels and observed that after MTX treatment, the varied ranges and percentage changes of hCG levels were similar in group 2 and group3, as shown in Table 2 B-A and (B-A)/A ($p = 0.219$ and $p = 0.273$, respectively). Three days after curettage, the hCG percentage changes were also similar among the 3 groups as shown in Table 2 C/B ($p = 0.674$).

The outcomes of the treatment are shown in Table 3. There were no significant differences in intraoperative blood loss and rates of retained products of conception among the 3 groups ($p = 0.066$ and $p = 0.658$, respectively). Duration of hospitalisation was significantly shorter in group 1 ($p<0.001$).

Data comparing patients who underwent MTX therapy with patients who did not is displayed in Table 4. The outcomes of the treatment are the same when we further divided the MTX group according to mode of administration; by intramuscular injection or by intravenous injection. There were no significant differences in intraoperative blood loss and rates of retained products of conception among MTX patients and patients who were not treated with MTX ($p = 0.051$ and $p = 0.437$, respectively). Duration of hospital stay was significantly shorter in the group that did not receive MTX ($p<0.001$).

Discussion

In this study, the efficacy of MTX use before curettage in managing CSP was assessed. The clinical outcomes of the three groups (groups 1 to 3) assessed in this study were similar, with intraoperative blood loss of 39.83 ± 16.96 ml, 55.33 ± 44.19 ml and 42.86 ± 22.68 ml, respectively. Assuming the lack of retained products of conception as a clinical success, we observed success rates of 97.9, 95.7 and 92.9%, respectively. We also found that using MTX before curettage, either by intramuscular or intravenous injection, could significantly prolong the hospital-stay duration of patients.

Table 2 Human chorionic gonadotropin levels (mIU/ml) in patients not treated with MTX (Group 1), treated with MTX by intramuscular injection (Group 2) or treated with MTX by intravenous injection (Group 3)

	Mean ± SD/Rate			*P* value
	Group 1(*n* = 47)	Group 2(*n* = 46)	Group 3(*n* = 14)	
A:Before MTX treatment	–	44,603.28 ± 38,615.27	25,648.86 ± 16,125.92	0.080
B:After MTX treatment or before curettage	31,163.48 ± 28,626.86	37,712.91 ± 23,880.85	31,005.21 ± 23,029.37	0.196
C:Three days after curettage	2838.68 ± 3.10	4434.98 ± 4.90	3263.46 ± 2.93	0.077
B-A	–	9664.21 ± 8993.10	22,506.29 ± 36,916.63	0.219
(B-A)/A	–	0.27 ± 0.213	1.33 ± 3.451	0.273
C/B	0.085 ± 0.04	0.084 ± 0.05	0.79 ± 0.04	0.674

Table 3 Comparison of outcomes for patients not treated with MTX (Group 1), treated with MTX by intramuscular injection (Group 2) or treated with MTX by intravenous injection (Group 3)

	Mean ± SD/Rate			*P* value
	Group 1(*n* = 47)	Group 2(*n* = 46)	Group 3(*n* = 14)	
Intraoperative blood loss (ml)	39.83 ± 16.96	55.33 ± 44.19	42.86 ± 22.68	0.066
Pregnancy tissue retained, n (%)	1(2.1%)	2(4.3%)	1(7.1%)	0.658
Hospital stay (days)	7.00 ± 2.29	9.59 ± 2.46	13.86 ± 3.88	<0.001

CSP can be classified into several subtypes based on different conditions, such as the degree of invasion of the amniotic sac, gestational age at diagnosis, positive fetal heart beat and myometrial thickness of the lower segment. The optimal management of CSP is unclear and a variety of therapeutic strategies are being used, with presently no clearly defined protocol consensus. Özkan Özdamar et al. demonstrated that in appropriate CSP cases, ultrasound-guided suction curettage appears to be a reliable treatment option. [12]. Jurkovic D. also considered suction curettage as an effective method for the treatment of CSP which was associated with a lower risk of blood transfusion and hysterectomy [13]. Nonetheless, several studies have reported that suction curettage should not be considered as an optimal first line of therapy [9, 14]. Different patients with a wide range of conditions who visit diverse doctors are definitely treated differently. The same situation occurs in our hospital. In the present study, we analyzed 107 patients with similar basic and clinical characteristics who underwent ultrasound-guided suction curettage. Before curettage, some patients were treated with MTX, either by intramuscular or intravenous injection.

Systemic and local MTX are two of the most widely used forms of management for CSP. Previous studies comparing the two treatments showed conflicting results likely due to differences in study design, supplementary treatments and various definitions of response [15, 16]. A recent review [2] showed that almost every fourth woman treated with systemic MTX required additional treatment, and severe complications occurred in 13% of them. Therefore, one may wonder whether chemotherapy using MTX is truly justified. Our present study showed similar outcomes among the three groups studied. Even though patients underoging MTX treatment, had elevated hCG levels after the initial dose, 3 days after curettage, the hCG percentage change was also the same whether patients were treated with MTX or not. In theory, MTX may take some time to cause trophoblastic cytolysis. In addition, MTX half-life is short, making it difficult for MTX to reach the sac and embryo [17]. Owing to of these setbacks, trophoblastic cells in CSP may be insensitive to MTX. Another possibility is that not enough time was given after the MTX treatment to observe a responsive effect. In consideration of these possibilities that may confound the effects of MTX, we further analyzed the outcomes of the 3 groups.

Massive hemorrhage is a major complication of CSP. In this study, the means of intraoperative blood loss were similar in all three groups. Only 1 patient in group 2 reported a blood loss of more than 300 ml and subsequently underwent a laparoscopy. None of the patients suffered from uterine rupture and devastating hemorrhage. Perhaps, our results differed from other reports, because of differences in the selection criteria used when determining which patients could be treated with suction curettage.

Table 4 Comparison basic clinical characteristics and outcomes of patient not treated by MTX or treated by MTX

	Mean ± SD/Rate		*P* value
	Not treated by MTX (*n* = 47)	treated by MTX (*n* = 60)	
Age (years)	32.04 ± 6.283	31.85 ± 5.544	0.867
Gestational age at diagnosis (days)	52.68 ± 11.664	49.37 ± 10.096	0.119
Fetal heart beat positive, n (%)	15(31.9%)	26(43.3%)	0.299
B:After MTX treatment or before curettage (mIU/ml)	31,163.48 ± 28,626.86	52,841.27 ± 41,148.83	0.003
C:Three days after curettage (mIU/ml)	2838.68 ± 3.10	4161.63 ± 4.52	0.090
C/B	0.085 ± 0.04	0.082 ± 0.05	0.856
Intraoperative blood loss (ml)	39.83 ± 16.96	52.37 ± 40.2	0.051
Pregnancy tissue retained, n (%)	1(2.1%)	3(5.0%)	0.437
Hospital stay (days)	7.00 ± 2.29	10.58 ± 3.35	<0.001

Retention of products of conception after CSP treatment is a major concern for both patients and their physicians, as it may adversely influence menstruation and any future fertility wishes. In this present study, among the 3 groups, respectively 1 (2.1%), 2 (4.3%), and 1 (7.1%) patients, reported retained products of conception and required further treatment. These findings revealed no significant differences between the 3 groups. Our hospital records have no instances where only MTX was used to treat CSP and as a result, we could not assess the outcomes of standalone MTX treatment. Hua Yang [18] reported that conservative MTX treatment achieved satisfactory therapeutic effects, similar to uterine artery embolization (UAE) group, but the recovery time was significantly longer than that of the curettage group. In our study, the duration of hospitalization was also significantly longer in the MTX groups. Therefore, based on our results, MTX administration before curettage has no obvious remedial effects in patients managed with ultrasound-guided suction curettage and has an additional side effect of prolonging hospital-stay.

This studying is primarily limited by its retrospective nature. However, it would have been ethically inappropriate to compare our results with a control group because some of these procedures would need to be thouroughly explained before approval of patients which would induce various sorts of bias and interference originating from the authors, hospital personnel or patients. Another limitation we wish to disclose is that subsequent fertility outcomes of the different treatment groups was unfeasible in the present setting and hence not investigated.

Conclusions

In conclusion, all the CSP patients treated with ultrasound-guided suction curettage reported satisfactory results. Besides, the use of MTX before curettage had no significant effects on intraoperative blood loss or retention of pregnancy tissue. Concurrently, the duration of hospital stay of patients treated with MTX was significantly prolonged.

Abbreviations

CSP: Cesarean scar pregnancy; hCG: human chorionic gonadotropin; MTX: methotrexate; UAE: uterine artery embolization

Authors' contributions

YL conducted the experimental design. SW collected the data. XYM and SW analyzed the data and discussed the results. SW wrote the paper. RB and YL revised the manuscript. All authors have read and approved the final manuscript.

Competing interests

The authors declare that they have no competing interests.

References

1. Rotas MA, Haberman S, Levgur M. Cesarean scar ectopic pregnancies: etiology, diagnosis, and management. Obstet Gynecol. 2006;107(6): 1373–81.
2. Birch PK, Hoffmann E, Rifbjerg LC, Svarre NH. Cesarean scar pregnancy: a systematic review of treatment studies. Fertil Steril. 2016;105(4):958–67.
3. Giampaolino P, Della Corte L, Venetucci P, D'Antuono F, Morra I, Nappi C, et al. Treatment of asymptomatic uterine rupture of caesarean scar pregnancy in patient with advanced gestational age: case report. J Obstet Gynaecol. 2017:1–2.
4. Tanaka T, Hayashi H, Kutsuzawa T, Fujimoto S, Ichinoe K. Treatment of interstitial ectopic pregnancy with MTX: report of a successful case. Fertil Steril. 1982;37(6):851–2.
5. Di Spiezio Sardo A, Vieira MDC, Laganà AS, Chiofalo B, Vitale SG, Scala M, et al. Combined systemic and Hysteroscopic intra-amniotic injection of methotrexate associated with Hysteroscopic resection for cervical pregnancy: a cutting-edge approach for an uncommon condition. Eurasian J Med. 2017;49(1):66–8.
6. Haimov-Kochman R, Sciaky-Tamir Y, Yanai N, Yagel S. Conservative management of two ectopic pregnancies implanted in previous uterine scars. Ultrasound Obstet Gynecol. 2002;19(6):616–9.
7. Litwicka K, Greco E. Caesarean scar pregnancy: a review of management options. Curr Opin Obstet Gynecol. 2011;23(6):415–21.
8. Uludag SZ, Kutuk MS, Ak M, Ozgun MT, Dolanbay M, Aygen EM, et al. Comparison of systemic and local MTX treatments in cesarean scar pregnancies: time to change conventional treatment and follow-up protocols. Eur J Obstet Gynecol Reprod Biol. 2016;206:131–5.
9. Seow KM, Huang LW, Lin YH, Lin MY, Tsai YL, Hwang JL. Cesarean scar pregnancy: issues in management. Ultrasound Obstet Gynecol. 2004;23(3): 247–53.
10. Jurkovic D, Hillaby K, Woelfer B, Lawrence A, Salim R, Elson CJ. First-trimester diagnosis and management of pregnancies implanted into the lower uterine segment cesarean section scar. Ultrasound Obstet Gynecol. 2003; 21(3):220–7.
11. Stovall TG, Ling FW, Gray LA. Single-dose MTX for treatment of ectopic pregnancy. Obstet Gynecol. 1991;77(5):754–7.
12. Özdamar Ö, Doğer E, Arlıer S, Çakıroğlu Y, Ergin RN, Köpük ŞY, et al. Exogenous cesarean scar pregnancies managed by suction curettage alone or in combination with other therapeutic procedures: a series of 33 cases and analysis of complication profile. J Obstet Gynaecol Res. 2016; 42(8):927–35.
13. Jurkovic D, Knez J, Appiah A, Farahani L, Mavrelos D, Ross JA. Surgical treatment of cesarean scar ectopic pregnancy: efficacy and safety of ultrasound-guided suction curettage. Ultrasound Obstet Gynecol. 2016;47(4): 511–7.
14. Ayoubi JM, Fanchin R, Meddoun M, Fernandez H, Pons JC. Conservative treatment of complicated cesarean scar pregnancy. Acta Obstet Gynecol Scand. 2001;80(5):469–70.
15. Peng P, Gui T, Liu X, Chen W, Liu Z. Comparative efficacy and safety of local and systemic MTX injection in cesarean scar pregnancy. Ther Clin Risk Manag. 2015;11:137–42.
16. Cok T, Kalayci H, Ozdemir H, Haydardedeoglu B, Parlakgumus AH, Tarim E. Transvaginal ultrasound-guided local MTX administration as the first-line treatment for cesarean scar pregnancy: follow-up of 18 cases. J Obstet Gynaecol Res. 2015;41(5):803–8.
17. Kutuk MS, Uysal G, Dolanbay M, Ozgun MT. Successful medical treatment of cesarean scar ectopic pregnancies with systemic multidose MTX: single-center experience. J Obstet Gynaecol Res. 2014;40(6):1700–6.
18. Yang H, Li S, Ma Z, Jia Y. Therapeutic effects of uterine artery embolisation (UAE) and MTX (MTX) conservative therapy used in treatment of cesarean scar pregnancy. Arch Gynecol Obstet. 2016;293(4):819–23.

9

Is anemia an independent risk factor for postpartum depression in women who have a cesarean section?

Nirmala Chandrasekaran[1*], Leanne R De Souza[1], Marcelo L Urquia[2], Beverley Young[3], Anne Mcleod[4], Rory Windrim[5] and Howard Berger[1]

Abstract

Background: The symptoms of anemia and depression are very similar suggesting that there may be an association between the two entities. The aim of this study is to assess whether postpartum anemia (PPA) is an independent risk factor for de novo postpartum depression (PPD)in women undergoing elective cesarean section.

Methods: Women after an uncomplicated term cesarean section were recruited and their hemoglobin and iron status were measured on day 3–5 post section and again at 6 weeks. Postpartum depression was screened using the Edinburgh Postnatal Depression Scale (EPDS) and functional capacity was assessed with the RAND 12-item Health survey.

Results: One hundred and three women completed the study. The incidence of probable postpartum depression (PPD) as defined by EPDS score ≥ 10 was 17% at 6 weeks. There was no difference in hemoglobin or iron status in women who had PPD compared to those without (OR-0.69; 95% CI-0.15-2.49). Similarly, there was no significant association between low hemoglobin and maternal functional status (OR -1.03; 95% CI-0.34 - 2.94).

Conclusions: Neither anemia or low iron stores were found to be an independent risk factors for postpartum depression or decreased postpartum functional capacity in women who undergo an elective cesarean section.

Keywords: Anemia, Iron stores, Cesarean section, Postpartum depression, Functional status

Background

Postpartum anemia (PPA) is a serious health condition affecting approximately 27% of North American women during the early postpartum period (puerperium). Among women with PPA, an estimated 50% are also iron deficient, wherein iron stores are depleted while hemoglobin could be normal or low [1–3]. Maternal consequences of anemia are well known and include cardiovascular symptoms like palpitations and dizziness, fatigue, reduced physical and mental performance, reduced immune function, reduced peripartum blood reserves and increased risk of blood transfusion [4].

Postpartum depression (PPD) is one of the most common conditions in the postnatal period affecting between 10 and 15% of women [5]. The causes of postpartum depression remain unclear and risk factors include a family or personal history of depression before pregnancy, low income, poor social support, poor interfamilial relationships, low self-esteem, parental stress, unwanted or unplanned pregnancy and recent stressful life events in a woman's life [6, 7]. Up to 50% of women with PPD will go on to develop PPD in subsequent pregnancies, and their offspring are at increased risk of impaired psychological and intellectual development [8, 9]. The classic symptoms associated with PPD are depressed mood, anxiety, anhedonia, appetite and sleep disturbances, physical agitation, fatigue, feelings of worthlessness and

* Correspondence: chandrasekan@smh.ca
[1]Department of Maternal and Fetal Medicine, St Michaels Hospital, 30 Bond street, Toronto, ON M5B 1W8, Canada
Full list of author information is available at the end of the article

excessive guilt, decreased concentration and recurrent thoughts of death or suicidal ideation [10].

Symptoms of PPD are common to those found in women with PPA. Whether a causal pathway relates PPD and PPA, is unknown, however identifying a physiological link between these two conditions may help identify women at increased risk of PPD. Such an association has been suggested in the literature but there are few studies that specifically address the association between postpartum anemia and postpartum depression [11–13]. Furthermore the association between PPA and maternal functional status, defined by an individual's ability to perform normal daily activities required to meet basic needs, fulfill usual roles, and maintain health and well-being has not been previously studied in the context of developing PPD.

Moreover, some studies show that women who undergo cesarean delivery could potentially be at increased risk of developing PPD possibly due to perceived pain and immobility of recovery, stress response to surgery and perceived failure to undergo vaginal birth as potential reasons for the association. A meta-analysis of the effects of cesarean delivery on the risk of PPD concluded that although the risk of PPD was higher with both elective and emergency Cesarean sections compared to vaginal delivery, no statistically significant association was identified for elective section and PPD [14].

We aimed to determine whether anemia and iron deficiency, or the combination of these, are independent risk factors for newly diagnosed postpartum depression and decreased functional capacity in women who deliver by elective cesarean section.

Methods

The study was approved by the Research and Ethics board (REB) of St Michaels Hospital (REB #08–155). Informed written consent was obtained from all the women that agreed to participate in the study.

All women 18 years of age or older, with a full term, singleton pregnancy (37–41 weeks' gestation), undergoing elective Caesarean section were eligible to enroll in the study. Emergency Caesarean sections were excluded to avoid potential obstetric confounders associated with adverse labor and delivery experiences. Women were excluded from the study if they had symptomatic anemia necessitating blood transfusion, significant fetal anomalies, preexisting severe chronic maternal illness (e.g. cardiac disease with functional class >II, chronic renal failure), preexisting maternal depression or other psychiatric illness, preexisting hemoglobinopathy (e.g. thalassemia, sickle cell disease) or confounding social factors (e.g. single parent or no fixed address).

The primary outcome for our study was the incidence of probable postpartum depression determined by the Edinburgh postpartum depression scale (EPDS). The secondary outcomes were the association of PPD with measures of iron stores, measured by hemoglobin and soluble transferrin receptor and functional status measured by the RAND test.

Eligible women were approached within 24 h of delivery and followed prospectively for 6 weeks. Baseline demographic (age, ethnicity, gestational age) and clinical data (use of prenatal vitamins or iron supplements and any medical comorbidities) were collected, followed by venous blood collection for hemoglobin (gm/dl), ferritin (ng/ml) and soluble transferrin receptor (mg/L) levels. The intention to breastfeed was documented. Anemia was defined as hemoglobin < 110 g/l as described by the World Health Organization (WHO, 2007) [15]. A venous blood draw was repeated at 3 weeks postpartum to assess hemoglobin and ferritin levels. Women identified with anemia were prescribed iron supplements, with compliance monitored using a pill counter. At 6 weeks postpartum, a thyroid function test was administered to exclude postpartum thyroiditis as a potential confounder.

Functional status was assessed by administering the RAND 36-item health survey (SF-36). The RAND is a validated questionnaire that evaluates 8 health concept sub scales that include physical functioning, bodily pain, role limitations due to physical health problems, role limitations due to personal or emotional problems, emotional well-being, social functioning, energy/fatigue, and general health perceptions that may affect quality of life [16, 17]. From these 8 individual subscales, 2 overall scores were generated: physical health component (PCS) and mental health component (MCS). The scoring for the 8 domains and the 2 overall components are based on a 0–100 General Health Rating index scale, with a higher value corresponding to a higher quality of life [16].

The EPDS was administered at enrollment, 24 h after elective Cesarean section and again at 3 and 6 weeks postpartum. A score of ≥10 on the EPDS was considered positive for postpartum depression, as this has previously been shown to be highly sensitive for the detection of minor depression. Despite its intended use as a screening tool, the EPDS is widely accepted as a validated method to detect postpartum depression and the cut off threshold score of 10, readily identifies all cases of major depression with a negative predictive value of 99.7% [18–21]. Patients with a score ≥ 10 in the EPDS or > 2 in question 10 (thoughts of self-harm), were referred to a staff psychiatrist for the administration of the gold standard diagnostic tool - the Structured Clinical Interview for DSM-III-R (SCID, nonpoint version) and treatment if deemed necessary.

A lactation consultant contacted each woman at 2, 4 and 6 weeks postpartum to inquire about the frequency of breastfeeding or bottle-feeding and supplementation with formula among women who were breastfeeding. Women who reported rare supplementation with formula were coded as predominantly breastfeeding. Among those who reported exclusive bottle feeding, the number of weeks of any breastfeeding was recorded.

Statistical analysis

Previous studies indicate approximately 13% of women are diagnosed with major or minor PPD [5]. Using a 13% incidence of PPD among non-anemic patients, a sample size of 100 women would detect a 2.8-fold increase in PPD (37%) or higher in the defined anemic group (hemoglobin < 110), with a statistical power of 80% and alpha 0.05. This magnitude of increased risk is similar to the risk observed for other accepted risk factors for PPD [e.g. History of psychiatric disease OR 3.1 (2.3–4.2; Social isolation OR 3.6 (1.9–7.0)] [22] and would thus be a clinically significant effect size. This sample size also offers 80% power to detect a 50% increase in mean EPDS score.

Fisher's exact test was used to test the association between categorical variables and PPD and a T-test assessed continuous variables. We also used exact logistic regression to obtain odds ratios with 95% confidence intervals. Linear regression was used for the comparison of means between groups.

Given the lower than expected incidence of anemia in the study cohort, data were stratified according to the lowest quartiles to enable a comprehensive description of the effects of hemoglobin and iron status on functional capacity and postpartum depression. In multivariable analyses, we controlled for maternal age at delivery, parity, prenatal intake of vitamins and continuation of breastfeeding, each collected at 6 weeks postpartum. Data was analyzed with SAS 9.4 (SAS Institute Inc., Cary, NC).

Results

A total of 248 women were recruited for the study, with 145 lost to follow-up (Fig. 1). The excluded women were not demographically different from the study group (data not shown). Demographic characteristics of the 103 women are as listed in Table 1. There were no statistical differences in the baseline characteristics of women who screened positive for PPD and those who did not have any indication of PPD (Table 1).

The incidence of probable postpartum depression in our study population was 17% at 6 weeks postpartum. There were 14 women (13%) who were anemic prior to the Cesarean section. There were no cases of anemia identified at the 6-week follow-up visit. Patients who scored > 10 on EPDS and > 2 on question 10 (self-harm) were referred to a psychiatrist. Not all patients accepted the referral. The 3 patients who accepted the referral had the diagnosis confirmed and were commenced on SSRIs.

Anemia indices and PPD

The incidence of postpartum depression was not different in anemic vs. non-anemic mothers (Table 2).

There was no statistical difference in hemoglobin, ferritin and soluble transferrin receptor levels between women who had a positive screen for PPD and those who did not have PPD according to EPDS scores.

To assess a possible effect of acute blood loss on PPD, we calculated the change in pre-operative hemoglobin values to those at 6 weeks' post-partum (ΔHb). There was no significant association between ΔHb and the presence of PPD (Table 2). There were also no significant differences in the thyroid stimulating hormone levels between the women with and without a positive screen for post-partum depression.

Functional capacity as assessed by the RAND score did not significantly differ between the two groups (Table 2) and, scores on the RAND showed no relation to the scores on the EPDS.

Anemia indices and postpartum functional capacity

There is no established cut off threshold values for RAND scores. Therefore, we compared the lowest RAND score quartile to the upper three quartiles. As indicated in Table 3, there was no correlation between either the hemoglobin or the iron store indices with measures of functional status.

Exact binary logistic regression analysis showed that neither anemia nor iron status independent predictor of postpartum depression or post-partum functional status (Table 2).

Discussion

We found that neither anemia nor iron stores measured postpartum are associated with postpartum depression or functional status postpartum.

The biological association between PPD and PPA could be attributed to iron deficiency rather than decreased hemoglobin levels. Iron is critical for adequate myelination, neurotransmitter metabolism and function, and neuronal cellular and oxidative processes and through these processes, may contribute to the development of clinical depression [23]. The association between anemia and poor functional status is well established in the non-pregnant population and has been attributed to poor muscle oxygenation and reduced exercise tolerance. To date, there have been no studies that evaluated this association in the pregnant population.

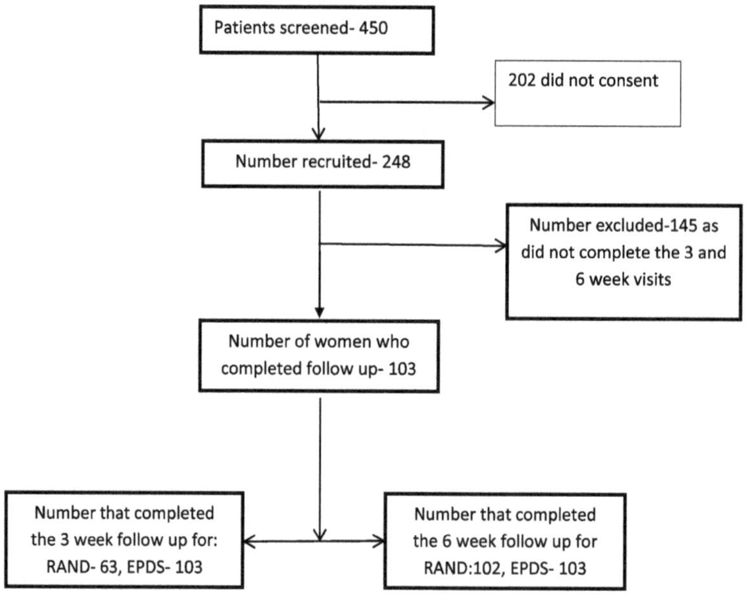

Fig. 1 Flow chart of the recruitment process

While iron deficiency and anemia have been related to poor cognition, depression and reduced functional capacity in the non-pregnant population, there have been conflicting results in studies examining pregnant populations. In one study [11], the authors used the Center for Epidemiological Studies-Depressive Symptomatology Scale (CES-D) to screen for symptoms of depression on day 28 postpartum and reported that hemoglobin concentration on day 7 to be negatively correlated with self-reported depressive symptoms on day 28, however this study had a relatively small sample size and did not measure iron status or thyroid function. In contrast, other research reported no correlation between low hemoglobin levels and high Edinburgh test for post-partum depression (EPDS) scale [12]. Possible cohort effects may impede extrapolation of study findings as those with low hemoglobin were also more likely to have had an abnormal delivery and a consequent propensity for

Table 1 Characteristics of the study population

Maternal characteristics	EPDS ≥10 at any visit (PPD = yes)	EPDS < 10 at any visit (PPD = no)	*p*-value**
N (%)	18(17.5%)	85 (82.5%)	
Age: mean (SD)	34.1 (4.1)	34.9 (4.3)	0.46
Nulliparous (%)	2/18 (11%)	31/85 (36%)	0.17
Number of previous livebirths or stillbirths: mean (SD)	0.7 (0.8)	0.9 (0.8)	0.36
Gestation weeks at delivery: mean (SD)	38.9 (0.6)	38.8 (0.9)	0.72
Less than 13 years of education, N (%)	3 (16.7)	4 (4.7)	0.11
Ethnicity (non-White) *$N = 102$	10 (55.6)	36 (42.9)	0.44
Pregnancy complications (GDM, PIH, IUGR and Preeclampsia)	6 (33.3)	23 (27.1)	0.58
Smoking during pregnancy *$N = 102$	0 (0.00)	1 (1.19)	1.00
alcohol use during pregnancy *$N = 102$	5 (27.8)	9 (10.7)	0.07
Illegal Drug use during pregnancy*$N = 102$	0 (0.00)	1 (1.19)	1.00
Birth weight: N, mean (SD)	3334 (401)	3370 (470)	0.76
BMI: N; mean (SD)	25.9 (6.9)	25.6 (5.5)	0.84
Prenatal Vitamins (%)	12 (66.7)	60 (70.6)	0.78
Breastfeeding (%)	15 (83.3)	76 (89.4)	0.44

*Indicates total N, excluding missing/unknown values for row characteristics (1 subject in the PPD = yes group)
**Fisher's test for proportions, 2-sided

Table 2 Associations between anemia indicators, functional status and postpartum depression

Maternal characteristics	N	EPDS > = 10 at any visit (PPD = yes N = 18)	EPDS < 10 at any visit (PPD = no N = 85)	Odds Ratio[a] (q1 vs. rest) or mean differences (95% CI)	Adjusted Odds Ratio[b] (q1 vs. rest) or mean differences (95% CI)
Anemia indicators					
HGB quartile 1 at pre-c/section), N (%)	103	3 (16.67)	27 (31.76)	0.43[a] (0.07 to 1.72)	0.44[b] (0.08 to 1.74)
HGB quartile 1 at visit 1 N (%)	101	3 (16.67)	24 (28.92)	0. 50[a] (0.08 to 1.98)	0.53[b] (0.09 to 2.12)
Mean HGB at pre-c/ section (SD)	103	124.0 (9.9)	119.2 (9.2)	4.8 (−0.4 to 10.0)	4.6 (−0.2 to 9.5)
Mean HGB at visit 1 (SD)	101	109.4 (9.6)	105.2 (9.7)	4.2 (−0.4 to 10.0)	3.8 (−1.3 to 8.8)
HGB quartile 1 at visit 3, N (%)	103	4 (22.22)	25 (29.41)	0.69[a] (0.15 to 2.49)	0.73[b] (0.15 to 2.82)
Mean HGB at visit 3 (SD)	103	133.4 (8.1)	129.0 (8.1)	4.4 (0.2 to 8.5)*	4.2 (0.1 to 8.2)*
Delta Hgb_visit 1 - Hgb_presection (note 1)	101	– 13.9 (9.0)	−14.0 (8.3)	−0.1 (– 6.7 to 6.5)	– 1.1 (– 6.9 to 4.7)
Delta Hgb_visit 3 - Hgb_presection (note 2)	103	8.1 (9.8)	10.0 (8.9)	1.9 (−3.6 to 7.4)	−1.0 (– 7.2 to 5.3)
Delta Hgb_visit 3-Hgb visit 1 (note 2)	101	22.7 (11.09)	24.1 (9.2)	1.4 (−4.4 to 7.2)	– 0.2 (– 6.8 to 6.3)
Ferritin quartile 1 at visit 1, N (%)	103	6 (33.33)	20 (23.53)	1.62[a] (0.44 to 5.42)	1.80[b] (0.46 to 6.60)
Mean ferritin at visit 1 (SD)	103	48.8 (27.7)	46.7 (25.4)	2.12 (−11.2 to 15.4)	0.9 (– 12.7 to 14.4)
Ferritin quartile 1 at visit 3, N (%)	103	3 (16.67)	23 (27.06)	0.54[a] (0.09 to 2.18)	0.52[b] (0.09 to 2.20)
Mean ferritin at visit 3 (SD)	103	54.9 (41.0)	42.7 (29.6)	12.3 (−4.1 to 28.7)	13.1 (−3.5 to 29.7)
Soluble transferrin receptor quartile 1 at visit 1, n (%)	103	3 (16.67)	24 (28.24)	0.51[a] (0.09 to 2.05)	0.46[b] (0.08 to 1.87)
Mean Soluble transferrin receptor at visit 1 (SD)	103	1.21 (0.33)	1.14 (0.43)	0.1 (−0.1 to 0.3)	0.1 (– 0.1 to 0.3)
Rand, quartile 1 at visit 3, n (%)	102	8 (44.44)	19 (22.35)	2.75[a] (0.82 to 9.04)	3.24[b] (0.92 to 11.70)
Exclusive Breastfeeding at visit 3, n (%)	103	10 (55.56)	59 (69.41)	0.55 (0.17 to 1.82)	0.39*
Rand mean score at visit 3 (SD)	102	83.7449 15.1247	89.1667 13.1908	−5.4 (−12.4 to 1.6)	−5.8 (−12.7 to 1.1)

*P-value < 0.05; [a]Unadjusted Odds ratio; [b]Odds ratio adjusted for age, parity, prenatal vitamins, breastfeeding at week 6

PPD regardless of degree of anemia. A randomized control trial demonstrated an improvement in emotional and cognitive measures at 9 months postpartum in iron treated anemic women but not in placebo controls [13]. A study examining risk factors for postpartum psychosis demonstrated anemia in 51.4% of cases with postpartum psychosis. However, there is no information about the incidence of anemia in a control group of women without postpartum psychosis. These results are most likely not applicable to the postpartum population in developed countries and cannot be extrapolated to patients with PPD.

Another study illustrates no relation between maternal iron stores and postpartum depression [24]. The incidence of postpartum depression in this population was significantly higher (> 20%) and again the authors did not control for hemoglobin. Some authors have suggested that anemia, but not iron deficiency is associated with a higher incidence of postnatal depression [25]. But this study was limited by a small sample size. Also, the incidence of PPD was significantly lower (5.5%) compared to what is quoted in the literature. A similar finding was reported in a recent study from Saudi Arabia by Alharbi et al. [26].They found that anemia but not iron deficiency is a significant risk factor for postpartum depression, but this study had a higher than normal incidence of PPD (33%) and the investigators did not control for confounders like traumatic delivery or history of preexisting depression.

In a recent nested cohort study, the authors demonstrate a positive association between anemia at

Table 3 Associations between anemia indicators and postpartum functional status

Maternal characteristics	N	RAND Quartile 1 at visit 3 (n = 27)	RAND Quartiles 2, 3 and 4 at visit 3 (N = 76)	Odds Ratio[a] (q1 vs. rest) or mean differences (95% CI)	Adjusted Odds Ratio[b] (q1 vs. rest) or mean differences (95% CI)
Anemia indicators					
HGB quartile 1 at pre-csection, N (%)	103	8 (29.63)	22 (28.95)	1.03[a] (0.34 to 2.94)	1.13[b] (0.37 to 3.28)
Mean HGB (pre-csection) (SD)	103	120.3 (11.16)	119.9 (8.84)	0.4 (−4.6 to 3.9)	0.1 (−4.2 to 4.4)
HGB quartile 1 at visit 1, N (%)	101	7 (25.93)	20 (27.03)	0.95[a] (0.29 to 2.80)	1.01[b] (0.30 to 3.12)
Mean HGB at visit 1 (SD)	101	105.9 (8.88)	105.9 (10.16)	0.01 (−4.4 to 4.4)	0.04 (−4.6 to 4.5)
HGB quartile 1 at visit 3, N (%)	103	10 (37.04)	19 (25.00)	1.75[a] (0.61 to 4.92)	2.44[b] (0.76 to 8.00)
Mean HGB at visit 3 (SD)	103	129.2 (9.20)	130.0 (7.89)	−0.8 (−2.9 to 4.5)	−1.8 (−5.4 to 1.7)
Delta Hgb_visit 1 - Hgb_presection (note 1)	101	−14.4 (7.9)	−13.9 (8.6)	−0.5 (−4.3 to 3.2)	− 0.3 (− 4.2 to 3.5)
Delta Hgb_visit 3 - Hgb_presection (note 2)	103	8.9 (11.2)	10.1 (8.1)	−1.2 (−5.2 to 2.8)	− 1.9 (−6.0 to 2.2)
Delta Hgb_visit 3-Hgb visit 1 (note 2)	101	23.3 (7.9)	24.2 (10.0)	−0.9 (−5.2 to 3.3)	−1.9 (− 6.2 to 2.4)
Ferritin quartile 1 at visit 1, N (%)	103	5 (18.52)	21 (27.63)	0.60[a] (0.16 to 1.91)	0.77[b] (0.19 to 2.70)
Mean ferritin at visit 1 (SD)	103	50.4 (26.1)	45.9 (25.7)	4.5 (−6.9 to 16.0)	5.0 (−6.9 to 16.8)
Ferritin quartile 1 at visit 3, N (%)	103	5 (18.52)	21 (27.63)	0.60[a] (0.16 to 1.91)	0.71[b] (0.18 to 2.39)
Mean ferritin at visit 3 (SD)	103	50.5 (35.2)	42.8 (30.8)	7.7 (−6.5 to 21.9)	5.5 (−9.2 to 20.2)
Soluble transferrin receptor quartile 1 at visit 1, n (%)	103	8 (29.63)	19 (25.00)	1.26[a] (0.41 to 3.65)	1.26[b] (0.41 to 3.65)
Mean Soluble transferrin receptor at visit 1 (SD)	103	1.1 (0.3)	1.2 (0.5)	−0.1 (−0.3 to 0.1)	−0.1 (−0.2 to 0.1)

[a]Unadjusted Odds ratio; [b]Odds ratio adjusted for age, parity, prenatal vitamins, breastfeeding at week 6

discharge from the maternity ward and the development of PPD symptoms, even after controlling for plausible confounders such as previous psychological contact, experience of delivery, mood during pregnancy and no exclusive breastfeeding at 6 weeks postpartum (OR = 2.29, 95%CI = 1.15–4.58) [27].

Anemia has been shown to be a possible risk factor for reduced functional status and is well studied in cardiac, elderly and cancer patients but there are no studies addressing this issue in pregnant patients.

The strengths of this study include the use of a prospective study design, limiting the cohort to women who had an elective Caesarean section which eliminated potential obstetric confounders that have known associations with postpartum depression. The exclusion of women with preexisting depression was a strength as this is a known risk factor and permitted the determination of de novo postpartum depression in a cohort of low risk women. We also controlled for the continuation of breast feeding as there is evidence that there is reduced risk of PPD in women who continue to breast feed [28]. In addition, we controlled for thyroid function - a well-known confounder for postpartum depression. The use of soluble transferrin receptor levels allowed us to more accurately define true iron deficiency. This is first study to our knowledge that explored the effects of anemia and iron status on functional scores in Obstetric population.

Our limitations include a potential selection bias as only 103 out of the 248 women recruited completed the planned follow up. The incidence of anemia and iron deficiency in our population was lower than expected, thereby limiting the variability in the exposure and an ability to detect significant effects, if they exist. We attempted to overcome this by analyzing hemoglobin using the lowest quartile values. There is the possibility of an association between maternal anemia (or iron deficiency) and the risk of developing PPD, but this association will manifest only at certain threshold values. Given that all anemic women post Cesarean section were treated with iron supplements, there were no anemic patients at the 6 weeks visit when the second EPDS was administered. The results reported herein are applicable only to women undergoing elective Cesarean sections and it is possible that there would be different results in women having CS in labour or vaginal delivery which need to be explored further. Finally, there is also a possibility that the women who did not complete the 3 and 6 weeks follow up might have been affected by postpartum depression that the study did not capture.

Conclusion

We did not find any evidence of an association between postpartum anemia and postpartum depression, despite this association occurring in the non-pregnant population. Further research is needed to ascertain why iron status relates to these symptoms in some contexts but not in others.

Abbreviations

EPDS: Edinburgh Postnatal Depression Scale; PPA: Postpartum anemia; PPD: Postpartum depression

Acknowledgements

We thank all the women that agreed to participate in the study.

Funding

This study was funded by Canadian Foundation for Women's Health (The Garfied Weston award grant received by Dr. Berger).

Authors' contributions

NC was involved in data collection and writing the manuscript, LD was involved in recruitment and revising the manuscript critically, MU was involved in statistical support. Authors BY, AM, RW were involved in conceiving the idea and initiation of the proposal. Author HB was the principle investigator of the study that was involved in conception, design and approval of the final manuscript. All authors participated in the editing of manuscript and have given their final approval for publication.

Consent for publication

N/A

Competing interests

HB is a member of the editorial board (section editor) of the journal.

Author details

[1]Department of Maternal and Fetal Medicine, St Michaels Hospital, 30 Bond street, Toronto, ON M5B 1W8, Canada. [2]Li Ka Shing Knowledge Institute, St Michael's Hospital, Toronto, Canada. [3]Perinatal Mental Health Program, Mount Sinai Hospital, Toronto, Canada. [4]Sunnybrook Health Sciences, Toronto, Canada. [5]Mt Sinai Hospital, Toronto, Canada.

References

1. Recommendations to prevent and control iron deficiency in the United States. Centers for Disease Control and Prevention. MMWR Recomm Rep. 1998;47(RR-3):1–29.
2. Bodnar LM, Siega-Riz AM, Miller WC, et al. Who should be screened for postpartum anemia? An evaluation of current recommendations. Am J Epidemiol. 2002;156(10):903–12.
3. Bodnar LM, Scanlon KS, Freedman DS, et al. High prevalence of postpartum anemia among low-income women in the United States. Am J Obstet Gynecol. 2001;185(2):438–43.
4. Breymann C. Iron deficiency and anaemia in pregnancy: modern aspects of diagnosis and therapy. Blood Cells Mol Dis. 2002;29(3):506–16.
5. O'Hara MW, Swain AM. Rates and risk of postpartum depression - a meta-analysis. International Review of Psychiatry. 1996;8(1):37–54.
6. Evagorou O, et al. Cross cultural approach of postpartum depression: manifestation, practices applied, risk factors and therapeutic interventions. Psychiatr Q. 2016;87:129–54.
7. Nielsen FD, Videbech P, Hedegaard M, et al. Postpartum depression: identification of women at risk. BJOG. 2000;107(10):1210–7.
8. Caplan HL, Cogill SR, Alexandra H, et al. Maternal depression and the emotional development of the child. Br J Psychiatry. 1989 Jun;154:818–22.
9. Cogill SR, Caplan HL, Alexandra H, et al. Impact of maternal postnatal depression on cognitive development of young children. Br Med J (Clin Res Ed). 1986;292(6529):1165–7.
10. The diagnostic and statistical manual of mental disorders, 4th ed.:DSM-IV. 4th ed. Washington, D.C.: American Psychiatric Association, 1994.
11. Corwin EJ, Murray-Kolb LE, Beard JL. Low hemoglobin level is a risk factor for postpartum depression. J Nutr. 2003;133(12):4139–42.
12. Paterson JA, Davis J, Gregory M, et al. A study on the effects of low haemoglobin on postnatal women. Midwifery. 1994;10(2):77–86.
13. Beard JL, Hendricks MK, Perez EM, et al. Maternal iron deficiency anemia affects postpartum emotions and cognition. J Nutr. 2005;135(2):267–72.
14. Hui X, Ding Y, Ma Y, Xin X, Zhang D. Cesarean section and risk of postpartum depression: a meta-analysis. J Psychosom Res. 2017;97:118–26 https://doi.org/10.1016/j.jpsychores.2017.04.016.
15. Candio F, Hofmeyr GJ. Treatments for iron deficiency anemia in pregnancy. RHL commentary. The WHO reproductive health library. Geneva: WHO; 2007.
16. Ware JE Jr, Gandek B. Overview of the SF-36 health survey and the international quality of life assessment (IQOLA) project. J Clin Epidemiol. 1998;51(11):903–12.
17. Stewart AL, Hays RD, Ware JE Jr. The MOS short-form general health survey. Reliability and validity in a patient population. Med Care. 1988;26(7):724–35.
18. Navarro, P., Ascaso, C., Garcia-Esteve, et al 2007. Postnatal psychiatric morbidity: a validation study of the GHQ-12 and the EPDS as screening tools. Gen. Hosp. Psychiatry 29, 1–7.
19. Boyd RC, Le HN, Somberg R. Review of screening instruments for postpartum depression. [review] [92 refs]. Archives of Women's. Mental Health. 2005;8(3):141–53.
20. Cox JL, Holden JM, Sagovsky R. Detection of postnatal depression. Development of the 10-item Edinburgh postnatal depression scale. Br J Psychiatry. 1987;150:782–6.
21. Harris B, Huckle P, Thomas R, et al. The use of rating scales to identify post-natal depression. Br J Psychiatry. 1989;154:813–7.
22. Murray L, Carothers AD. The validation of the Edinburgh post-natal depression scale on a community sample. Br J Psychiatry. 1990;157:288–90.
23. Beard JL, Connor JR. Iron status and neural functioning. Annu Rev Nutr. 2003;23:41–58.
24. Armony-Sivan R, Shao J, Li M, et al. No relationship between maternal Iron status and postpartum depression in two samples in China. J Pregnancy. 2012;2012:521431.
25. Goshtasebi A, Alizadeh M, Gandevani SB. Association between maternal anaemia and postpartum depression in an urban sample of pregnant women in Iran. J Health Popul Nutr. 2013;31(3):398–402.
26. Alharbi AA, Abdulghani H. Risk factors associated with postpartum depression in the Saudi population. Neuropsychiatr Dis Treat. 2014;10:311–31.
27. Eckerdal P, Kollia N, Löfblad J, et al. Delineating the association between heavy postpartum Haemorrhage and postpartum depression. PLoS One. 2016;11(1):e0144274. https://doi.org/10.1371/journal.pone.0144274.
28. Nam JY, et al. The synergistic effect of breastfeeding discontinuation and cesarean section delivery on postpartum depression: a nationwide population-based cohort study in Korea. J Affect Disord. 2017;218:53–8 https://doi.org/10.1016/j.jad.2017.04.048.

10

Effects of music intervention during caesarean delivery on anxiety and stress of the mother a controlled, randomised study

Philip Hepp[1,2*], Carsten Hagenbeck[2], Julius Gilles[2], Oliver T. Wolf[3], Wolfram Goertz[4], Wolfgang Janni[5], Percy Balan[2], Markus Fleisch[1], Tanja Fehm[2] and Nora K. Schaal[6]

Abstract

Background: Stress and anxiety during pregnancy and childbirth have negative consequences for both mother and child. There are indications that music has a positive effect in this situation. The present study investigates the influence of music during the caesarean on anxiety and stress of the expectant mother.

Methods: The SAMBA study is a single-centre, controlled, randomized study including 304 patients. Women in the intervention group heard music via loudspeakers from one of four self-selected genres. The control group had standard treatment without music. The caesarean was performed in regional Anesthesia. At admission, at skin incision, during skin suture and two hours after completion of surgery, different subjective (State-Trait Anxiety Inventory, visual analogue scale for anxiety) and objective parameters (salivary cortisol/amylase, heart rate, blood pressure) were collected. Mixed-factorial Analysis of variances as well as independent sample t-tests were applied for data analysis.

Results: At skin suture, significantly lower anxiety levels were reported in the intervention group regarding State anxiety (31.56 vs. 34.41; $p = .004$) and visual analogue scale for anxiety (1.27 vs. 1.76; $p = .018$). Two hours after surgery, the measured visual analogue scale for anxiety score in the intervention group was still significantly lower (0.69 vs. 1.04; $p = .018$). The objective parameters showed significant differences between the groups in salivary cortisol increase from admission to skin suture (12.29 vs. 16.61 nmol/L; $p = .043$), as well as systolic blood pressure (130.11 vs. 136.19 mmHg; $p = .002$) and heart rate (88.40 vs. 92.57/min; $p = .049$) at skin incision.

Conclusions: Music during caesarean is an easy implementable and effective way of reducing stress and anxiety of the expectant mother.

Keywords: Caesarean, Anxiety, Stress, Music intervention

Background

Almost one in three women delivers by caesarean in Germany. Thus it is the most common abdominal surgery and one of the most common operations. Although the circumstances in almost all cases give cause for joy, it is also a feared event, which is associated with a significant level of stress for the patient [1, 2]. Studies have shown adverse effects of maternal stress on the foetus and on psychological development later in life [3, 4]. In addition, it is known that increased levels of stress and anxiety can negatively affect pain perception and the usage of analgesics postoperatively [5, 6] as well as the new mothers lactation [7, 8]. In view of the limited pharmacological options of intervention for pregnant women, the need for alternative, low-risk approaches to positively influence anxiety and stress arises.

In this regard, the positive effect of music on anxiety and stress is one of the oldest treatment approaches.

* Correspondence: science@dr-hepp.de
[1]Clinic for Gynecology and Obstetrics, Helios University Hospital Wuppertal, University Witten/Herdecke, Heusnerstr 40, 42283 Wuppertal, Germany
[2]Clinic for Gynecology and Obstetrics, Heinrich-Heine-University, Düsseldorf, Germany
Full list of author information is available at the end of the article

Even Asclepius attributed a healing power to music [9]. Its positive influence in various medical interventions across all disciplines has been repeatedly examined [10–13]. Supported by a recent review by Hole et al. in the Lancet, these results also drew the attention of the wider public [14].

Nevertheless, data for music during caesarean are sparse and inconclusive [15]. Two randomized studies examining the influence of music during the pre-operative waiting time could show a positive influence of music on non-validated questionnaires as well as heart rate and heart rate variability as a surrogate for stress and anxiety. In part, this effect could still be detected six hours after the caesarean [16, 17]. A Cochrane analysis [15] investigating the effect of music during the procedure could only identify one randomized study that was able to show a positive effect of music intervention on heart rate at the end of the caesarean in 64 participants [18]. Due to their study design, no further conclusions on subjective and objective perception of anxiety were possible. Another study examined the influence of music during caesarean delivery under general anesthesia on postoperative pain and could not show any effect [19].

Therefore, the aim of the present study is to systematically examine the anxiolytic and stress reducing effect of a music intervention during the caesarean on the wake patient using validated questionnaires and a comprehensive set of objective measurements (salivary cortisol/amylase, blood pressure and heart rate).

Methods

The *SAMBA* (**S**ectio Caesarea und die **A**uswirkung von **M**usik**B**egleittherapie auf **A**nxiolyse; English: Caesarean and the effect of music intervention on anxiety) study is a single-centre, controlled, randomized trial conducted at the University Hospital Dusseldorf, Germany. The study adheres to the CONSORT guidelines.

Ethics, consent and permissions

The study protocol was approved by the ethics committee of the Medical Department of the Heinrich-Heine-University in Dusseldorf (No.: 3625) in accordance with the declaration of Helsinki and registered in the German registry for clinical trials (DRKS00007840) and with the WHO (Universal Trial Number U1111–1173-3204). Upon reasonable request the study protocol can be obtained via email from the corresponding author. All eligible patients gave informed written consent prior to participation.

Participants

From March 2015 to August 2017, pregnant women with an indication for primary caesarean in regional anesthesia and adequate German language comprehension were recruited.

We only included patients with normal hearing abilities. Additionally, the patients were only included when no serious comorbidities (according to the physician's assessment) were present, no significantly increased surgical risk (e.g. placental disturbances) were identified preoperatively and only if no serious condition of the foetus was known. Furthermore, only patients without any generalized anxiety disorder or other serious mental alterations were included in the study.

Outcomes, measuring instruments and procedure

The impact of music during caesarean delivery on anxiety and stress measured by State-Trait Anxiety Inventory (STAI), a visual analogue scale depicting anxiety (VAS-A) as well as on salivary cortisol and alpha-amylase were pre-specified as primary outcome measures.

To measure subjective anxiety, STAI and VAS-A were used. The STAI is an introspective inventory comprising 40 self-report items pertaining to anxiety [20]. It distinguishes between two questionnaires with 20 items each, one measuring anxiety perceived in the current situation (STAI-state) and the other evaluating a general tendency towards anxiety (STAI-trait). Participants are asked to give a response to each item on a 4-point Likert scale. A total value is calculated (possible range 20–80 for each questionnaire). Higher scores reflect higher levels of anxiety. The VAS-A comprises a 10 cm line, on which the participant marks her current degree of anxiety with the left end of the line being labelled "no anxiety" and the right end being labelled "maximum anxiety". For analysis the marking is then measured in mm from the left end.

Saliva samples were collected in order to determine cortisol and alpha-amylase levels as objective measures of stress. Salivary cortisol is a marker of the activation of the hypothalamic-pituitary-adrenal axis, whereas salivary alpha-amylase is an indirect marker of the autonomic activity [21]. For the saliva samples, patients had to thoroughly insalivate a cotton swab. The saliva samples were kept frozen at – 18 degrees until analysed, following the methods described elsewhere [22]. Heart rate and blood pressure values were taken from the anaesthesia records.

After inclusion, the computer-assisted randomization took place and divided the patients into the music group vs. control group in the ratio of one to one. Women in the music group chose their preferred music genre from lounge, classical, jazz, and meditation music.

The participating women filled in the STAI-trait when they came to the routine surgical preparation appointment 7 to14 days before the caesarean. At admission on the day of the scheduled caesarean, the VAS-A, the STAI-state and the first saliva sample were taken during the routine cardiotocogram. There was no routine preoperative medication in either group. Intraoperative, the parameters blood pressure and heart rate were recorded at skin incisions and suture. During skin suture, a second saliva sample was obtained and the patient answered the STAI-state questionnaire and the VAS-A. At the end of post-operative monitoring two hours after skin suture, a third saliva sample was taken. Furthermore, the participant answered the STAI-state questionnaire and VAS-A for a third time. Additionally, questions were asked about the music experience. Figure 1 shows the study procedure with the measurement time points schematically.

Intervention

For the music group, the music intervention started when the participant entered the operating theatre. The music was played on a CD player (TEAC CR-H 500 CD receiver) using a speaker system from Cambridge Audio 300. The participant was presented with music continuously in a standardized volume determined on the device and measured at the participants' head of 55 dB (A). All music titles had a slow tempo of 60–80 bpm in common and followed the recommendations made by Nilsson [23]. The music pool contained 60 songs. 15 tracks were each assigned to one of the 4 different genres of music. The control group received no music.

Statistical analysis

The statistical software package SPSS 24 (IBM Inc., Armonk, NY) was used for all data analyses. The group affiliation was coded and therefore the analysis was performed blind. In order to check for differences in environmental parameters between groups, which could influence the results, we compared the time of the procedure (morning vs. afternoon) using a chi-square-test and the length of the surgery with an independent sample t-test.

To compare the subjective course of anxiety on the day of the caesarean, two 2 × 3 mixed-factorial ANOVAs with the between-subject factor *group* (music group vs control group) and the within-subject factor *measurement time point* (admission, skin suture, 2 h post-surgery) and the dependent variables STAI-state and VAS-A were calculated. If sphericity was not met, a correction of the degrees of freedom according to Greenhouse-Geisser was carried out. For the objective variables heart rate and systolic and diastolic blood pressure, 2 × 2 mixed-factorial ANOVAs were used with the factors *group* and *measurements time point* (skin incision and skin suture). In addition, direct group comparisons were performed with independent-samples t-tests. Amylase values were logarithmized analogously to the generally accepted approach [24].

An a-priori power analyses for sample-size estimation was calculated using G*Power (HHU, Düsseldorf, Germany) [25]. Given an expected small to medium effect size (d = 0.35), a power of 85% and an alpha-error of .05 the required (to be analysed) sample-size is 296 (148 per group).

Results

We screened and informed 412 patients about study participation. Sixty-two patients had to be excluded from further participation because they no longer fulfilled the inclusion criteria at the time of intervention (three had delivered spontaneously, 18 had an indication for caesarean preterm, 41 had a secondary caesarean (for example because of premature rupture of membranes)). Forty-five women did not take part due to technical difficulties (reconstruction of the operation theatre). One patient discontinued the study prematurely. In total 304 participants completed the study in accordance with the protocol (Fig. 2). The patients had a mean age of 33.6 years (range: 18–47 years) and a mean gestation age of 268.5 days. The data revealed that the two groups did not differ regarding the time of the procedure (morning vs. afternoon) [$\chi^2(1, 301) = 0.75$, $p = .388$] nor on the duration of the procedure [$t(290) = 1.36$, $p = .175$].

An overview of the descriptive data of the music and control group and the main results is given in Table 1.

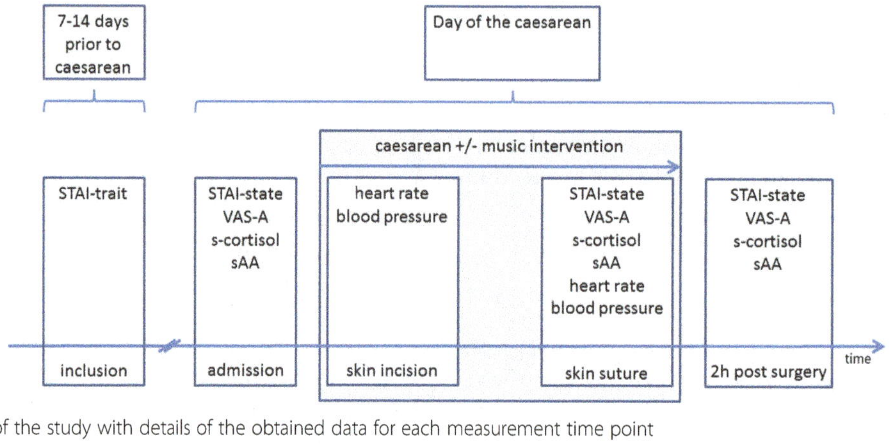

Fig. 1 Flow chart of the study with details of the obtained data for each measurement time point

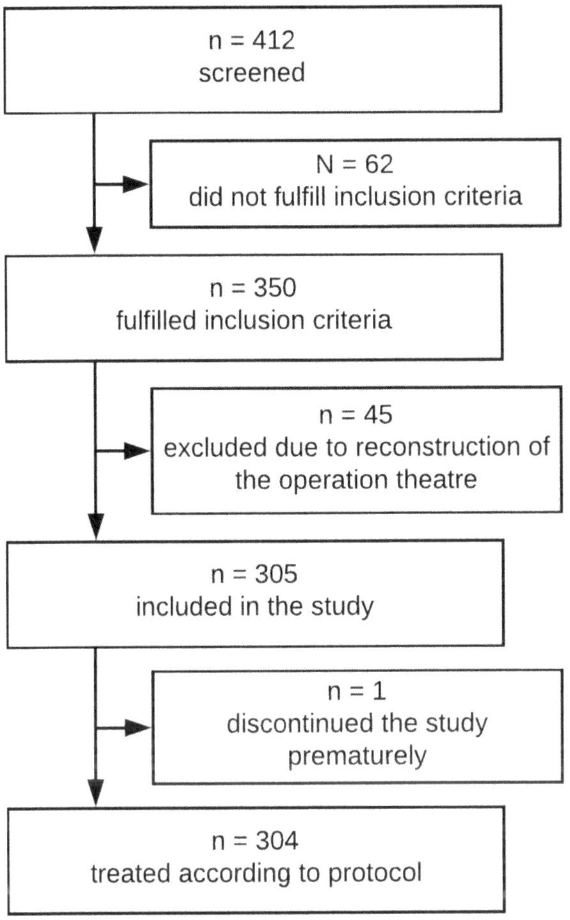

Fig. 2 Participant flow chart

Subjective parameters

For the STAI-state, significant main effects were found for the factors *measurement time point* [F (1.78, 451.28) = 454.35, p < .001] and *group* [F (1.254) = 4.12, p = .043]. The interaction was not significant [F (1.78, 451.28) = 1.47, p = .230]. Post-hoc comparisons showed that the two groups did not differ on admission (p = .593). At skin suture the music group showed significantly less anxiety compared to the control group [t (254) = 2.88, p = .004, mean difference = 2.72, 95% CI (0.76, 4.67), d = 0.36]. 2 h after surgery there was no significant difference (p = .140) (Fig. 3a).

For the VAS-A, the factors *measurement time point* [F (1.39, 301.32) = 378.50, p < .001] and *group* [F (1.217) = 4.51, p = .035] showed significant effects, whereas no interaction was present [F (1.39, 301.32) = 0.17, p = .847]. A post-hoc t-test showed that the level of anxiety in the two groups did not differ at admission (p = .349). At skin suture [t (217) = 2.39, p = .018, mean difference = 0.49, 95% CI (0.08, 0.89), d = 0.32] and 2 h post-surgery [t (217) = 2.38, p = .018, mean difference = 0.35, 95% CI (0.06, 0.64), d = 0.32] there were significant differences in favour of the music group (Fig. 3b).

Objective parameters

Cortisol increase from admission to skin suture was significantly lower in the music group than in the control group [t (181) = 2.04, p = .043, mean difference = 4.32, 95% CI (0.14, 8.49), d = 0.30] (Fig. 4a). The decrease in cortisol from skin suture to 2 h post-surgery did not differ significantly between the two groups [t (193) = 1.53, p = .121, mean difference = 3.30, 95% CI (− 0.95, 7.55), d = 0.22]. The increase in amylase from admission to skin suture and decrease to 2 h after surgery did not differ between the two groups (p-values > .165).

For systolic blood pressure, significant main effects were found for *group* [F (1,270) = 4.73, p = .030] and *measurement time point* [F (1,270) = 132.58, p < .001] and a significant interaction revealed [F (1,270) = 8.57, p = .004]. At skin incision the mean systolic blood pressure was significantly lower in the music group (M = 130.11 mmHg) than in the control group (M = 136.19 mmHg) [t (270) = 3.18, p = .002, mean difference = 6.35, 95% CI (2.59, 10.11), d = 0.39] (Fig. 4b). There was no difference at skin suture (p = .981). For the diastolic blood pressure value, no significant group differences were found (p-values > .197).

Also for heart rate significant effects of the factors *group* [F (1,266) = 4.51, p = .035] and *measurement time point* [F (1,266) = 104.99, p < .001] were revealed. There was no significant interaction [F (1,266) = 0.55, p = .457]. Post-hoc comparisons showed that at skin incision the heart rate was significantly lower in the music group (M = 88.40) than in the control group (M = 92.57) [t (269) = 1.98 p = .049, mean difference = 4.13, 95% CI (0.02, 8.24), d = 0.24]. At skin suture, the groups did not differ significantly (p = .141) (Fig. 4c).

Acceptance of music intervention

Of the participants in the music group 95.5% stated that they would listen to music again at a possible next caesarean. Eighty-six percent were satisfied with the choice of music. In addition, 89.7% said that the music made the situation more enjoyable and 73.4% thought the music had calmed them.

Discussion

Overall, the study shows, in subjective as well as objective dimensions, an anxiety and stress reducing effect of music during caesarean.

While both groups showed high baseline values for STAI-state and VAS-A without significantly differing from each other at admission, the subjective anxiety drop in both, STAI-state and VAS-A, was significantly higher in the music group and resulted in significantly lower anxiety scores compared to the control group at

Table 1 Overview of characteristics and results

	Music group	Control group	*P* value
Number	154	150	
Age [years]	33.5 ± 5.4 (18–47)	33.7 ± 5.4 (21–44)	.883
Gestational Age [days]	269	268	.231
Time of procedure [morning/evening]	81/73	70/77 (3 N/A)	.388
Duration of procedure [mins]	43.0	41.6	.175
STAI-Trait	36.39 ± 8.45	37.14 ± 8.74	.474
STAI-State I	47.54 ± 10.40	48.28 ± 11.79	.593
STAI-State II	31.56 ± 6.30	34.41 ± 9.23	**.004**
STAI-State III	29.54 ± 5.91	30.91 ± 7.14	.140
VAS-A I [cm]	4.83 ± 2.61	5.18 ± 2.89	.349
VAS-A II [cm]	1.27 ± 1.20	1.76 ± 1.78	**.018**
VAS-A III [cm]	0.69 ± 0.88	1.04 ± 1.29	**.018**
C-increase I to II [nmol/L]	12.29 ± 12.15	16.61 ± 16.14	**.043**
C-decrease II to III [nmol/L]	− 13.77 ± 13.05	−17.07 ± 16.80	.128
sAA-increase [ln] I to II	1.58 ± 1.40	1.76 ± 1.24	.414
sAA-decrease II to III	−0.31 ± 1.27	−0.57 ± 1,10	.165
RR sys skin incision [mmHg]	130.11 ± 14.97	136.19 ± 16.57	**.002**
RR sys II [mmHg]	121.42 ± 12.89	121.58 ± 13.00	.981
RR dia skin incision [mmHg]	70.82 ± 9.35	72.77 ± 10.55	.106
RR dia II [mmHg]	64.65 ± 9.61	64.99 ± 9.21	.764
HR skin incision [1/min]	88.40 ± 16.23	92.57 ± 18.26	**.049**
HR II [1/min]	77.97 ± 13.91	80.51 ± 14.23	.141

N/A: data not available; I: at admission; II: at skin suture; III: 2 h post-surgery; VAS-A: Visual Analogue Scale for Anxiety; C: salivary cortisol; sAA: salivary alpha amylase; RR sys: systolic blood pressure; RR dia: diastolic blood pressure; HR: heart rate
Note: bold values indicate a significant difference between groups

skin suture. The shown positive effect of music on these subjective measures for anxiety and stress is in line with previous studies investigating the effect of music in the context of caesarean and other medical procedures [11, 13, 14, 16, 23, 26]. One of these studies showed a persisting positive effect for six hours [16]. Our data support this observation insofar that women in the music group had significantly lower scores on the VAS-A for another two hours after skin suture. This effect was not found for the STAI-state. It is likely that the STAI-state is less appropriate than the VAS-A in the obstetrical environment due to the duration of the survey?

In terms of objective parameters, the music group showed a significantly lower increase in salivary cortisol

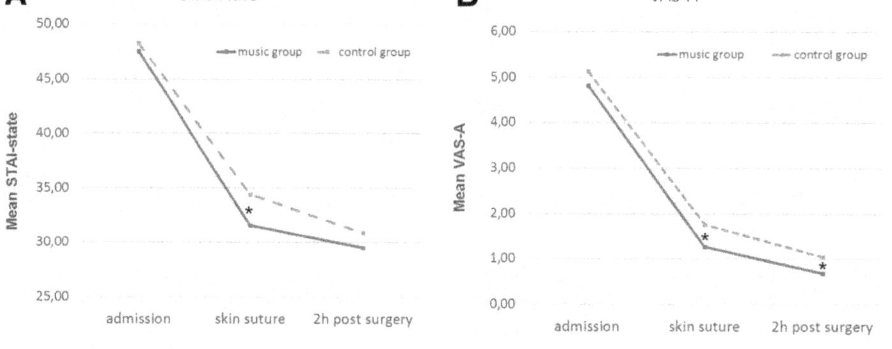

Fig. 3 The subjective course of anxiety for both groups. **a** For the STAI-state scores the music group displayed significantly lower anxiety levels at skin suture than the control group. **b** For the VAS-A scores anxiety levels of the music group are significantly below the control group at skin suture and remain lower two hours after the caesarean. * $p < .05$

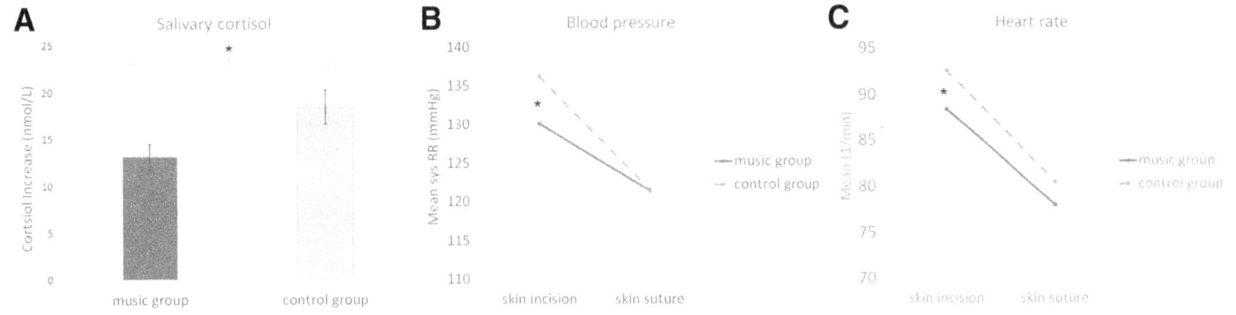

Fig. 4 Objective Measures. **a** The increase of salivary cortisol from admission to skin suture is significantly higher in the control group than the music group. **b** The music group show significantly lower systolic blood pressure at skin incision. **c** Heart rate is significantly lower in the music group than the control group at skin incision

than the control group from admission to skin suture. Saliva cortisol measures the impact of a stressor with a latency of about 30 min [27]. In this respect, the measurement at skin suture represents a large part of the objective stress sensation during the operation [2]. Therefore, the present result reflects that the music group also objectively experiences reduced stress levels during the caesarean. A lowering effect of music on cortisol could also be shown in studies in other medical fields [28].

A comparable effect could not be found for salivary amylase. Whereas cortisol represents the activity of the hypothalamic-pituitary-adrenocortical axis, salivary amylase represents the activation of the sympathetic nerve system [29]. In line with previous work on stress during surgical procedures, our study shows no measurable difference in salivary amylase between the groups [30, 31]. This might be an indication that there are unrecognized factors, which impede a reliable interpretation of the salivary amylase during surgical procedures.

A variety of studies have examined the influence of music on the cardiovascular system [32]. In addition to a direct impact on the dopaminergic mesolimbic reward centre [33], an interaction of the external musical rhythm with the internal body rhythms of heart and respiratory rate as a main carrier of the effect of music is debated [34–36]. Thereby, the value of systolic blood pressure and heart rate is well documented as objective parameters reflecting stress and anxiety [32]. In the present study, the music group showed significantly lower heart rate and systolic blood pressure levels at skin incision. This took place on average 18 min after the patient had been admitted to the operating room and the start of the music intervention. Therefore, we would argue that the calming effect of music on the expectant mother was already present at skin incision. In the case of skin suture, however, no significant difference was detectable. At this time, the new-born was usually already in the arms of the mother, so that pulse and blood pressure are certainly subject to an undetermined bias.

Besides the positive influence of music on the measured stress and anxiety of patients, the high acceptance of the intervention should also be noted. Ninety-six percent of women in the intervention group would want to hear music again during a possible repeated caesarean, regardless of any therapeutic effects. The positive response of the women regarding the music intervention alone are gratifying and should encourage the use of music in obstetrics and further research in this area.

A limitation of the study is the lack of opportunity to gain an even more comprehensive picture of the course of anxiety during caesarean through measuring more time points. For example a measurement of anxiety levels just before the women enters the operating theatre would be desirable as this time point may be the most anxious time for the women. This is partially compensated by the fact that the different measuring instruments used in this study have different latencies and thus cover a large period of time around the intervention. Additionally, in order to ensure a trial close to normal conditions of a caesarean and the needs of the woman, we decided not to use headphones, in contrast to other studies [18]. Naturally, this impeded blinding of the study staff. Using group blinded analysis and application of objective parameters such as saliva cortisol, this disadvantage was accounted for as far as possible. Another limitation which could have influenced the study results is the lack of data on the relationship and role of the nurses and other health professionals in usual interaction and information sharing with the woman during and after procedure.

We would like to emphasize that with a large sample of 304 participants and several measurement time points throughout the day of the caesarean as a strength of the study. This is the first study in this area of research that has the necessary power to detect even small effect sizes.

Conclusions

In view of the results, the present study should have implications for clinical practice. Music is a simple, inexpensive, effective and safe intervention that can be easily implemented in everyday clinical practice. Therefore, it would be desirable if the possibility to listen to music could be routinely offered to women giving birth by caesarean. However, further research should consider the impact of music on the surgical team. Although previous work showed adverse effects only for high volumes and complex interventions [37], this has not been investigated explicitly in the context of caesarean.

In conclusion, the results of the present study show that music during caesarean has an anxiety and stress soothing effect on the wake patient. Implementation in clinical routine therefore seems advisable.

Abbreviations

ANOVA: Analysis of variance; C: Salivary cortisol; CONSORT: Consolidated Standards of Reporting Trials; HR: Heart rate; Pts: Patients; RR dia: Diastolic blood pressure; RR sys: Systolic blood pressure; sAA: Salivary alpha amylase; SD: Standard deviation; STAI: State-Trait Anxiety Inventory; VAS-A: Visual analogue scale for anxiety

Acknowledgements

We'd like to thank the dedicated team of midwives of the department of gynaecology and obstetrics of the Heinrich-Heine-University Düsseldorf.

Funding

The study was funded by a research grant from the Anton-Betz-Foundation.

Authors' contributions

PH and NKS managed the project. PH, CH, WG, WJ and NKS conceived and designed the study. CH, JG, PB lead the acquisition of data. PH, JG and NKS analysed the data. PH, OTW, WG, WJ, MF, TF, NKS interpreted the data. JG, PB, and MF provided administrative, technical and logistic support. PH and NKS drafted the manuscript. All authors revised the manuscript critically for important intellectual content and approved the final version of the manuscript.

Competing interests

All authors declare that they have no competing interests.

Author details

[1]Clinic for Gynecology and Obstetrics, Helios University Hospital Wuppertal, University Witten/Herdecke, Heusnerstr 40, 42283 Wuppertal, Germany. [2]Clinic for Gynecology and Obstetrics, Heinrich-Heine-University, Düsseldorf, Germany. [3]Department of Cognitive Psychology, Institute of Cognitive Neuroscience, Faculty of Psychology, Ruhr-University Bochum, Bochum, Germany. [4]Musikerambulanz, Heinrich-Heine-University, Düsseldorf, Germany. [5]Clinic for Gynecology and Obstetrics, University Hospital Ulm, Ulm, Germany. [6]Department of Experimental Psychology, Heinrich-Heine-University, Düsseldorf, Germany.

References

1. Blüml V, Stammler-Safar M, Reitinger AK, Resch I, Naderer A, Leithner K. A qualitative approach to examine women's experience of planned cesarean. J Obstet Gynecol Neonatal Nurs. 2012;41:E82 90. https://doi.org/10.1111/j.1552-6909.2012.01398.x.
2. Hepp P, Hagenbeck C, Burghardt B, Jaeger B, Wolf OT, Fehm T, et al. Measuring the course of anxiety in women giving birth by caesarean section: a prospective study. BMC Pregnancy Childbirth. 2016;16:113. https://doi.org/10.1186/s12884-016-0906-z.
3. Mulder EJH, Robles de Medina PG, Huizink AC, den Bergh BRH V, Buitelaar JK, GHA V. Prenatal maternal stress: effects on pregnancy and the (unborn) child. Early Hum Dev. 2002;70:3–14 http://www.ncbi.nlm.nih.gov/pubmed/12441200. Accessed 15 Oct 2017.
4. O'Donnell KJ, Glover V, Barker ED, O'Connor TG. The persisting effect of maternal mood in pregnancy on childhood psychopathology. Dev Psychopathol. 2014;26:393–403. https://doi.org/10.1017/S0954579414000029.
5. Good M. Effects of relaxation and music on postoperative pain: a review. J Adv Nurs. 1996;24:905–14 http://www.ncbi.nlm.nih.gov/pubmed/8933249. Accessed 15 Oct 2017.
6. Powell R, Scott NW, Manyande A, Bruce J, Vögele C, Byrne-Davis LM, et al. Psychological preparation and postoperative outcomes for adults undergoing surgery under general anaesthesia. In: Powell R, editor. Cochrane Database of Systematic Reviews. Chichester: John Wiley & Sons, Ltd; 2016. p. CD008646. https://doi.org/10.1002/14651858.CD008646.pub2.
7. Dewey KG. Maternal and fetal stress are associated with impaired lactogenesis in humans. J Nutr. 2001;131:3012S–5S http://www.ncbi.nlm.nih.gov/pubmed/11694638. Accessed 15 Oct 2017.
8. Grajeda R, Pérez-Escamilla R. Stress during labor and delivery is associated with delayed onset of lactation among urban Guatemalan women. J Nutr. 2002;132:3055–60 http://www.ncbi.nlm.nih.gov/pubmed/12368395. Accessed 15 Oct 2017.
9. Conrad C. Music for healing: from magic to medicine. Lancet (London, England). 2010;376:1980–1 http://www.ncbi.nlm.nih.gov/pubmed/21171230. Accessed 15 Oct 2017.
10. Goertz W, Dominick K, Heussen N, Vom dahl J. Music in the cath lab: who should select it. Clin Res Cardiol. 2011;100:395–402. https://doi.org/10.1007/s00392-010-0256-1.
11. Smolen D, Topp R, Singer L. The effect of self-selected music during colonoscopy on anxiety, heart rate, and blood pressure. Appl Nurs Res. 2002;15:126–36 http://www.ncbi.nlm.nih.gov/pubmed/12173164. Accessed 14 Oct 2015.
12. Koelsch S, Fuermetz J, Sack U, Bauer K, Hohenadel M, Wiegel M, et al. Effects of music listening on cortisol levels and Propofol consumption during spinal anesthesia. Front Psychol. 2011;2:58. https://doi.org/10.3389/fpsyg.2011.00058.
13. Angioli R, De Cicco NC, Plotti F, Cafà EV, Dugo N, Damiani P, et al. Use of music to reduce anxiety during office hysteroscopy: prospective randomized trial. J Minim Invasive Gynecol. 2014;21:454–9. https://doi.org/10.1016/j.jmig.2013.07.020.
14. Hole J, Hirsch M, Ball E, Meads C. Music as an aid for postoperative recovery in adults: a systematic review and meta-analysis. Lancet. 2015;386:1659–71. https://doi.org/10.1016/S0140-6736(15)60169-6.
15. Laopaiboon M, Lumbiganon P, Martis R, Vatanasapt P, Somjaivong B. Music during caesarean section under regional anaesthesia for improving maternal and infant outcomes. Cochrane Database Syst Rev. 2009: CD006914. https://doi.org/10.1002/14651858.CD006914.pub2.
16. Li Y, Dong Y. Preoperative music intervention for patients undergoing cesarean delivery. Int J Gynaecol Obstet. 2012;119:81–3. https://doi.org/10.1016/j.ijgo.2012.05.017.
17. Kushnir J, Friedman A, Ehrenfeld M, Kushnir T. Coping with preoperative anxiety in cesarean section: physiological, cognitive, and emotional effects of listening to favorite music. Birth. 2012;39:121–7. https://doi.org/10.1111/j.1523-536X.2012.00532.x.
18. Chang S, Chen C. Effects of music therapy on women's physiologic measures, anxiety, and satisfaction during cesarean delivery. Res Nurs Health. 2005;28:453–61. https://doi.org/10.1002/nur.20102.
19. Reza N, Ali SM, Saeed K, Abul-Qasim A, Reza TH. The impact of music on postoperative pain and anxiety following cesarean section. Middle East J Anaesthesiol. 2007;19:573–86 http://www.ncbi.nlm.nih.gov/pubmed/18044285. Accessed 15 Oct 2017.
20. Laux L, Glanzmann P, Schaffner P, Spielberger CD. Das State-Trait-Angstinventar (STAI) (Beltz-Test). Beltz Test GmbH: Göttingen; 1981.
21. Strahler J, Skoluda N, Kappert MB, Nater UM. Simultaneous measurement of salivary cortisol and alpha-amylase: application and recommendations. Neurosci Biobehav Rev. 2017;83:657–77. https://doi.org/10.1016/j.neubiorev.2017.08.015.

22. Schoofs D, Wolf OT. Are salivary gonadal steroid concentrations influenced by acute psychosocial stress? A study using the Trier social stress test (TSST). Int J Psychophysiol. 2011;80:36–43. https://doi.org/10.1016/j.ijpsycho.2011.01.008.
23. Nilsson U. The anxiety- and pain-reducing effects of music interventions: a systematic review. AORN J. 2008;87:780–807. https://doi.org/10.1016/j.aorn.2007.09.013.
24. Petrakova L, Doering BK, Vits S, Engler H, Rief W, Schedlowski M, et al. Psychosocial stress increases salivary alpha-amylase activity independently from plasma noradrenaline levels. PLoS One. 2015;10:e0134561. https://doi.org/10.1371/journal.pone.0134561.
25. Faul F, Erdfelder E, Buchner A, Lang A-G. Statistical power analyses using G*power 3.1: tests for correlation and regression analyses. Behav Res Methods. 2009;41:1149–60. https://doi.org/10.3758/BRM.41.4.1149.
26. Ikonomidou E, Rehnström A, Naesh O. Effect of music on vital signs and postoperative pain. AORN J. 2004;80:269–74, 277–8. http://www.ncbi.nlm.nih.gov/pubmed/15382598 Accessed 15 Oct 2017.
27. Khalfa S, Bella SD, Roy M, Peretz I, Lupien SJ. Effects of relaxing music on salivary cortisol level after psychological stress. Ann N Y Acad Sci. 2003;999:374–6 http://www.ncbi.nlm.nih.gov/pubmed/14681158. Accessed 15 Oct 2017.
28. Zengin S, Kabul S, Al B, Sarcan E, Doğan M, Yildirim C. Effects of music therapy on pain and anxiety in patients undergoing port catheter placement procedure. Complement Ther Med. 2013;21:689–96. https://doi.org/10.1016/j.ctim.2013.08.017.
29. van Stegeren AH, Wolf OT, Kindt M. Salivary alpha amylase and cortisol responses to different stress tasks: impact of sex. Int J Psychophysiol. 2008;69:33–40.
30. Orbach-Zinger S, Ginosar Y, Elliston J, Fadon C, Abu-Lil M, Raz A, et al. Influence of preoperative anxiety on hypotension after spinal anaesthesia in women undergoing caesarean delivery. Br J Anaesth. 2012;109:943–9. https://doi.org/10.1093/bja/aes313.
31. Sadi H, Finkelman M, Rosenberg M. Salivary cortisol, salivary alpha amylase, and the dental anxiety scale. Anesth Prog. 2013;60:46–53. https://doi.org/10.2344/0003-3006-60.2.46.
32. Koelsch S, Jäncke L. Music and the heart. Eur Heart J. 2015;36:3043–9. https://doi.org/10.1093/eurheartj/ehv430.
33. Koelsch S. Brain correlates of music-evoked emotions. Nat Rev Neurosci. 2014;15:170–80. https://doi.org/10.1038/nrn3666.
34. Bernardi L, Porta C, Casucci G, Balsamo R, Bernardi NF, Fogari R, et al. Dynamic interactions between musical, cardiovascular, and cerebral rhythms in humans. Circulation. 2009;119:3171–80 http://www.ncbi.nlm.nih.gov/pubmed/19569263. Accessed 22 Oct 2017.
35. Bernatzky G, Kreutz G. Musik und Medizin Chancen für Therapie, Prävention und Bildung. Vienna: Springer; 2015.
36. Thaut MH, McIntosh GC, Hoemberg V. Neurobiological foundations of neurologic music therapy: rhythmic entrainment and the motor system. Front Psychol. 2014;5:1185. https://doi.org/10.3389/fpsyg.2014.01185.
37. Weldon S-M, Korkiakangas T, Bezemer J, Kneebone R. Music and communication in the operating theatre. J Adv Nurs. 2015;71:2763–74. https://doi.org/10.1111/jan.12744.

11

Magnitude and determinants of surgical site infecion among women underwent cesarean section in Ayder comprehensive specialized hospital Mekelle City, Tigray region, Northern Ethiopia, 2016

Tsehaynesh Aslake Wendmagegn*, Gerezgiher Buruh Abera, Weyzer Tilahun Tsehaye, Kibrom Brhanu Gebresslasie and Berhe Girmay Tella

Abstract

Background: Surgical site infection (SSI) is an infection that occurs after surgery within 30 days in the part of the body where the surgery took place. Some of the common symptoms are: drainage of cloudy fluid from the surgical wound, pain or tenderness, localized swelling, redness, and raised body temperature. Lack of data on surgical site infection among women who underwent cesarean section (C/S) initiated us to undertake this paper which is targeted to assess the magnitude and determinants of SSI among women who underwent cesarean section.

Methods: Retrospective document review study design was conducted among mothers who underwent cesarean section in Ayder Comprehensive, Specialized Hospital (ACSH) from September 2014 –January 2016. Mother's charts were selected using systematic random sampling technique. Data were cleaned using EPI info version 3.5.1 and analyzed using SPSS version 20. Descriptive statistics, Bivariate, and multivariable logistic regression were conducted to summarize the data.

Result: A total of 206 medical records of women who underwent C/S in ACSH comprehensive specialized hospital were reviewed. The mean age was 27 years (± 5 year). The magnitude of surgical site infection was 11.7%. Premature rupture of membrane (PROM), prolonged labor, rural setting, human immune deficiency Virus, chorioaminities and blood loss showed significant association [(AOR = 8.818 95%CI (21.71–35.816)], [AOR = 16.17, 95%CI (2.850–91.819), [AOR = 5. 666,95%CI (1.568–20.483)], [AOR = 6.982,95%CI (1.382–35.269), [AOR = 16.17,95%CI (2.850–91.819)] and [AOR = 0. 097,9%CI (0.017–0.569)] respectively.

Conclusion: The magnitude of post C/S infection in this study 11.7%. PROM, prolonged labor, residence, HIV, Chorioaminities and blood loss are considered to be an independent risk factor.

Keywords: Women, Cesarean section, Ayder, Hospital, Surgical site infection, Tigray, Northern Ethiopia

* Correspondence: tsehayaslake@gmail.com
School of Nursing, College of Health Sciences, Mekelle University, Mekelle, Ethiopia

Background

The surgical site infection (SSI) case was identified using the definition provided by the Center of Disease Control (CDC) United States of America (USA) which states that infection is regarded as SSI if it occurs within 30 days of the procedure and has at least one of the following sign and symptoms: purulent drainage from the wound, pain or tenderness, localized swelling, redness, malodor and fever [1].

Among the obstetrical and gynecological surgeries, cesarean section is the most common which attributes to short time consequences like SSI that in turn increases maternal morbidity, prolongs hospital stay and increase medical costs [2].

Approximately 18.5 million cesarean sections are performed yearly worldwide. About 40% of the countries have C/S rates < 10%, about 10% have C/S rates between 10 and 15%, and approximately 50% have C/S rates of > 15%. Majority of the countries that did 18.5 million C/S were from Africa (68.5%) and remaining (29.6%) were from Asia, Latin America and the Caribbean. Due to the worldwide continuous rise in the incidence of cesarean deliveries, the number of women with surgical site infection is expected to increase. The SSI after cesarean section causes physical, psychological and economic burden to the woman, her family and in the community [3]. The rate of C/S in published series in different areas of Ethiopia ranges 14.23–27.6% [4, 5].

The maternal infection following delivery increases by eight-fold when delivered by cesarean section than vaginal delivery. Based on studies related to SSI following caesarean section, the proportion of the SSI ranges from 3 to 15% [6].

Based on the surgical wound classification, cesarean section is a clean contaminated type of surgery where procedure- related chances of infection are less likely to occur, but infection after cesarean section is still a major problem in our setup. The majority of the problem arises from preventable causes, which, if addressed would significantly reduce rates of wound infection.

Identifying risk factors for post-cesarean surgical-site infections (SSIs) could contribute to a decrease in maternal morbidity.

Only one study has been done in Ethiopia to give a picture of a post-cesarean section SSI. Based on the findings of a study on the Surgical Site Infection done in Jimma University, Ethiopia 2010, the SSI among cesarean section cases was 66 (8.55%) [7]. As infection continues to be a common postoperative complication in the study area, and no previous study has been done, there is a need to assess the magnitude and factors contributing to surgical site infection. Thus, this study aims to assess the magnitude and determinants of SSI following cesarean section.

Methods

Retrospective medical record review study was conducted among mothers underwent C/S from 2014 to 2016 at ACSH, Mekelle city to determine the magnitude and determinants of SSI following C/S delivery.

Mekelle is the capital city of Tigray region and the largest city in northern Ethiopia, at a distance of 783 km from Addis Ababa. It has a population of more than 323,000 among these populations, there are 110,788 females, 104,758 males, 26,536 under five, 60,998 women in reproductive age (15–49 years) and 78,770 < 15 years age [8]. Mekelle has one public referral hospital (ACSH) and three general hospitals namely (Mekelle Hospital, Quiha Hospital and Northern Command Hospital) which are public government hospitals.

ACSH commenced rendering its referral and non-referral services since 2008 to 8 million people in its catchment areas of the Tigray, Afar and Southeastern parts of Amhara Regional States and currently it provides antenatal, delivery and post natal services. It provides a broad range of medical services to both in and out patients of all age groups. As such, the Hospital can be designated as the most advanced medical facility, by all accounts, in the Northern part of the country and that it stands as the second largest hospital in the nation. It has a total capacity of about 500 inpatient beds in four major departments and other specialty units and 84 beds in obstetrics & gynecology department. The obstetrics & gynecology department has 51 staff (5 gynecologist, 7 residents, 18 midwifery and 21 nurses) and is also used as a teaching hospital for the College of Health Sciences, Mekelle University. Annually, ACSH has 2500 deliveries per year; of this, 660 are C/S deliveries [9]. In ACSH, the medical doctors range from resident one up to senior gynecologist specialists. Routinely used antibiotics are Ceftriaxone (as prophylaxis & treatment), Ampicillin and Metronidazole.

The sample size was calculated using the single population proportion formula based on the following assumptions, 95% confidence interval with a 4% margin of error, the expected proportion of post C/S infection taken from a study done in Jimma university hospital which was (P) 8.5% [7]

$$N = \frac{(Za/_2)^2 P\ (1\text{-}P) = Za/_2 = 1.96 \text{ at CI of } 95\%}{d^2}$$

$$N = \frac{6(1.96)2\ \ 0.85(0.915)N = 187}{(0.04)2}$$

By adding 10% contingency for charts with incomplete information the final sample size was 206.

Sampling procedure

Within the time of September 2014–January 2016, about 923 charts with C/S were found. Systematic sampling technique was used to select 206 charts with cesarean section from records since September 2014–January 2016 in ACSH. By dividing the source population to sample size the kth has been calculated, which was 4. A random number was selected from 1 up to 4 with the lottery method; which was 2 as the first sample chart. The next sample was taken every k^{th} interval provided that for an incomplete chart, we consider the next to be included.

Charts of mothers who underwent cesarean section elsewhere, then referred to ACSH were excluded.

Data collection procedure and tool

The data were collected from medical records of the 206 selected charts by trained 2 BSc Nurses using structured check list. The checklist was adapted by reviewing different literature of similar studies done on the magnitude and determinant factors of SSI. In this study, socio-demographic characteristic as well as obstetric history, pre-operative and intra-operative, duration of hospital stay, maternal preexisting medical condition variables were considered. The pre-operative events include (Indication for c/s, Prophylaxis taken, Length of days stay in hospital) and intraoperative events included (type of C/S, duration of operation, estimated blood loss and type of incision).The data collection process was supervised by 1BSc nurse who has previous experience in data collection.

Data quality control

Data collectors and supervisor were carefully trained about the objective of the study, the meaning of each, alternative answers and blank spaces and when to skip as necessary. The checklist was also carefully designed and prepared in English language and was used for data collection. Before the actual data collection, the checklist was pre tested with 10% similar population at Mekelle hospital. Based on the pre-test, the checklist was assessed for its clarity, completion, and the time necessary. During the actual data collection, a supervisor was in place to oversee all activities, and the collected data were reviewed and checked for completeness and consistency by the principal investigator on a daily basis.

Data management and analysis

Data were coded, entered, checked and cleaned using Epi info version 3.5.1 and exported to SPSS version 20 statistical software package for analysis. Descriptive statistics were computed to determine the proportion of post cesarean section wound infection. Bivariate and multivariable logistic regression was also computed to assess statistical association between the outcome variable and independent variables. Factors that were ≤ 0.2 significant level in the bivariate logistic regression analysis were considered in the multivariable logistic regression analysis. Odds ratios with 95% Confidence Interval (CI) and p value (< 0.05) were computed to assess the presence and degree of statistical association between dependent and independent variables.

Ethical considerations

Ethical clearance was obtained from Mekelle University College of Health Sciences, Research Review Committee, and written permission was obtained from the Medical Director of ACSH to support the research. All the information obtained from the medical record was held with confidentiality and used only for the intended purpose.

Results

Two-hundred six medical records were reviewed in this study. The finding of this thesis includes demographic data, patient's obstetric character, operation related factors, and the results of post cesarean section infection and factors that contributing to surgical site infection.

Socio demographic data

The mean age of study participants was 27 years ±standard deviation (SD) =5 and 175 (85%) of the study participant within the age group ranged 20–34. The minimum and maximum age of mothers was (15 & 45 years) respectively. Of the total study participants 139 (67.3%) of women who underwent C/S were from urban areas (Table 1).

Obstetric characteristic of respondents

More than half 109 (52%) of study participant were multiparous and 8 (7.3%) of them was developed SSI.

Table 1 Socio-demographic characteristics of the Women who underwent c/s in Ayder referral hospital, Mekelle, Tigray, Northern Ethiopia, 2016 (*N*=206)

Variables	Category	Post c/s SSI				Total (%)
		Yes		No		
		N	%	N	%	
Age	≤19	0	0%	7	100.0%	7(3.4%)
	20–34	18	10.3%	157	89.7%	175(85%)
	≥35	6	25%	18	75.0%	24(11.6%)
Residence	Rural	14	20%	53	79.1%	67(32.5%)
	Urban	10	7.2%	129	92.8%	139 (67.5%)
Ethnicity	Tigray	22	11.1%	176	88.9%	198(96.1%)
	Amhara	0	0%	3	100.0%	3(1.5%)
	Afar	2	40%	3	60.0%	5(2.4%)

Almost all the study participants 196 (95.1%) had antenatal care (ANC) follow up & from those 20 (10.2%) were developed SSI. About 172 (83.5%) of study participants had no history of abortion. 44 (21%) of the participants had a history of previous C/S and 5 (11%) of them developed SSI (Table 2).

Indication for cesarean section

For 79 (38.2%) of the study participants, the indication for cesarean section was non-reassurance fetal heart beat (NRFHB). For 9 (4.3%), indication was post term (Fig. 1).

Operation related characteristics

Only 13 (6.3%) of the procedure was elective, and none of these participants developed SSI. About 192 (93.2%) of the study participant had less than 1000 ml intra operative blood loss and only 3% of the skin incision was longitudinal (Table 3).

Qualification of persons performed cesarean section

For 87 (42%) of women who underwent cesarean section, the procedure was performed by Resident two (R_2) (second year resident in 4 year obstetrics and gynecology training program). Four cesarean sections (1.9%) were performed by senior specialists (obstetrics and gynecology specialist) (Fig. 2).

Magnitude SSI

From the total of 206 study participants who underwent cesarean section in Ayder Comprehensive Specialized Hospital, 24 (11.7%) of them had post C/S infection (Fig. 3).

Preexisting medical condition

The minimum and maximum preoperative hemoglobin label was 8.2 mg/dl-16 mg/dl, respectively, with their mean 13 mg/dl &SD 1.4. About 183 (88.8%) of the study participant were non-reactive for HIV. More than 95% (203) of study participant had no history of diabetes mellitus (DM) (Table 4).

Determinants of post caesarean section infection

Bivariate logistic regression

During bivariate logistic regression analysis, those variables which had ≤0.2 significance level were considered in multivariable logistic regression. Out of twenty-five independent variables, thirteen variables, namely age, residence, anemia, and ANC follow up. Parity, chorioaminities,

Table 2 Distribution of indication for cesarean section among women who underwent c/sin Ayder referral hospital, Mekelle, Tigray, Northern Ethiopia, 2016 (*N*=206)

Variables	Category	SSI				Total (%)
		YES		NO		
		N	%	N	%	
Parity	Primipara	10	(12.8%)	68	(87.2%)	78(37.9)
	multi para	8	(7.3%)	101	(92.7%)	109(52.9)
	Grand multi para	6	(31.6%)	13	(68.4%)	19(9.2)
ANC follow up	Yes	20	(10.2%)	176	(89.8%)	196(95.1)
	No	4	(40.0%)	6	(60.0%)	10(4.9)
Gestational age at c/s	Preterm	2	(11.1%)	16	(88.9%)	18(8.8)
	Term	21	(12.4%)	148	(87.6%)	169(82)
	Post term	1	(5.3%)	18	(94.7%)	19(9.2)
PROM	Yes	12	(37.5%)	20	62.5%	32(16.0)
	No	12	(6.9%)	162	93.1%	174(84.0)
Prolonged labor	Yes	17	(25.8%)	49	74.2%	66(32)
	No	7	(5.0%)	133	(95.0%)	140(68)
Chorioaminities	Yes	8	(66.7%)	4	(33.3%)	12(5.8)
	No	16	(8.2%)	178	(91.8%)	194(94.2)
Previous c/s	Yes	5	(11.4%)	39	(88.6%)	44(21.4)
	No	19	(11.7%)	143	(88.3%)	162(78.6)
History of abortion	Yes	4	(11.8%)	30	(88.2%)	34(16.5)
	No	20	(11.6%)	152	(88.4%)	172(83.5)

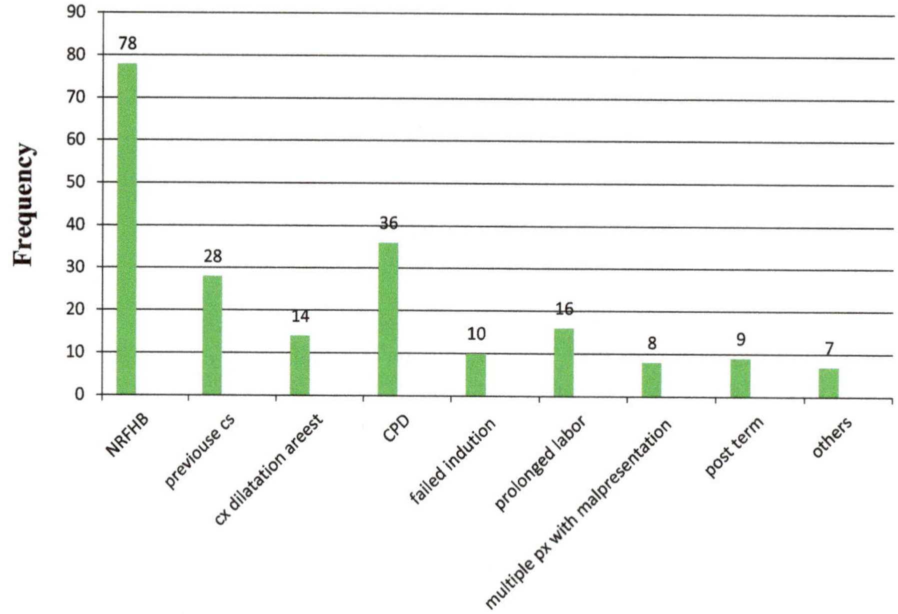

Fig. 1 Distribution of indication for cesarean section among women who underwent surgery in Ayder comprehensive specialized hospital, Mekelle, Tigray, Northern Ethiopia, 2016 ($N = 206$)

PROM, prolonged labor, blood loss, length of hospital stay, DM, HIV and duration of operation had shown an association in bivariate analysis with p-value less than 0.2, and those variables were entered into multivariable analysis.

Multivariable logistic regression

After entering the 13 variables in the multivariable logistic regression analysis simultaneously, Rural setting, PROM, prolonged labor chorioaminities, HIV and blood loss had shown a significant association with p value< 0.05.

Accordingly, women who were from rural area were 5.6 times more likely to develop post C/S infection than those from an urban area [AOR = 5.666, 95%CI: (1.568–20.483, p = 008)].

The odds of developing post c/s infection among women who had a history of PROM were 8.8 times higher than those who had not [(AOR = 8.818, 95%CI: (21.71–35.816, p = 0.002)].

Table 3 Distribution of operation related characteristics among women who underwent C/S in Ayder referral hospital, Mekelle, Tigray, Northern Ethiopia, 2016 (N= 206)

Variables	Category	SSI				Total (%)
		YES		NO		
		N %		N	%	
Type of c/s	Elective	0	(0.0%)	13	(100.0%)	13(6.3%)
	Non elective	24	(12.4%)	169	(87.6%)	193(93.7%)
Type of incision	Longitudinal	0	(0.0%)	3	(100.0%)	3(1.5%)
	Transverse	24	(11.65%)	179	(86.89%)	203(98.5%)
Time taken for operation	<30	0	(0.0%)	2	(100.0%)	2(1%)
	30–60	19	(9.8%)	174	(90.2%)	93(93.7%)
	>60	5	(45.5%)	6	(54.5%)	11(5.3%)
Amount of blood loss	<1000	20	(10.4%)	172	(89.6%)	192(93.2%)
	≥1000	4	(28.6%)	10	(71.4%)	14(6.8%)
Length of stay	≤7	18	(9.4%)	173	(90.6%)	191(92.7%)
	>7	6	(40.0%)	9	(60.0%)	15(7.3%)

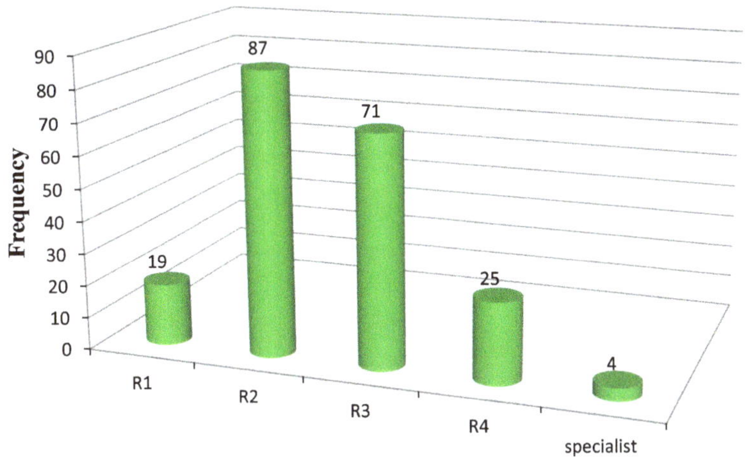

Fig. 2 Qualification distribution of person who perform the procedure on women who underwent c/s in Ayder comprehensive specialized hospital, Mekelle, Tigray, Northern Ethiopia, 2016($N = 206$)

Furthermore, women who had chorioaminities were sixteen times [(AOR = 16.17, 95%CI: (28.50–91.819, $p = 0.002$)] more likely to have post C/S infection.

Women who had prolonged labor were six times [(AOR = 6.064, 95%CI: (1.676–21.949, $p = 0.006$)] more likely to develop post C/S infection. Similarly, HIV positive women are seven times [(AOR = 6.982, 95%CI: (1.382–35.269, $p = 0.019$)] more likely to have post c/s infection than HIV negative women.

Finally, those women who had blood loss less than 1000 ml were almost 90% [(AOR = 0.097,95% CI: (0.017–0.569, $p = 0.01$)] less likely to have post C/S infection than those women who had blood loss greater than 1000 ml (Table 5).

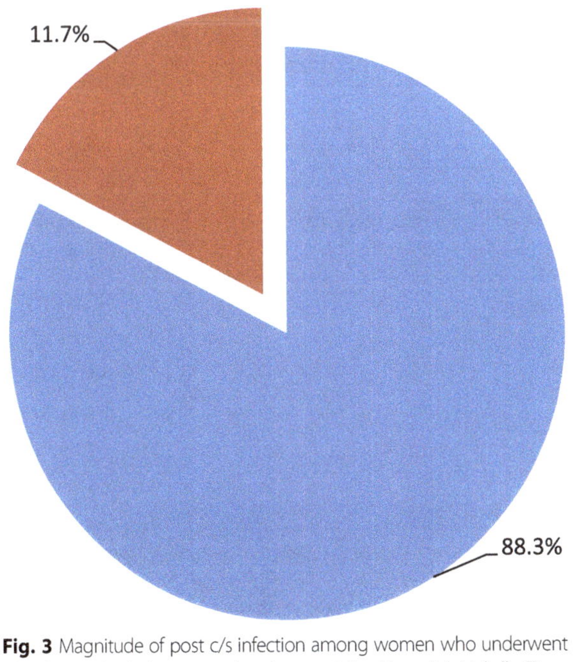

Fig. 3 Magnitude of post c/s infection among women who underwent c/s infection in Ayder comprehensive specialized hospital, Mekelle, Tigray, Northern Ethiopia, 2016, ($N = 206$). Legend: With SSI and with no SSI

Discussion

Medical records were reviewed to find out the magnitude and associated factors of post-cesarean section infection (S.S.I) on women who underwent C/S ACSH. A total of 206 (193 non-elective and 13 elective) were eligible for analysis.

This study indicated that 24 (11.7%) of the study participant had SSI. This figure is higher than the result reported from different studies which revealed that the rate of SSI in US hospitals was 4.1%, in New Zealand 5%, in Brazil 1.44%, China 0.7%, Pakistan 5.8%, Estonian university 6.2%, Saudi Arabia 4–2.4%, and in Nizwa, Oman 2.66%. This discrepancy could be due to the difference in socioeconomic status and health care delivery system [10–13, 14–17].

Similarly, in this study the magnitude of SSI has also shown higher from the studies conducted in England, Nigeria and Jimma which, the rate of post C/S infection was 9.6, 9.3 and 8.55% respectively [7, 18, 19]. This variation might be due to the difference in study area and study participants. However, the results are approximately similar to those from studies conducted in Dhulikhel Hospital, Nepal and Tanzania in which the rates of post c/s infection were 12.6 and 10.9% respectively [20, 21].

This study found a number of factors associated with SSI following C/S. Women who had premature rupture

Table 4 Frequency distribution of pre-existing medical condition of women who underwent c/s in Ayder referral hospital, Mekelle, Tigray, Northern Ethiopia, 2016 (*N*=206)

Variables	Category	SSI				Frequency	Percent (%)
		Yes		No			
		N	(%)	N	(%)		
Anemia	Yes	4	(25%)	12	(75%)	16	7.8%
	No	20	(10.5%)	170	(89.5%)	190	92.2%
Hypertension	Yes	3	(16.7%)	15	(83.3%)	18	8.7%
	No	21	(11%)	167	(89%)	188	91.3%
DM	Yes	2	(66.7%)	1	(33.3%)	3	1.5%
	No	22	(10.8%)	181	(89.2%)	203	98.5%
HIV	Reactive	5	(41.7%)	7	(58.3%)	12	5.8%
	Non-reactive223	17	(9.3%)	166	(90.7%)	183	88.8%
	Unknown status	2	(18%)	9	(82%)	11	5.3%
Immunosuppressive drug	Yes	0	(0%)	2	(100%)	2	1%
	No	24	(11.8%)	180	(88.2%)	204	99%
Pre op Hgb label	<11 mg/dl	3	(13%)	20	(87%)	23	11.2%
	11mg/dl	21	(11.5%)	162	(88.5%)	183	88.8%

of membrane are six times more likely to develop post C/S infection than those who had not. [AOR = 6.064, CI: (1.676–21.949)]. This finding is in line with the study conducted in US hospitals [OR = 3.0; 95% CI, (3.24–3.5)] and Nigeria (OR = 4.45) [10, 19]. This association could be due to the fetal membrane acting as a barrier to infection. However, when the fetal membrane is ruptured early, it loses its protective effect and microorganisms found in the vagina may easily migrate. This may expose the mother for SSI. This finding was also supported by

Table 5 Bivariate and Multivariable logistic regression analysis of post c/s infection among women underwent C/S in Ayder referral hospital, Mekelle, Tigray, Northern Ethiopia, 2016 (*N*=206)

Variable	Category	SSI		COR (95%CI)	AOR (95% CI)
		YES	NO		
Residence	Rural	14	53	3.408(1.424-8.152)*	5.666(1.568-20.483)**
	Urban	10	129	1	1
ANC follow up	Yes	20	176	0.199(0.044-0.656)*	0.220(0.2-2.4)
	NO	4	6	1	1
Parity	Primi	10	68	1.857(0.697-4.943)	1.967(0.535-7.230)
	Multi	8	101	1	1
	Grand multi	6	13	5.827(1.745-19.459)*	9.554(1.519-60.075)**
PROM	Yes	12	20	8.1(3.211-20.432)*	8.818(2.171-35.816)**
	No	12	162	1	1
Prolonged labor	Yes	17	49	6.592(2.577-16.861)*	6.064(1.676-21.949)**
	No	7	133	1	1
Chorioaminities	Yes	8	4	22.25(6.035-82.026)*	16.17(2.850-91.819)**
	No	16	178	1	1
HIV	Reactive	5	7	6.975(1.995-24.38)*	6.982(1.382-35.269)**
	Non reactive	17	166	1	1
	Unknown	2	9	2.17(0.433-10.871)	6.979(0.58-83.908)
Blood loss	<1000	22	169	0.26(0.081-0.832)	0.097(0.017-0.569)**
	>=1000	5	10	1	1

**p*-value <0.05 in bivariate analysis ***p*-value <0.05 in multivariable analysis

other studies conducted in Brazil, China, Nepal and Sub-Saharan Africa [12, 13, 20, 22].

The other factor that showed significant association were women who had chorioaminities was sixteen times more likely to have SSI following c/s than those who had not. [AOR = 16.17, 95%CI: (28.50–91.8190] This is also consistent with a study conducted in an Estonian university hospital revealing that women who had chorioaminities were 8.8 times more likely to have post C/S infection (OR, 8.8; 95%CI, 1.1–69.6) [15]. This variation might be related to socioeconomic difference between the countries. Another study conducted in Jimma as also shown significant association [7].

In this study, a rural setting has shown significant association. Women from rural areas were five times more likely to have post C/S infection than those women from urban areas. [(AOR = 5.666, 95% CI: 1.568–20.483)]. This could be due limited access to hygienic materials and poorer hygiene for women living in rural areas when compared to those in urban areas. However, a study conducted in a US urban setting showed significant association with post C/S infection [10].

This study also found that prolonged labor prior to surgery had shown a significant association with SSI following C/S. Women who had prolonged labor were six times more likely to have SSI than those who had not. Similar finding were also reported from a study conducted in New Zealand [11]. This relationship between duration of labor and SSI may be due to increased exposure time where infection can be acquired and to the fact that as duration of labor increase, number of vaginal examinations also increased. Studies conducted in Brazil, China and Tanzania [12, 13, 21] shown that post C/S infection had significant association with frequent vaginal examination.

The other factor that showed significant association was blood loss. Women with intra-operative blood loss of less than 1000 ml were 90% less likely to have SSI than those who had blood loss of more than 1000 ml [(AOR = 0.097,95% CI: 0.017–0.569)]. This finding is consistent with a study conducted in US revealing that women with excessive blood loss were 2.4 times [(OR, 2.42; 95% CI, 2.34–2.49)] more likely to develop post C/S infection [10]. This finding is also supported by a study conducted in Jimma [7]. This association could be due to excessive blood loss associated with poor control and tissue damage due to prolonged retraction, leading to use of extra sutures which may reduce local resistance mechanism.

Finally, the HIV status of women had shown a significant association. HIV positive women had about seven times more likely to have post C/S infection than those HIV negative women [(AOR = 6.982, CI: 1.382–35.269)]. However, other studies did not show its association.

In this study, the age of the mother, ANC follow up, parity, emergency C/S, skin incision, duration of operation, and skill of the person who performs the procedure had no significant association with post c/s infection. However, it is difficult to conclude that those variables are not totally important.

Conclusions

The magnitude of post C/S infection in this study is high. PROM, chorioaminities, prolonged labor, HIV status, residence and blood loss had shown significant association with post C/S infection.

In this study age of the mother, ANC follow up, parity, emergency c/s, skin incision, duration of operation, and skill of the person who perform the procedure had no significant association with post C/S infection. However, it is difficult to conclude that those variables are not totally important. A small sample was there to show statistical significance.

Based on the finding, the following recommendations are forwarded:

- ❖ Increased awareness, development, and strict implementation of protocol should be done by all the health care professionals in order to minimize and prevent the infection rate after cesarean section
- ❖ Post-operative antibiotics should be given to patients who underwent cesarean section, especially those who are at risk of post cesarean section infection i.e. sero positive, PROM, chorioaminities
- ❖ Evaluate and improve pre, intra and post-operative care through further training and supervision involving more qualified person to decrease post caesarean section infection.
- ❖ Infection prevention procedure in order to reduce the risk of wound infection should be followed appropriately
- ❖ Further prospective study with a large sample size should be conducted.

Abbreviations

ACSH: Ayder comprehensive, specialized hospital; AOR: Adjusted odds ratio; C/S: Cesarean section; CI: Confidence interval; DM: Diabetes mellitus; OR: Odds ratio; PROM: Premature Rapture of Membrane; SSI: Surgical site infection

Acknowledgments

I would like to say thank you to my friends and coworker for their support by providing constructive comments and sharing their experience during the process of doing this thesis.

My appreciation also goes to the supervisor and data collectors for their kind participation in this study.

Funding

This study benefited from neither source of funding nor sponsorship, either from the public, private or not-for-profit sectors. Availability of data and materials supporting the conclusions of this article are not included within the manuscript because of confidentiality.

Authors' contributions

TA Conceived and designed the study. TA, GB, KB, WT and BG analyzed and interpreted the data, and drafted the manuscript. TA Critically reviewed and revised the manuscript. All authors approved the final manuscript.

Competing interests

The authors declare that they have no competing interests.

References

1. Whiting P, Rutjes AWS, Reitsma JB, Bossuyt PMM, Kleijen J. The development of QUADAS: a tool for the quality assessment of studies of diagnostic accuracy included in systematic reviews. BMC Med Res Meth. 2003;3:25.
2. Olsen MA, Butler AM, Willers DM, et al. Risk factors for surgical site infection after low transverse cesarean section. Infect Control Hosp Epidemiol. 2008; 9(4):77–84.
3. Gibbons L, J M Belizán, J ALauer, A P Betrán, M Merialdi and F Althabe. The Global Numbers and Costs of Additionally Needed and Unnecessary Caesarean Sections Performed per Year Background Paper, Overuse as a Barrier to Universal Coverage; World Health Report .2010. p. 30.
4. Moges A, Wondafresh B, Mulgeta G. Prevalence and outcome of cesarean section in attat hospital Gurage, SNNPR, Ethiopia. imedpub journals. 2015;7 no.4:8. available at: http://www.archivesofmedicine.com/medicine/prevalence-and-outcome. Accessed Dec 2015.
5. Kahsay S, Berhe G, Gebremariam A. et al. Determinants of Caesarean Deliveries and its Major Indications in Adigrat Hospital, Northern Ethiopia. Epidemiology Sunnyvale. 2015;5(3):5-6.
6. Newlin C, Kuehl TJ, Pickrel A, Cawyer CR, Jones RO. Cesarean section incision complications and associated risk factors: a quality assurance project. Open J Obstet Gynecol. 2015;5:789–94.
7. Demisew A, Tefera B, Fitsum A. Surgical site infection rate and risk factors among obstetric cases of Jimma University Specialized Hospital, Southwest Ethiopia. Ethiop J Health Sci. 2010;21(2):95–96.
8. Central Statistical Agency [Ethiopia]. Population Projection of Ethiopia for All Regions at Wereda Level from 2014–2017. Addis Ababa: Central Statistical Agency; 2013.
9. Official website of Mekelle University. URL: http://www.mu.edu.et/chs/index.php/ayder-referral-hospital. Accessed Dec 2015.
10. Goff S, Pekowps Ayrunun J, et al. Patterns of obstetric infection rate in large sample of US hospitals. Am J Obstet Gynecol. 2013;208:456.e1–13.
11. Marcus G, Deirdre R, Grace J, et al. Post-caesarean section surgical site infection rate and risk factors New Zerland Med J. 2011;124(1339):32-33.
12. Farret T. Risk factors for surgical site infection following cesarean section in a Brazilian Women's Hospital. Braz J Infect Dis 2014;19(2):114-5.
13. Shi PG, Hong XG, Hong ZZ, et al. Morbidity and risk factors for surgical site infection following cesarean section in Guangdong Province. China J Obstet Gynecol Res. 2012;38(3):509–51.
14. Anila A Surgical Site Infection in Obstetrics Practice. J Surg Pakistan Int. 2013;18(2):68-69.
15. Piret M, Katrin L, Aira P, et al. Surgical-site infections following cesarean section .National center for biotechnology. Med J. 2005;26:5.
16. Nada AA, Jehan MA, Muayed MY, et al. Significant reduction in the post cesarean delivery surgical site infection rate after use of prophylactic antibiotics in Madinah Maternity hospital, Saudi Arabia. Life Sci J. 2014;11(7): 833–9.
17. Dhar H, Al-Busaidi, Rathi B et. al. A study of post-caesarean section wound infections in a regional referral hospital, Oman. Sultan Qaboos Univ Med J. 2014; 14(2):212-3.
18. Wloch C, Wilson J, Lamagni T, et.al. Risk factors for surgical site infection following caesarean section in England: international Journal of Obstetrics and Gynecology © RCOG. BJOG. 2012,119(11):1324–33.
19. Onyema AO, Comfort NA, Ifeanyichukwu UE, et al. Determinants of post-caesarean wound infection in Nnewi, Nigeria. Brit J Med Med Res. 2015;5(6): 767–74.
20. Shrestha S, Shrestha R, Shrestha B, et al. Incidence and Risk Factors of Surgical Site Infection Following Cesarean Section at Dhulikhel Hospital. Kathmandu Univ Med J. 2014;46(2):113–6.
21. Filbert JM, Stephen EM, Mariam MM et. al. Incidence and predictors of surgical site infections following caesarean sections at Bugando Medical Centre, Tanzania. 2014; 3(25). Published online 2014 Aug 11. doi: https://doi.org/10.1186/2047-2994-3-25. PMCID: PMC4131772.
22. Kathryn CR, Miguel T. Title Original Scientific Report. World J Surg. 2015; 39(2):350–5.

12

'If I do 10–15 normal deliveries in a month I hardly ever sleep at home.' A qualitative study of health providers' reasons for high rates of caesarean deliveries in private sector maternity care in Delhi, India

Alison Peel[1], Abhishek Bhartia[2], Neil Spicer[3] and Meenakshi Gautham[3*]

Abstract

Background: Although the overall rate of caesarean deliveries in India remains low, rates are higher in private than in public facilities. In a household survey in Delhi, for instance, more than half of women delivering in private facilities reported a caesarean section. Evidence suggests that not all caesarean sections are clinically necessary and may even increase morbidity. We present providers' perspectives of the reasons behind the high rates of caesarean births in private facilities, and possible solutions to counter the trend.

Methods: Fourteen in-depth interviews were conducted with high-end private sector obstetricians and other allied providers in Delhi and its neighbouring cities, Gurgaon and Ghaziabad.

Results: Respondents were of the common view that private sector caesarean rates were unreasonably high and perceived time and doctors' convenience as the foremost reasons. Financial incentives had an indirect effect on decision-making. Obstetricians felt that they must maintain high patient loads to be commercially successful. Many alluded to their busy working lives, which made it challenging for them to monitor every delivery individually. Besides fearing for patient safety in these situations, they were fearful of legal action if anything went wrong. A lack of context specific guidelines and inadequate support from junior staff and nurses exacerbated these problems. Maternal demand also played a role, as the consumer-provider relationship in private healthcare incentivised obstetricians to fulfil patient demands for caesarean section. Suggested solutions included more support, from either well-trained midwives and junior staff or using a 'shared practice' model; guidelines introduced by an Indian body; increased regulation within the sector and public disclosure of providers' caesarean rates.

Conclusions: Commercial interests contribute indirectly to high caesarean rates, as solo obstetricians juggle the need to maintain high patient loads with inadequate support staff. Perceptions amongst providers and consumers of caesarean section as the 'safe' option have re-defined caesareans as the new 'normal', even for low-risk deliveries. At the policy level, guidelines and public disclosures, strong initiatives to develop professional midwifery, and increasing public awareness, could bring about a sustainable reduction in the present high rates.

Keywords: Caesarean section rates, Private sector, Qualitative interviews, Delhi, India

* Correspondence: Meenakshi.gautham@lshtm.ac.uk
[3]Department of Global Health and Development, Faculty of Public Health and Policy, London School of Hygiene and Tropical Medicine, London, UK
Full list of author information is available at the end of the article

Background

Caesarean section can be a life-saving intervention during deliveries where the mother or baby is at significant risk of adverse outcome. Many high maternal mortality regions struggle to provide safe and timely caesarean sections in such circumstances [1], yet women worldwide are increasingly undergoing procedures for which there is little clinical justification [2]. These 'unnecessary' caesarean sections have been associated with increased maternal risk of severe morbidity and even mortality [3, 4]. High rates of caesarean sections also have economic repercussions on patients and their families, as financial costs for the procedure are higher than for vaginal birth and a longer period of hospitalization is necessary. This is especially true in low- and middle-income countries where medical care is often purchased 'out-of-pocket' [5]. It is widely accepted, including by the World Health Organization (WHO), that caesarean deliveries should only be undertaken where medically necessary [3, 4, 6, 7].

Caesarean section rates vary widely across the globe, ranging from as low as 1% in parts of Sub-Saharan Africa to 30% in the USA and 45% in Brazil [5]. Following debate over the most appropriate rates of caesarean sections at national and regional levels, the WHO issued a statement in 2015 recommending that every effort should be made to provide caesarean sections to women *in need,* rather than striving to achieve specific population-level rates [6]. At the facility-level, it is recommended the 'Robson classification' system be used as it allows for comparison of caesarean rates within and across different risk groups of women [6, 8].

A wide variety of explanations have been proposed for rising caesarean rates, ranging from medical and demographic factors to changing patient expectations and provider practices. Repeat caesareans are an important contributor to high rates, as previous caesarean delivery pre-empts need for the procedure in successive deliveries. The risk of morbidity increases with each procedure [9].

Studies in multiple settings have found high rates of caesarean sections associated with non-medical factors. Higher caesarean rates are consistently associated with delivery by private providers, and thus have often been linked to financial incentives [10–19]. Research in private facilities has also shown that both planned and unplanned caesarean sections, including some emergency ones, are more likely to occur on weekdays or during daylight hours [20–22]. It is possible that elective procedures account for many of these daytime caesareans, and that some emergency caesareans may be held over until day staff come on duty, rested and alert, to ensure better outcomes. However, these studies [20–22] also suggest that physician factors, including convenient timing of deliveries and desire for increased leisure time, are significant predictors of caesarean sections. Obstetricians' fears of complaints and legal action have also been indicated as determinants of caesarean delivery [23–27], and it has been suggested that providers perceive fewer risks, both legal and medical, associated with caesarean versus vaginal deliveries [4, 26]. Another concept frequently cited in literature is the influence of patient-related factors, such as maternal request for caesarean section. Maternal demand could be motivated by a number of non-medical factors including fear of vaginal birth, need for control, and cultural acceptability of the procedure [28]. One study in the UK suggested that doctors perceived maternal request as the most important factor driving caesarean rates, although few actually reported receiving a large number of requests or performing caesareans on request themselves [26].

The Indian context

India has made significant progress in improving maternal health, with the current maternal mortality ratio almost half of what it was in 2000 [29]. As mortality rates fall and increasing numbers of women gain access to formally trained maternity care providers, improving quality of care is becoming a priority for policy-makers. Indeed, some data suggest that quality of care is generally poor, though variable, in both the public and private healthcare sectors [30]. The private sector currently accounts for more than 70% of primary healthcare in India following rapid growth in recent decades [31]. This expansion has been accompanied by very little regulation or quality assurance, and insufficient standardisation of treatments, protocols and pricing. Private medical insurance is becoming increasingly common, although a large proportion of people still pay for care 'out-of-pocket' and are vulnerable to financial impoverishment if they require expensive surgeries or medication [32].

Private providers play a significant role in maternity care in India, accounting for 48% of institutional childbirths in urban areas and 24% in rural areas [31]. In Delhi, as in many other large cities in India, the vast majority of deliveries in the private sector are undertaken by obstetricians, who typically operate fee-for-service solo practices. There is very little practice of midwifery in urban hospitals and obstetricians often assume the role of the primary carer during deliveries, with limited support from other healthcare staff, especially midwives [33]. The size and structure of private sector facilities varies widely, from small nursing homes to large hospitals that are part of multi-national corporate chains [14].

Although the overall rate of caesarean deliveries in India is around 17%, rates have risen rapidly over the last ten years from 8.5% in 2005–06 to 17.2% in 2015–16 [34], driven particularly by increases in the private sector and in urban areas. Data collected over 2 years in the city of Chennai in south India indicated a caesarean rate of 47% in private healthcare [18]. Other studies have reported that women in the states of Kerala, Goa, Andhra Pradesh, Bihar, Gujarat, Karnataka, Punjab, Uttar Pradesh, Delhi, Maharashtra, and Tamil Nadu are far more likely to deliver by caesarean if they receive private care [11, 13, 15]. A community-based household survey indicated that 54% of women delivering in the private sector in Delhi underwent caesarean section, compared with a 24% rate in the public sector [14]. Although rates were not classified according to women's risk-status, this figure appears to indicate overuse of the procedure.

A small number of studies have presented data that begin to explain *why* caesarean section rates in the Indian private sector are higher than in the public sector. An analysis of supplier-induced demand in Madhya Pradesh and Gujarat [35] found that direct economic incentives led to increases in caesarean rates whilst financial disincentives led to decreasing rates. This suggests that private obstetricians induce maternal demand for caesarean section due to profit-making motives. Other studies have identified a positive correlation between maternal educational level and likelihood of caesarean delivery in private facilities, suggesting that maternal demand also plays a role, particularly amongst women with a higher level of education [15, 17]. Despite these findings, one of the studies [15] suggests that rising rates of caesarean delivery are more a result of supply factors (relating to the obstetrician) than maternal demand.

A number of studies reporting high rates of caesarean sections in the private healthcare sector in India have hypothesized that these reflect financial incentives, time pressures, the custom of solo practice, fear of litigation, maternal request, and use of intensive foetal monitoring [13, 14, 18]. However, it was not within the remit of the studies to test these hypotheses, and so the evidence remains lacking. No studies have explored providers' perspectives of the reasons for high caesarean rates in their private practices in India. The small quantity of data generated in other settings, especially high-income countries, may not be applicable to the Indian private sector. Our study sought to explore the perspectives of private healthcare professionals involved in maternity care in Delhi on reasons for high caesarean section rates, and solutions to reverse the trend of high rates in private maternity care in Delhi. The study is among the first to explore provider-side perspectives on this issue in the Indian setting.

Methods

Study setting

The study was located in Delhi and its neighbouring suburbs of Gurgaon and Ghaziabad, all in the National Capital Region (NCR) of India. Maternity care is delivered by a wide range of private and public facilities that vary greatly in size, structure, and staffing arrangements in these three settings. There are more than 560 private hospitals and nursing homes in Delhi alone [36]. Women of high socio-economic status are more likely to pay for private maternity care, with more than 80% attending private facilities. A substantial proportion of middle and low socio-economic status women (40 and 16%, respectively) also opt for private maternity care. Caesarean sections are more common in private facilities, where the rate is 54% compared with 24% in the public sector [14]. Our study focused on private maternity care providers in this setting. We collaborated with a private medical hospital and research institute based in South Delhi.

Study design

Fourteen in-depth qualitative interviews were conducted during July and August 2015. We approached key informants who could offer insights from the perspective of a private sector maternity care provider. To get an all-round providers' perspective, we purposively selected practicing obstetricians and a small number of other healthcare professionals with involvement in maternity care - two paediatricians, the manager of a private maternity hospital and a 'doula' or birth companion, who is professionally trained to provide physical, emotional and educational support to the mother. This gave us the opportunity to compare and contrast the perspectives of obstetricians with those of other professionals with good knowledge of the sector.

The majority of study participants worked in South Delhi, with an additional participant working in East Delhi and two in other cities in the NCR, Gurgaon and Ghaziabad. As the sector is highly diverse, we selected providers from secondary and tertiary facilities of different sizes, with capacity for performing caesarean sections: small hospitals or nursing homes (< 50 beds), medium-sized hospitals (50–150 beds), and a large corporate hospital (> 150 beds). These included a mix of multi-specialty and super specialty private hospitals where a normal delivery can cost upwards of INR 40,000 (US$ 615), and a caesarean section in a super luxury room can be priced as high as INR 12,00,000 (US$ 18,461). These were amongst the more high-end private hospitals in the NCR, serving the wealthiest socio-economic sections of the population, who would typically seek only private sector maternity care.

With the help of our collaborating research institute, we drew up an initial list of 19 potential respondents and contacted them for interviews. Ten agreed to an interview during the period that the primary researcher was available, and with the help of these respondents, we identified and interviewed an additional four who agreed.

The interviews were conducted using an interview guide that explored participants' professional status and background, perceptions of current caesarean section rates in the private sector, awareness of guidelines regarding rates, reasons they attributed to high rates, and their suggested solutions for reducing rates.

Confidentiality was maintained by conducting the interviews in private rooms at participants' workplaces or homes. Interviews were audio-recorded where permission was given. In the case of three participants where permission was not given, detailed hand-written notes were taken. All interviews were carried out in English by a single interviewer.

Analysis

All audio-recorded interviews were transcribed. Transcripts and interview notes were coded manually using a coding frame developed both from concepts that emerged in the data and those found in the existing literature, for example financial incentives. Data were organised into matrices for each major topic to help systematize analysis, identify patterns in the data, and compare participants. A final list of key themes and sub-themes emerging from interviews was identified.

Results

Perceptions of caesarean rates in Delhi private sector

Most respondents were of the view that caesarean section rates in the private maternity homes they visited were unjustifiably high and that a substantial proportion of procedures were performed without clear medical need. Two obstetricians believed that rates could be as high as 90% in the different hospitals where they practiced. Others cited rates of 15–50% in their facilities. Most respondents acknowledged that, as high caesarean section rates were rarely discussed within the healthcare community, practitioners were unlikely to know precise facility-level or even personal rates and little self-auditing occurred in private hospitals.

> "It's not part of the Indian medical environment right now to really critically analyse their outcomes and compare it to standards." (Hospital chief executive)

Reasons for high rates of caesarean sections

Three groups of themes emerged in our analysis of participants' explanations for high caesarean rates in the Delhi and NCR private sector: provider-related, system-related, and patient-related factors. These are presented in the following sections.

Provider-related factors

Personal convenience The majority of respondents said that providers' convenience, in terms of time spent and timing of deliveries, was the most important consideration for doctors. Vaginal deliveries could involve more than 12 h of labour and occur at inconvenient times, particularly during the night. Caesareans allowed doctors to exercise control over the duration and timing of delivery so that they had more time for personal and professional activities.

> "One normal delivery costs me at least a night, sometimes 2 nights. If I do 10-15 normal deliveries in a month I hardly ever sleep at home. If I do 15 caesareans I'm not home late for coffee." (Private sector obstetrician)

Concerns about decision-making Many respondents spoke about the pressure of an obstetrician's demanding workload, which meant that doctors were unable to commit their full attention to every delivery because they were pre-occupied by other concerns or a lack of sleep. This could affect decision-making regarding deliveries.

> "Supposing one is awake the whole night for 2 days, the third night one will have a tendency to take weak decisions." (Private sector obstetrician)

Another common theme was the pressure of having sole responsibility for a delivery (due to the norm of working alone), and having to make difficult, subjective decisions about the safest option for a patient.

> "Decision-making is very tough. For caesarean anybody can make decision, but how long you have to wait for a normal delivery is very difficult to assess". (Private sector obstetrician)

Some spoke about fearing for the safety of patients and their babies during deliveries. This fear could lead them to decide in favour of a caesarean section earlier than necessary.

> "Whatever I was trained in just goes away...suddenly I think I have to give her a live baby" (Private sector obstetrician)

Fear of legal action by patients emerged as another important challenge to doctors' decision-making. Respondents explained that, according to the existing laws, if anything goes wrong the sole legal responsibility lies with the obstetrician. Therefore, they considered caesarean as the safer option for avoiding litigation, as one described it, a caesarean was *"a more comfortable and assured path..."* (Private sector obstetrician).

Some respondents suggested that use of technologies such as 'cardiotocography' machines for continuous foetal heart rate monitoring could also be increasing the frequency of decisions for caesarean deliveries. They described doctors panicking or becoming *"hyper"* when they saw decelerations in foetal heartrate, leading them to perform a caesarean section even though the labour may have progressed normally.

Training and continuing medical education Some interviewees explained that waiting for normal labour to progress might seem counterintuitive to doctors because of the training they have received. They argued that doctors are trained for pathological events and therefore they are predisposed to intervene, even during a physiologically normal birth.

> "Doctors are not trained for sitting and watching and waiting, they are trained to intervene...they are people who need to jump in when something is going wrong" (Private sector paediatrician)

Aside from this, the providers interviewed thought that the initial training for obstetrics was adequate, although some expressed concern about obstetricians not updating themselves on current knowledge later in their careers. Although interviewees stated that continuing medical education was available for obstetricians, they indicated that many would not attend due to heavy workloads, or a perceived lack of need for additional training.

> "Most of us don't do trainings, we just run our own clinics and the basic idea is the financial situation is fine, and if you're sensible enough, then you don't do any harm to your patients" (Private sector obstetrician)

Respondents believed that, due to a lack of continuing medical education, some obstetricians were unaware of current evidence-based guidelines and performed unnecessary caesareans as a result.

Non-compliance with guidelines was also an issue. Many obstetricians reported working in hospitals where a set of standard guidelines were available. However, one protested that there is little compulsion for visiting consultants to follow guidelines.

> "You cannot enforce the guidelines on them... if we force them they will not bring the patient to the hospital, so hospital will lose those number of clients." (Private sector obstetrician)

As we report further on, respondents also expressed concerns over a lack of guidelines that were appropriate to the setting.

In addition, it emerged that many obstetricians associated little risk with caesarean deliveries. Respondents spoke about caesareans having become routine procedures, with doctors thinking of them as *"no big deal"*. Nevertheless, they also described adverse consequences associated with medically unindicated caesarean sections and believed that all obstetricians would be aware of these from their training. One respondent attempted to explain the disparity between these viewpoints:

> "We all know what we're doing, but of course the mind is between knowing and using that knowledge" (Professor of obstetrics).

Some respondents reasoned that a vaginal delivery may appear more risky to obstetricians as there were more 'unknowns' compared with a caesarean section.

Commercial interests A few respondents mentioned financial incentives as a reason for high caesarean section rates in the private sector. However, they placed less weight on this than the other reasons. This could be because they felt uncomfortable admitting to monetary incentives in interviews, or because the financial benefits of caesarean deliveries affected them only indirectly.

Many respondents referred to hospitals, rather than individual doctors, being financially motivated. Several described how, in their experience, corporate hospitals were often run in a way where doctors were encouraged to take on as many patients as possible in order to generate revenue.

> "[Hospitals] see the business that you are doing. They will not see how many caesareans or normal deliveries you're doing...the doctor is under pressure to have more patients because that's her power, her importance in the institution is what she brings to the hospital." (Private sector obstetrician)

It was also reported that patients paid more for caesarean than vaginal delivery, due to additional charges for operating theatre rent, anaesthetists, and other necessary arrangements. Some suggested that these dis-incentivised facilities to decrease caesarean rates.

> "Hospitals earn about 30-50% more revenue as the result of a caesarean delivery compared to a normal delivery. And almost all of the additional revenue is additional margin. So, hospitals have a clear financial incentive to not mind a high caesarean section rate." (Hospital chief executive)

In contrast, some other interviewees were insistent that commercial incentives played no part in doctors' decisions to perform caesarean sections.

> "No no no no no! ...the charges [fees charged by doctors] for caesarean and normal delivery are almost at one. So that is never a reason." (Private sector obstetrician)

This assertion that doctors' fee for both modes of delivery were the same or very similar was reiterated by several respondents. Many emphasised that obstetricians *"don't do it for money but to save time".*

> "An obstetrician would rather do a caesarean and go and save time, maximise the benefit of the time spent to do more deliveries, see more OPD patients." (Private sector paediatrician)

Even those who believed that financial incentives played a role stated that time was a more important factor. However, this was put into perspective by one obstetrician who pointed out that by attending to more patients in less time doctors could take on more clients and thus generate more revenue.

Furthermore, a number of other respondents indicated that the commercial nature of the private health sector's commercial nature prevents providers from lowering their caesarean rates. Doctors and hospital executives are compelled to maximise the number of patients they receive as it directly determines their income.

> "If you want to do always what is right for the patient but you reward clinicians on volumes there's a misalignment." (Hospital chief executive)

As obstetricians were unlikely to turn patients away even if their workload was high, there was always great pressure on their time. This was especially likely for doctors visiting multiple hospitals, as one respondent described of an obstetrician she knew:

> "She did clinics and had women waiting in labour at all of the hospitals. She was getting calls continuously. It's that sort of life, very hectic. That will increase caesarean rates." (Private sector paediatrician)

The norm of solo practice in the sector exacerbated this problem, as obstetricians could not rely on other doctors to assist them when they were short of time, unlike in a 'shared' practice.

System-related factors

Some interviewees believed that the structure of the private sector could be partially to blame for high caesarean rates. They emphasised lack of regulation as an important systemic factor. There were no government requirements for reporting on maternity care in the private sector, and some believed that this could be a reason for high rates.

> "If I'm an obstetrician with a 70% caesarean rate I can go on that way for the next 30 years. Nobody will find out." (Hospital chief executive)

Many respondents believed that obstetricians would be less likely to perform unnecessary caesareans if they knew their practice was being monitored.

Some respondents also pointed to the lack of clinical guidelines for making decisions about caesarean sections issued by an Indian body. Indeed, several obstetricians reported using guidelines from other countries and some expressed concern about their use in an Indian setting. Others mentioned that the Federation of Obstetric and Gynaecological Societies of India issues a limited number of guidelines relating to caesarean sections, but these were not comprehensive and awareness of them was low amongst obstetricians.

Poor support systems were also cited as a cause of high caesarean rates. Respondents said that the standards of support from junior and nursing staff in the private sector varied greatly.

> "The nurses are not trained in midwifery, they are not taking part in the antenatal period...I think they are underutilised, which is a big problem" (Private sector obstetrician)

One obstetrician explained that *"...as a result* [of poor support], *all of the decision-making responsibility flows straight up to the consultant" (private sector obstetrician),* highlighting the additional pressure on doctors caused by these inadequate support systems.

Patient-related factors

Respondents reported that caesareans frequently occur because of patient demand, sometimes scheduled beforehand, but often requested during the process of labour. Many expressed that caesarean sections were perceived as the 'normal' mode of delivery amongst women.

> "Caesarean has become the new normal. Chances are my friends, my mum, more people that I know have had caesarean deliveries rather than normal deliveries." (Hospital chief executive)

Respondents perceived that women viewed caesarean as an *"easy way out"* of the pain of labour, and spoke about women hearing accounts of traumatic experiences, through either word of mouth or the media, which led them to request caesarean deliveries. A couple of respondents also observed a link between fear of labour and women's bodies, saying that this led to the body not responding well to natural birth, so that a caesarean was necessary. Other patient-related factors included the convenience of a *"short-cut"* delivery and desire to schedule deliveries on auspicious dates.

Some respondents expressed concern about the sources from which patients obtained their information on deliveries, which they perceived to be primarily peer groups and family. Several stated that women did not fully understand the risks of a caesarean delivery, or that women perceived caesarean to be a safer choice than normal delivery. Many thought that counselling of patients by doctors, where the relative risks and benefits of delivery methods were explained, was often insufficient or entirely lacking.

Obstetricians often agreed to patients' demands and performed caesareans even though they were not medically necessary. This was attributed to the time and effort required to change a patient's mind.

> "The easiest approach is that I do what the patient is saying...the more I try to explain the more time is used...I might as well give her a date for caesarean in 5 minutes" (Private sector obstetrician)

Others spoke about patients who insisted on a caesarean delivery in spite of counselling, and felt that they could not *"force"* a woman to have a natural delivery. Some respondents said that patients' families put pressure on doctors to intervene during labour. Consumer-provider type relationships in the private sector implied that obstetricians were willing to satisfy patients' demands for caesarean sections. If they refused to perform a procedure the patient could easily go to a doctor who was more willing, and this would result in loss of patients. *"It's a demand and supply kind of thing"* said one private sector obstetrician, emphasising that private sector clients have more power to make demands than in the public sector because they are paying customers.

In addition to ideas about patient's expectations and choices, interviewees spoke about lifestyle changes, such as women having babies later in life or being more sedentary and overweight, which were related to the higher socio-economic status of patients using the private sector. Previous caesareans were another reason, as women were likely to require a caesarean section if they had had one previously, due to the increased risks of complications. One interviewee stated that vaginal birth after caesarean was *"almost zero"* in the private sector in Delhi.

Possible solutions to high caesarean rates

The most frequently mentioned solution was improved counselling by doctors, in order to reduce patient demand for caesareans.

> "Shaping women's attitudes and behaviour is a very important aspect of this challenge if we actually want to solve the caesarean problem." (Hospital chief executive)

Many respondents called for better education of pregnant women about the vaginal delivery process, the risks associated with caesarean sections, and maximising the chances of a natural delivery. This would help women cope with labour pains and could be imparted during existing sessions, such as antenatal workshops.

Acknowledging the present lack of guidelines, several respondents suggested that standardised evidence-based guidelines, issued by an Indian body and tailored to the Indian setting, would be effective in reducing caesarean rates. They expressed that guidelines should be introduced at the institutional level at the least, and that doctors should be encouraged to follow them. One obstetrician, who managed the mother and child unit of a hospital, stated that introducing standard guidelines had been the most effective method for lowering numbers of caesarean deliveries in their facility.

A number of respondents believed that regulation would be important for enforcing these guidelines. Some suggested the possibility of a higher-level regulatory body auditing caesarean rates and imposing penalties where unnecessary procedures were being performed. Others thought that promoting transparency could begin to tackle the problem.

> "If, as part of a professional code of conduct, I was required to disclose it [my caesarean rate], now suddenly women would know...there would be an incentive for everyone in the system to start rectifying the situation." (Hospital chief executive)

Another solution was to improve support for obstetricians from other medical staff. Respondents emphasised that nurses should receive training to provide more 'hands-on' support during labour. Some respondents suggested an expanded role for midwives as the primary carers in low-risk deliveries. A counter argument was that patients in private hospitals might not feel comfortable if they were attended by a midwife rather than a doctor. Therefore, an additional suggestion for improving support was the idea of 'shared practice', where obstetricians could rely on each other for help with decision-making and performing deliveries.

Discussion

The present study identifies a number of important factors that may be driving high rates of caesarean sections in the private healthcare sector in Delhi and its neighbourhood. The rates reported by some respondents for facilities where they practiced varied from 15 to 50%, and a small number reported rates as high as 90%. As self- or facility-level auditing of caesarean sections was not commonly practiced in these facilities, these rates may be considered as estimates rather than precise figures. Even so, the figure of 50% is comparable to rates reported by two household surveys in Delhi: the National Family Health Survey-4 [34] that reported 43% caesarean births in the private sector and another household survey conducted at a similar time [14] that found 54% caesarean section births in the private sector. The higher rate of 90% reported by a small number of our respondents could be more facility specific and indicative of the substantial variation likely to exist across facilities. Similar variation can be seen in reported rates ranging from 50 to 99% in a study of private health facilities providing delivery care in the state of Uttar Pradesh, which borders Delhi [37].

The respondents we interviewed were generally of the opinion that unnecessary use of caesarean sections was an important issue in this sector. Key contributors were identified as: obstetrician convenience and time pressures, particularly owing to the high prevalence of solo obstetric practice; a perception of caesarean deliveries as the 'safe' option, both in terms of maternal health and protection from litigation; and financial pressures associated with running a successful clinic, or working for a commercial hospital. Other important reasons for high rates of caesarean deliveries included system-related factors, especially the lack of comprehensive guidelines tailored to the Indian setting, and lack of well-trained support staff such as midwives, as well as patient-related factors such as maternal and family related fears and demands. Interestingly, none of our respondents mentioned emergency referrals from smaller, more poorly-equipped private facilities or from government facilities as an important reason for the high caesarean rates. In a recent study in Uttar Pradesh [37], emergency referrals for caesarean sections were commonly reported by secondary and tertiary private facilities located on the outskirts of big cities and in smaller urban centres. Our study sample was quite different from these types of peri-urban facilities. Our respondents were all located within a metropolis, where most delivery facilities, private as well as public, have the capacity for performing caesarean sections and do not need to refer frequently. Moreover, the clientele at these facilities belonged to the wealthiest socio-economic groups who could afford pregnancy and delivery care at the best equipped private facilities from the very beginning.

Although respondents gave a variety of reasons for high caesarean rates, many of these can be retraced to the commercial nature of private sector practice that incentivises growing practices even to the point that time pressures interfere with the ability to provide quality care. Obstetricians must maintain their patient loads in order to run commercially viable practices, leading to immense pressures on their time. They must protect their patients from any adverse outcomes, and themselves from litigation. It is not possible to monitor every delivery to its normal conclusion, and so obstetricians may opt for caesarean deliveries in order to ensure patient safety and sufficient time to attend to all of their patients. As a result, caesarean section has come to be considered as the 'safe' option, in spite of the associated risks. A culture amongst obstetricians of performing caesarean sections, where 'caesarean is seen as the new normal,' reinforces this perception and may prevent providers from recognising high caesarean rates as abnormal or harmful. Furthermore, inadequate support systems, including very limited practice of midwifery in India, increase time pressures on obstetricians and the difficulty of decision-making regarding deliveries.

Maternal and family requests for caesarean section were also identified as a driver of caesarean rates. Providers perceived a culture where caesarean sections are considered an 'easy' option among women using private sector facilities. The apparent frequency with which obstetricians fulfil patients' requests for caesarean section reflects the provider-consumer type exchange between doctors and patients due to the commercial nature of their relationship. Doctors may feel obliged to fulfil patients' demands or refrain from taking a hard line during patient counselling in order to avoid losing that patient. Our data suggest that some women who request caesarean deliveries receive insufficient counselling regarding the associated risks, likely due to the pressures on obstetricians' time. Respondents did, however, identify physical factors, such as women postponing pregnancy until later in life or being overweight because they were leading more sedentary lifestyles, as a cause of rising caesarean rates, particularly amongst the high socio-economic status women who use private healthcare.

A lack of guidelines and regulation regarding caesarean sections amplify the effects of rising caesarean section rates, as obstetricians and institutions are not held accountable for their rates. The Indian government's most recent guidelines for dealing with obstetric complications were issued in 2005. These detail the complications for which a caesarean section may be necessary, but no thresholds for caesarean section are given and few associated risks are mentioned [38].

The solutions that respondents offered for reducing caesarean section rates reinforce these explanations. They suggested that the level of support from junior and nursing/midwifery staff be improved, by either expanding the roles of support staff or encouraging small groups of obstetricians to work in 'shared practice,' providing professional support to one another where necessary. Expanding the role of midwives to be the primary carers during normal deliveries, with support from obstetricians only when complications occur, could significantly reduce the time pressures on doctors and thus help avoid unnecessary caesareans. Unfortunately, midwifery remains an under-developed and under-recognised profession in India [33], with neither legislative support nor training standards for independent midwifery. The currently available training in midwifery, which is limited to a few months and combined with more general nursing training, has been found inadequate for preparing confident and competent midwives [39]. Greater policy support is required to promote midwifery in India, although this is likely to be met with initial resistance from providers and patients who are accustomed to doctors being present throughout the delivery. Other suggestions were that comprehensive caesarean section guidelines be made available from an Indian medical body, and that individual and institutional caesarean section rates undergo auditing and regulation. Some form of peer review within the sector, or regulation by an external body, could help to improve obstetricians' awareness of their own rates and incentivise them to only perform procedures in cases where they are truly necessary.

The present study adds depth to the current understanding of high caesarean rates in the Indian private sector. Our findings support results from previous studies both in Indian and non-Indian settings, which emphasise obstetrician time and convenience factors [20–22], fear of litigation [23–27], financial incentives [10–19], perceptions of low risk [4, 26], and maternal demand [26, 28] as important reasons for high caesarean section rates. In addition, the present study identifies some previously undocumented factors that may contribute to high caesarean rates in the Indian setting: a lack of appropriate guidelines on caesarean sections, and the culture of private sector obstetricians working in solo practice, often with insufficient support systems, particularly well-trained midwives. Furthermore, our analysis highlights the 'missing' link between caesarean sections and obstetricians' high practice volumes as a result of financial incentives in the private sector.

Limitations

The small sample size of this study, due to resource constraints and the difficulties in accessing busy obstetricians and other maternity healthcare providers, limits its generalisability. Our sample was also mostly limited to the higher end obstetricians and multi-speciality/super-specialty private hospitals that cater to wealthier, urban clients that can afford to pay a high fee for institutional deliveries in big city hospitals. The situation in smaller, less expensive private hospitals in peri urban and rural areas is likely to be quite different and needs to be explored through other studies. Another limitation was that we could not access any documented data on caesarean rates from the facilities and, therefore, the rates we present here are reported estimates. However, it is unlikely that this information would have been available in many cases, as the respondents themselves reported that little self-auditing occurred amongst providers. We have also shown that the estimates are comparable to rates reported in the published literature. Finally, we did not interview any patients in this study, as our focus was on providers' perceptions. Patients' perceptions could be very different, and especially useful for understanding the extent to which maternal requests play a role in this setting. Nonetheless, the providers' perceptions reported in this article are a valuable addition to the literature. We have reached out to an important and challenging group of providers and gathered rich and in-depth insights on a sensitive topic that will be useful for exploring caesarean reduction strategies, and designing further research around this important topic.

Conclusions

A complex relationship exists between high caesarean rates and the commercial nature of the private sector. Although there may be no direct link between providers' decisions for a caesarean section and financial gain, obstetric practice in the private sector is dependent on maintaining high patient loads. This can lead to doctors taking on more patients than they can feasibly manage, and opting for caesarean deliveries in order to ensure patient safety, as well as protection from litigation.

Reducing high rates of caesarean deliveries in the Delhi private sector will depend on the introduction of comprehensive caesarean section guidelines, including indications and thresholds for which the procedure should be performed, and public disclosure of the caesarean rate for individual obstetricians and hospitals. However, regulations and guidelines may be insufficient without a parallel strengthening of professional midwifery support for obstetricians, before, during and after childbirth, and improved patient counselling and awareness. As India's most prominent obstetric body, the Federation of Obstetrics and Gynaecological Societies of India could play an important role in steering a comprehensive and sustainable caesarean reduction strategy in the higher end private sector in India.

Abbreviations

NCR: National Capital Region; UK: United Kingdom; USA: United States of America; WHO: World Health Organization

Acknowledgements

We are grateful to all the healthcare providers who participated in the study and to Sitaram Bhartia for facilitating the study.

Funding

AP received student funding for travel and fieldwork from the London School of Hygiene and Tropical Medicine. MG was AP's student supervisor, and India

Country Coordinator of LSHTM's IDEAS project. This work was supported by IDEAS-Informed Decisions for Actions to improve maternal and newborn health (https://ideas.lshtm.ac.uk/) which is funded through a grant from the Bill and Melinda Gates Foundation to the London School of Hygiene and Tropical Medicine (Gates Global Health Grant Number: OPP1017031).

Authors' contributions

The study design was developed by AP and MG. AP conducted data collection and initial analysis, with support from MG and AB. AP, MG, NS and AB all had input into the interpretation and presentation of results. AP drafted the initial manuscript with critical inputs from MG. All authors critically reviewed the drafts, offered revisions and approved the final manuscript.

Competing interests

The authors declare that they have no competing interests.

Author details

[1]London School of Hygiene and Tropical Medicine, London, UK. [2]Sitaram Bhartia Institute of Science and Research, New Delhi, India. [3]Department of Global Health and Development, Faculty of Public Health and Policy, London School of Hygiene and Tropical Medicine, London, UK.

References

1. Ronsmans C, Holtz S, Stanton C. Socioeconomic differentials in caesarean rates in developing countries: a retrospective analysis. Lancet. 2006; 368(9546):1516–23.
2. Lavender T, Hofmeyr GJ, Neilson JP, Kingdon C, Gyte GM. Caesarean section for non-medical reasons at term. Cochrane Database Syst Rev. 2012;3(3): CD004660. https://doi.org/10.1002/14651858.CD004660.pub3.
3. Lumbiganon P, Laopaiboon M, Gulmezoglu AM, Souza JP, Taneepanichskul S, Ruyan P, et al. Method of delivery and pregnancy outcomes in Asia: the WHO global survey on maternal and perinatal health 2007-08. Lancet. 2010; 375(9713):490–9.
4. Souza JP, Gulmezoglu A, Lumbiganon P, Laopaiboon M, Carroli G, Fawole B, et al. Caesarean section without medical indications is associated with an increased risk of adverse short-term maternal outcomes: the 2004-2008 WHO global survey on maternal and perinatal health. BMC Med. 2010;8:71.
5. Gibbons LBJ, Lauer JA, Betran AP, Merialdi M, Althabe F. The Global Numbers and Costs of Additionally Needed and Unnecessary Caesarean Sections Performed per Year: Overuse as a Barrier to Universal Coverage. World Health Report Background Paper 30. Geneva: World Health Organization; 2010.
6. World Health Organisation. WHO statement on caesarean section rates. Geneva: WHO; 2015.
7. Vogel JP, Betran AP, Vindevoghel N, Souza JP, Torloni MR, Zhang J, et al. Use of the Robson classification to assess caesarean section trends in 21 countries: a secondary analysis of two WHO multicountry surveys. Lancet Glob Health. 2015;3(5):e260–70.
8. Betrán AP, Vindevoghel N, Souza JP, Gülmezoglu AM, Torloni MR. A systematic review of the Robson classification for caesarean section: what works, Doesn't work and how to improve it. PLoS One. 2014;9(6):e97769.
9. Marshall NE, Fu R, Guise JM. Impact of multiple cesarean deliveries on maternal morbidity: a systematic review. Am J Obstet Gynecol. 2011;205(3):262.e1–8.
10. Gomes UA, Silva AA, Bettiol H, Barbieri MA. Risk factors for the increasing caesarean section rate in Southeast Brazil: a comparison of two birth cohorts, 1978-1979 and 1994. Int J Epidemiol. 1999;28(4):687–94.
11. Padmadas SS, Kumar S, Nair SB, Kumari A. Caesarean section delivery in Kerala, India: evidence from a National Family Health Survey. Soc Sci Med. 2000;51(4):511–21.
12. Phadungkiatwattana P, Tongsakul N. Analyzing the impact of private service on the cesarean section rate in public hospital Thailand. Arch Gynecol Obstet. 2011;284(6):1375–9.
13. Mishra US, Ramanathan M. Delivery-related complications and determinants of caesarean section rates in India. Health Policy Plan. 2002;17(1):90–8.
14. Nagpal J, Sachdeva A, Sengupta Dhar R, Bhargava VL, Bhartia A. Widespread non-adherence to evidence-based maternity care guidelines: a population-based cluster randomised household survey. BJOG. 2015;122(2):238–47.
15. Leone T. Demand and supply factors affecting the rising overmedicalization of birth in India. Int J Gynaecol Obstet. 2014;127:157–62.
16. Roberts CL, Tracy S, Peat B. Rates for obstetric intervention among private and public patients in Australia: population based descriptive study. BMJ. 2000;321(7254):137–41.
17. Neuman M, Alcock G, Azad K, Kuddus A, Osrin D, More NS, et al. Prevalence and determinants of caesarean section in private and public health facilities in underserved south Asian communities: cross-sectional analysis of data from Bangladesh. India and Nepal BMJ Open. 2014;4(12):e005982.
18. Sreevidya S, Sathiyasekaran BW. High caesarean rates in Madras (India): a population-based cross sectional study. BJOG. 2003;110(2):106–11.
19. Lutomski JE, Murphy M, Devane D, Meaney S, Greene RA. Private health care coverage and increased risk of obstetric intervention. BMC pregnancy and childbirth. 2014;14:13.
20. Brown HS 3rd. Physician demand for leisure: implications for cesarean section rates. J Health Econ. 1996;15(2):233–42.
21. Burns LR, Geller SE, Wholey DR. The effect of physician factors on the cesarean section decision. Med Care. 1995;33(4):365–82.
22. Mossialos E, Allin S, Karras K, Davaki K. An investigation of caesarean sections in three Greek hospitals: the impact of financial incentives and convenience. Eur J Pub Health. 2005;15(3):288–95.
23. Fuglenes D, Oian P, Kristiansen IS. Obstetricians' choice of cesarean delivery in ambiguous cases: is it influenced by risk attitude or fear of complaints and litigation? Am J Obstet Gynecol. 2009;200(1):48.e1–8.
24. Belizan JM, Quaranta P, Paquez E, Villar J. Caesarean section and fear of litigation. Lancet. 1991;338(8780):1462.
25. Minkoff H. Fear of litigation and cesarean section rates. Semin Perinatol. 2012;36(5):390–4.
26. Weaver JJ, Statham H, Richards M. Are there "unnecessary" cesarean sections? Perceptions of women and obstetricians about cesarean sections for nonclinical indications. Birth. 2007;34(1):32–41.
27. Chaillet N, Dube E, Dugas M, Francoeur D, Dube J, Gagnon S, et al. Identifying barriers and facilitators towards implementing guidelines to reduce caesarean section rates in Quebec. Bull World Health Organ. 2007;85(10):791–7.
28. Fuglenes D, Aas E, Botten G, Oian P, Kristiansen IS. Why do some pregnant women prefer cesarean? The influence of parity, delivery experiences, and fear. Am J Obstet Gynecol. 2011;205(1):45.e1–9.
29. WHO, UNFPA, World Bank. Trends in maternal mortality: 1990 to 2013. Geneva: World Health Organisation; 2014.
30. Sharma G, Powell-Jackson T, Haldar K, Bradleya J, Filippi V. Quality of routine essential care during childbirth: clinical observations of uncomplicated births in Uttar Pradesh, India. Bull World Health Organ. 2017;95:419–29.
31. National Sample Survey Organization. Government of India. NSSO 71st round (Jan-Jun 2014). Report no. 574. Ministry of Statistics and Programme Implementation, Government of India: New Delhi; 2016.
32. National Commission on Macroeconomics and Health. Report of the national commission on macroeconomics and health. New Delhi: New Delhi: Ministry of Health and Family Welfare, Government of India; 2005.
33. Kumbhar K. Shunned for years, can trained midwives fix India's maternity mess? Quartz India. 2016. https://qz.com/629132/shunned-for-years-can-trained-midwives-fix-indias-maternity-mess. Accessed 23 March 2018.
34. IIPS. National Family Health Survey-4 (NFHS-4) 2015–16. India Factsheet. Government of India, 2015–16.
35. Bogg L, Diwan V, Vora KS, DeCosta A. Impact of alternative maternal demand-side financial support programs in India on the caesarean section rates: indications of supplier-induced demand. Maternal Child Health J. 2016;20(1):11–5.
36. Government of NCT of Delhi. Delhi Human Development Report 2006. New York, NY: Oxford University Press; 2006.
37. Goodman C, Gautham M, Iles R, Bruxvoort K, Subharwal M, Gupta S, Jain M. The nature of competition faced by private providers of maternal health services in Uttar Pradesh, India. A Report (unpublished). UK: London School of Hygiene and Tropical Medicine; 2017.
38. Guidelines for Pregnancy Care and Management of Common Obstetric Complications by Medical Officers. Maternal Health Division, DoFW, Minsitry of Health and Family Welfare, Government of India, New Delhi; 2005.

13

Prolonged operative time of repeat cesarean is a risk marker for post-operative maternal complications

Misgav Rottenstreich[†], Hen Y. Sela[†], Ori Shen, Rachel Michaelson-Cohen, Arnon Samueloff and Orna Reichman[*]

Abstract

Background: Repeat cesarean delivery (CD) accounts for approximately 15% of all annual deliveries in the US with an estimated 656,250 operations per year. We aimed to study whether prolonged operative time (OT; skin incision to closure) is a risk marker for post-operative maternal complications among women undergoing repeat CD.

Methods: We conducted a cross-sectional retrospective study in a single tertiary center including all women who underwent repeat CD but excluding those with cesarean hysterectomy. Prolonged OT was defined as duration of CD longer than the 90th percentile duration on record for each specific surgeon in order to correct for technique differences between surgeons. Bi-variate analysis was used to study the association of prolonged OT with each one of the following maternal complications: post-operative blood transfusion, prolonged maternal hospitalization (defined as hospitalization duration longer than 1 week post-CD), infection necessitating antibiotics, re-laparotomy within 7 days post-CD, and re-admission within 42 days post-CD. A multivariate regression analysis was performed controlling for maternal age, ethnicity, parity, number of fetus, gestational age at delivery, trial of labor after cesarean, anesthesia, and number of previous CDs. The adjusted odd ratio was calculated for each complication independently and for a composite adverse maternal outcome defined as any one of the above.

Results: A total of 6507 repeat CDs were included; prolonged OT was highly associated (P value < 0.000) with: post-operative blood transfusion (4.4% vs. 1.5%), prolonged hospitalization (8.4% vs. 4.0%), infection necessitating antibiotics (2% vs. 1%), and readmission (1.8% vs. 0.8%) when compared to control. The composite adverse maternal outcome was also associated with prolonged OT (20.2% vs. 11.2%, $p < 0.000$). These correlations remained statistically significant in the multivariate regression analysis when controlling for confounders.

Conclusions: Among women undergoing repeat CD, prolonged OT (reflecting CD duration greater than 90th percentile for the specific surgeon) is a risk marker for post-operative maternal complications.

Keywords: Repeat caesarean deliveries, Post-operative adverse maternal outcome, Operative time

Background

During the last three decades, the decrease in trial of labor after cesarean delivery (TOLAC), has been reflected in an inversely increased fraction of repeat cesarean deliveries (CD) [1, 2].

It is currently estimated that one-third of all CD in the United States are repeated CD and more than 90% of women who undergo CD will have a repeat procedure in subsequent pregnancies [3, 4].

Large observational studies have consistently shown that women who undergo repeat CD are at increased risk of dense adhesions and abnormal placentation [5–10]. These in turn make the surgical procedure and fetal extraction more challenging, prolong the time to delivery, and increase the risk of bowel or bladder injury [11–13] Both dense adhesions and abnormal placentation are associated with massive hemorrhage, disseminated intravascular coagulation, blood products transfusion, admission to

* Correspondence: orna.reich@gmail.com
[†]Misgav Rottenstreich and Hen Y. Sela contributed equally to this work.
Department of Obstetrics and Gynecology, Shaare Zedek Medical Center, Hebrew University, Jerusalem, Israel

intensive care unit (ICU), and in severe cases could result in maternal death [10].

A few studies have been published analyzing the association between CD operative time (OT) and maternal or neonatal complications [11, 14]. However, these studies combined primary and repeat CD and disregarded identification of the primary surgeon, a factor that can potentially influence OT due to differences in techniques between surgeons [15]. We aimed to study OT based on the individual surgeon's historical record of OT and post-operative maternal complications among women undergoing repeat CD. We defined prolonged OT as duration of CD surgery longer than the 90th percentile of that specific surgeon's recorded CD durations. Our primary aim was to ascertain whether there was a correlation between prolonged OT and (1) hemorrhage necessitating post-operative blood transfusion; (2) length of maternal hospitalization (3); infection necessitating administration of antibiotics (4); re-laparotomy within 7 days of CD; and (5) re-admission within 42 days of discharge.

Materials and methods

A retrospective cross sectional study was conducted at Shaare Zedek Medical Centre (SZMC), a university affiliated medical center, managing approximately 10% of all deliveries in Israel, with an average of 13,000 deliveries annually. National Health plans cover antenatal and peripartum care, and most deliveries (> 95%) are managed by this system. The study population included all women who underwent a repeat CD by an obstetrician who had performed at least ≥40 CD at SZMC between June 2005 and December 2014. Since hysterectomies occur in 0.6 cases/ 1000 deliveries and invariably prolong OT as well as being associated with higher maternal morbidity, we excluded all cases of hysterectomies regardless of indication.

The SZMC obstetrical database is continuously updated from the computerized electronic medical records (EMR)which are updated in real-time during labor and delivery. The EMR includes demographic characteristics, medical and obstetric history, and requisite descriptive variables as per the computerized surgical notes, such as inter-pregnancy interval, number of previous CD, elective CD versus TOLAC, type of anesthesia, OT (skin incision to closure), experience of the operating surgeon and presence of a third surgeon. Complications that were studied included (1) clinically significant hemorrhage defined as post-operative blood transfusion; (2) prolonged length of maternal hospitalization defined as length of stay following CD greater than 7 days (departmental protocol mandates discharge on day 5 post-operation); (3) infection necessitating antibiotics [including: Gentamycin, Amoxicillin/Clavulanate potassium, Ciprofloxacin and Cefazolin as markers for endometritis, wound infection, post-operative intra-abdominal infected collections and urinary tract infections]; (4) re-laparotomy within 7 days of the CD; and (5) re-admission within 42 days of discharge.

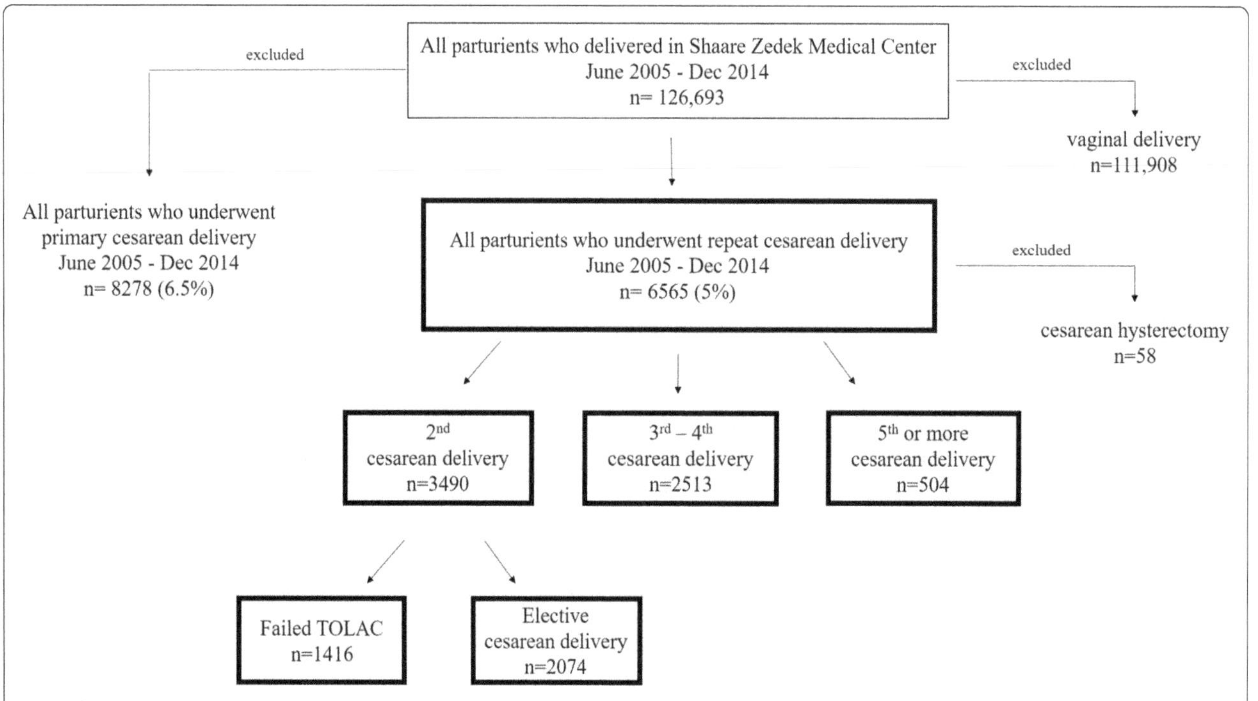

Fig. 1 flow chart of study population

Prolonged CD was defined as surgery where the OT was longer than the 90th percentile of CD durations on record for that specific surgeon. According to department policy an attending must be present at all CD; OT is attributed to the primary surgeon regardless of seniority. Bivariate analysis was performed for testing the association between prolonged CD and categorical variables using the χ^2 or Fisher exact test and continuous variables were analyzed by the Student's t-test as indicated. A multivariate regression analysis was performed controlling for confounders, and adjusted odds ratio were calculated. The sensitivity, specificity, positive and negative predictive value of prolonged OT for each complication and for the composite adverse outcome were calculated. Confidence interval of 95% and P value ≤0.05 were defined as statistically significant. All statistics were performed using the SPSS version 23. The study was approved by the SZMC IRB (# 0260–16).

Table 1 Sociodemographic and obstetrical characteristic of study population, distributed by length of surgery

		Length of cesarean surgery[a]		
		≤ 90th percentile	> 90thpercentile	*P* value
Age		33.0 ± 5.4	33.6 ± 5.3	< 0.000
Education	< 12 years	217 (4.1%)	52 (5.0%)	0.188
Ethnicity	Jew	4721 (86.7%)	894 (84.0%)	0.019
	Arab	722 (13.3%)	170 (16.0%)	
Parity	Multipara 2–5[c]	4150 (76.2%)	772 (72.6%)	0.010
	GMP 6–9	1029 (18.9%)	232 (21.8%)	
	GGMP≥10	264 (4.9%)	60 (5.6%)	
Interval from previous CD (months)[b]	< 12 months	434 (16.3%)	89 (16.5%)	
	12–24	1027 (38.5%)	184 (34.1%)	0.139
	> 24 months[c]	1206 (45.2%)	266 (49.4%)	
Number offetus	singleton	5204 (95.6%)	1032 (97%)	0.039
	multiple pregnancy	239 (4.4%)	32 (3.0%)	
Gestational week	term	4738 (87.1%)	838 (78.8%)	< 0.000
	preterm < 37	704 (12.9%)	226 (21.2%)	
Anesthesia	local	5246 (96.5%)	958 (90%)	< 0.000
	general	188 (3.2%)	106 (10.0%)	
Cesarean delivery	elective[c]	3219 (59.1%)	548 (51.5%)	
	elective in labor	94 (1.7%)	20 (1.9%)	< 0.000
	emergent	2126 (39.1%)	496 (46.6%)	
Number of CD	2[c]	3023 (55.5%)	467 (43.9%)	< 0.000
	3–4	2040 (37.5%)	473 (44.5%)	
	≥5	380 (7.0%)	124 (11.7%)	
Experience of surgeon	senior > 10 yrs. [c]	1709 (32.6%)	333(31.3%)	
	senior < 10 yrs.	430 (8.2%)	102 (9.6%)	0.289
	resident	3111 (59.3%)	629 (59.1%)	
Presence of a third surgeon in surgery	non-present	5443 (100%)	1052 (98.9%)	< 0.000
	present	0 (0%)	12 (1.1%)	
Fetal weight	macrosomia > 4000	354 (6.5%)	61 (5.7%)	
	AGA 2500–4000[c]	4468 (82.3%)	856 (80.5%)	
	LBW 1500–2500	523 (9.6%)	120 (11.3%)	0.059
	VLBW 1000–1500	60 (1.1%)	16 (1.5%)	
	ELBW < 1000	24 (0.4%)	10 (0.9%)	

GMP grand-multipara
[a]The 90th percentile was calculated individually for each surgeon
[b]missing data 3301 (50.7%)
[c]reference variable in the multivariate analysis

Results

During the study period, 14,875 CD were performed out of 126,693 total deliveries (11.6%). Of the CD 6507 (43.7%) were repeat CD. Approximately one-fifth of the study population, 1416 (22%) were repeat CD due to failed TOLAC (Fig. 1- flow chart). Fifty-nine obstetricians were included in the analysis: 23 board certified obstetrics and gynecology and 36 residents, with comparable numbers of CD (median of 200 and 190. respectively). Mean duration of CD ranged between surgeons with a minimum of 30 (±13) minutes to a maximum of 66 (±30) minutes. Demographic characteristics, medical and obstetric history, and clinical features of the study population stratified by OT are presented in Table 1. One-fifth of the study population 1293 (20%) was grand-multiparous (≥6 deliveries). Prolonged CD duration relative to expected CD duration per surgeon's history was highly associated (P value < 0.000) with: gestational age at delivery, general anesthesia, number of previous CDs, TOLAC; and presence of a third surgeon (Table 1). There was a strong association between prolonged CD and post-operative adverse maternal outcomes including post-operative blood transfusion (4.4% vs. 1.5%), prolonged hospitalization (8.4% vs. 4.0%), infection necessitating antibiotic treatment (2% vs. 1%) and readmission (1.8% vs 0.8%) (Table 2). These significant correlations remained in multivariate regression analysis controlling for confounders (Table 2). The sensitivity, specificity, positive and negative predictive values of prolonged OT for each of the post-operative maternal complications and for the combined composite complication is presented in Table 3. There was a high negative predictive value (NPV > 0.93) for all complications studied.

Discussion

This study confirms our hypothesis that prolonged CD defined as OT greater than the 90th percentile of CD durations on record for each surgeon, was associated with post-operative maternal complications including post-operative blood transfusion, prolonged maternal hospitalization, treatment with antibiotics and readmission. Therefore, prolonged CD can be seen as a **risk marker** for adverse maternal outcomes. Nonetheless, the low prevalence of these complications (Table 3), limits our predictive ability, i.e., which women with prolonged OT will actually suffer complications (positive predictive value of 0.02–0.20). On the other hand, OT within the surgeon's (<90th percentile) duration, can reassure women with a high degree of confidence that they probably are not at risk of the above complications.

Moreover, the negative predictive value for each one of the complications studied (0.93–0.99) implies that for women undergoing repeat CD within the surgeon's < 90th percentile duration, are less likely to suffer the adverse complications analyzed herein.

There are few studies regarding the effect of prolonged CD on maternal and fetal morbidity [11, 14]. These studies are limited as they grouped together primary and repeat CD and the later arbitrary defined prolonged operation as below and above 30 and 60 min [14]. As clinicians, we were concerned that defining OT as a fixed number without considering the surgeon who operated is problematic because of variability in techniques among surgeons regardless of seniority. In order to correct for the effect of the primary surgeon we defined prolonged CD as ≥90th percentile calculated individually for the primary surgeon. We attributed operative time to the primary surgeon who could have been a resident and not the attending physician. In addition, to minimize bias of confounders and modifications, we included only women undergoing repeat CD and not primary CDs that are by nature different than repeat CD [16].

There are some limitations inherent in this study. First, this is a retrospective, cross-sectional single center university hospital, yet we believe that for the research question addressed this methodology is equitable. Our study population with high parity may weaken external validity, yet it also enabled inclusion of a large number of parturients undergoing repeat CD: 2513 women underwent their 3rd or 4th CD and 504 parturient underwent their 5th CD or more.

Table 2 Post-operative maternal complications distributed by length of surgery, univariate and multivariate analysis[a]

	Univariate analysis (chi square)			Multivariate analysis (Adjusted Odds Ratio)	
	> 90th percentile	> 90th percentile	p value	aOR	95% CI
Post-operative blood transfusion	82 (1.5%)	47 (4.4%)	< 0.000	3.16	2.17–4.61
Prolonged length of hospitalization (≥ 7 days)	216 (4%)	89 (8.4%)	< 0.000	1.89	1.44–2.46
Rx with antibiotics[b]	393 (7.2%)	128 (12%)	< 0.000	1.59	1.28–1.98
Re- admission	42 (0.8%)	18 (1.8%)	0.004	1.94	1.10–3.44
Composite complication[c]	607 (11.2%)	215 (20.2%)	< 0.000	1.81	1.52–2.16

[a]multivariate analysis controlling for maternal age, ethnicity, parity, number of fetus, gestational age at delivery, urge of operation, anesthesia and number of cesarean delivery
[b]Rx with either Gentamycin, Augmentin, Ciprofloxacin, Cefazolin
[c]combining post-operative blood transfusion, prolonged length of hospitalization, treatment with antibiotics and readmission

Table 3 The sensitivity, specificity, positive and negative predictive value of prolonged cesarean delivery (> 90th percentile) to each one of the post-operative maternal complications

	sensitivity	specificity	PPV	NPV
Post-operative blood transfusion	0.36	0.85	0.15	0.99
Prolonged length of hospitalization[a]	0.29	0.84	0.08	0.96
Rx with antibiotics[b]	0.25	0.84	0.12	0.93
Re- admission	0.30	0.84	0.02	0.99
Composite post-operative complication[c]	0.26	0.85	0.20	0.89

PPV positive predictive value, *NPV* negative predictive value
[a]prolonged length of maternal hospitalization defined as discharge after 7 days or more
[b]Rx with either Gentamycin, Augmentin, Ciprofloxacin, Cefazolin
[c]combining post-operative blood transfusion, prolonged length of hospitalization, necessitating antibiotic treatment and readmission

Unfortunately body mass index which is an essential factor associated with maternal morbidity is not currently available in our computerized database such. Despite these limitations, the large study group along with the requisite variables that continuously updated in real time, decreases bias.

In conclusion, among women undergoing repeat CD, prolonged CD is a **risk marker** for post-operative maternal complications. In addition, OT < 90th percentile of the surgeon's on record CD duration has high NPV for adverse maternal outcome, implying **who will not** suffer the studied complications. We encourage surgeons and institutions to obtain OT of CD and calculate the 90th percentile for each surgeon. This will enable the surgeon, in case of OT within the normal limits (< 90th percentile), to reassure the patient and their family immediately after the CD that the risk of post-operative complication including blood transfusion or prolonged admission are very low.

Conclusions

Prolonged OT, beyond the surgeon's 90th percentile of on record CD durations, is a risk marker for post-operative maternal complications among women undergoing repeat CD. In case of prolonged OT, the surgeon may elect for more careful follow-up of the patient based on the local standard protocol.

Abbreviations

CD: Cesarean delivery; ICU: Intensive care unit; OT: Operative time; SZMC: Shaare Zedek Medical Centre; TOLAC: Trial of labor after cesarean delivery

Acknowledgements

We thank Rivka Farkash for maintaining the computerized data base.

Funding

No funding was used in the conduct of this study.

Authors' contributions

MR and HS made substantial contributions to conception and design, been involved in drafting the manuscript and revising it critically for important intellectual content. OR - made substantial contributions to conception and design and analysis and interpretation of data. Been involved in drafting the manuscript or revising it critically for important intellectual content. OC, OS, RM, AS been involved in drafting the manuscript and revising it critically for important intellectual content, given final approval of the version to be published. All authors read and approved the final manuscript.

Competing interests

The authors declare that they have no competing interests.

References

1. Ananth CV, Friedman AM, Keyes KM, Lavery JA, Hamilton A, Wright JD. Primary and repeat cesarean deliveries: a population-based study in the United States, 1979-2010. Epidemiol. 2017;28(4):567–74.
2. Edmonds JK, Hawkins SS, Cohen BB. Variation in vaginal birth after cesarean by maternal race and detailed ethnicity. Matern Child Health J. 2016;20(6): 1114–23.
3. Martin JA, Hamilton BE, Ventura SJ, Osterman MJK, Kirmeyer S, Mathews TJ, et al. Births: final data for 2009. Natl Vital Stat Rep. 2011;60(1):1–70.
4. Vaginal birth after cesarean: new insights manuscripts from an NIH Consensus Development Conference, March 8-10, 2010. Semin Perinatol. 2010;34(5):309-10.
5. Tulandi T, Agdi M, Zarei A, Miner L, Sikirica V. Adhesion development and morbidity after repeat cesarean delivery. Am J Obstet Gynecol. 2009;201(1): 56.e1–6.
6. Morales KJ, Gordon MC, Bates GW. Postcesarean delivery adhesions associated with delayed delivery of infant. Am J Obstet Gynecol. 2007; 196(5):461.e1–6.
7. Zia S, Rafique M. Intra-operative complications increase with successive number of cesarean sections: myth or fact? Obstet Gynecol Sci. 2014;57(3): 187–92.
8. Ioscovich A, Mirochnitchenko E, Halpern SH, Smueloff A, Grisaru-Granovsky S, Gozal Y, et al. Anesthetic considerations for high order cesarean sections: a prospective cohort study. Arch Gynecol Obstet. 2014;289(3):533–40.
9. Cook JR, Jarvis S, Knight M. Multiple repeat caesarean section in the UK: incidence and consequences to mother and child. A national, prospective, cohort study. BJOG. 2013;120(1):85–91.
10. Marshall NE, Fu R, Guise J-M. Impact of multiple cesarean deliveries on maternal morbidity: a systematic review. Am J Obstet Gynecol. 2011;205(3): 262.e1–8.
11. Rossouw JN, Hall D, Harvey J. Time between skin incision and delivery during cesarean. Int J Gynecol Obstet 2013;121(1):82–85. Available from: doi: 10.1016/j.ijgo.2012.11.008

12. Nisenblat V, Barak S, Griness OB, Degani S, Ohel G, Gonen R. Maternal complications associated with multiple cesarean deliveries. Obstet Gynecol. 2006;108(1):21–6.
13. Makoha FW, Felimban HM, Fathuddien MA, Roomi F, Ghabra T. Multiple cesarean section morbidity. Int J Gynaecol Obstet. 2004;87(3):227–32.
14. Doherty DA, Magann EF, Chauhan SP, Boyle ALO, Busch JM, Morrison JC. Factors affecting caesarean operative time and the effect of operative time on pregnancy outcomes. Aust N Z J Obstet Gynaecol. 2008;48(3):286–91.
15. Dodd JM, Anderson ER, Gates S, Grivell RM. Surgical techniques for uterine incision and uterine closure at the time of caesarean section. Cochrane database Syst Rev. 2014;7:CD004732.
16. Curtin SC, Gregory KD, Korst LM, Uddin SF. Maternal Morbidity for Vaginal and Cesarean Deliveries, According to Previous Cesarean History: New Data From the Birth Certificate, 2013. Natl Vital Stat Rep. 2015;64(4):1–13 back cover.

Longer travel time to district hospital worsens neonatal outcomes: a retrospective cross-sectional study of the effect of delays in receiving emergency cesarean section in Rwanda

Joseph Niyitegeka[1*†], Georges Nshimirimana[2†], Allison Silverstein[3,4], Jackline Odhiambo[5], Yihan Lin[3,6], Theoneste Nkurunziza[7], Robert Riviello[3,8], Stephen Rulisa[9], Paulin Banguti[1], Hema Magge[7,10,11], Martin Macharia[7], Regis Habimana[2] and Bethany Hedt-Gauthier[7,12]

Abstract

Background: In low-resource settings, access to emergency cesarean section is associated with various delays leading to poor neonatal outcomes. In this study, we described the delays a mother faces when needing emergency cesarean delivery and assessed the effect of these delays on neonatal outcomes in Rwanda.

Methods: This retrospective study included 441 neonates and their mothers who underwent emergency cesarean section in 2015 at three district hospitals in Rwanda. Four delays were measured: duration of labor prior to hospital admission, travel time from health center to district hospital, time from admission to surgical incision, and time from decision for emergency cesarean section to surgical incision. Neonatal outcomes were categorized as unfavorable (APGAR <7 at 5 min or death) and favorable (alive and APGAR ≥7 at 5 min). We assessed the relationship between each type of delay and neonatal outcomes using multivariate logistic regression.

Results: In our study, 9.1% (40 out of 401) of neonates had an unfavorable outcome, 38.7% (108 out of 279) of neonates' mothers labored for 12–24 h before hospital admission, and 44.7% (159 of 356) of mothers were transferred from health centers that required 30–60 min of travel time to reach the district hospital. Furthermore, 48.1% (178 of 370) of cesarean sections started within 5 h after hospital admission and 85.2% (288 of 338) started more than 30 min after the decision for cesarean section was made. Neonatal outcomes were significantly worse among mothers with more than 90 min of travel time from the health center to the district hospital compared to mothers referred from health centers located on the same compound as the hospital (aOR = 5.12, $p = 0.02$). Neonates with cesarean deliveries starting more than 30 min after decision for cesarean section had better outcomes than those starting immediately (aOR = 0.32, $p = 0.04$).

(Continued on next page)

* Correspondence: joeniyitegeka@gmail.com
†Equal contributors
[1]Department of Anesthesia, Critical Care and Emergency Medicine, School of Medicine and Pharmacy, College of Medicine and Health Sciences, University of Rwanda, P.O. Box 3286, Kigali, Rwanda
Full list of author information is available at the end of the article

(Continued from previous page)

Conclusions: Longer travel time between health center and district hospital was associated with poor neonatal outcomes, highlighting a need to decrease barriers to accessing emergency maternal services. However, longer decision to incision interval posed less risk for adverse neonatal outcome. While this could indicate thorough pre-operative interventions including triage and resuscitation, this relationship should be studied prospectively in the future.

Keywords: Emergency obstetric care, Rural health delivery, Maternal and newborn health, Neonatal mortality, Quality improvement, Sub-Saharan Africa

Background

Limited access to cesarean section contributes to poor neonatal and maternal outcomes worldwide [1–3]. The delays for cesarean delivery can be described using a "three delays" framework – first, the mother's delay in deciding to seek care; second, the mother's delay in presenting to the health center or hospital once her decision to seek care is made; and third, the delay in receiving care once at the facility [4, 5]. The negative effects of these delays on maternal and neonatal outcomes are often more pronounced in sub-Saharan Africa [6] due to multiple reasons. Cultural belief that traditional remedies are better than modern medicine, lack of family support, limited financial resources to seek care, lack of health insurance [7–10], substantial distances between the mother's home and health facilities and inadequate referral systems [7, 10], limited infrastructure to support cesarean deliveries [8–10], and inadequate human resources [8] hinder care seeking behavior.

In sub-Saharan Africa, cesarean section is the most performed major surgery, accounting for 10–50% of all surgical procedures provided at district hospitals [11]. An estimated one in seven cesarean sections in sub-Saharan Africa result in a neonatal death [12]. This is almost ten times greater than the 20 to 22 out of 1000 neonatal deaths following cesarean sections reported worldwide [13]. Among cesarean deliveries, emergency cesarean section requires timely access to and provision of quality care to prevent adverse maternal and neonatal outcomes. Delays in accessing care put both the mother's and newborn's lives in danger [2] when complications are not managed on time or worsen due to further delays. This has led to recommendations of timely intervention. For example, the American College of Gynecologists recommends that the decision-to-incision interval should be less than 30 min to promote optimal neonatal outcomes [14]. Although multiple factors can contribute to negative neonatal outcomes [15], understanding which delays drive these outcomes can help focus attention on where preventative interventions are needed.

Rwanda is a low-income country in sub-Saharan Africa, with a neonatal mortality ratio of 20 per 1000 live births [16]. The maternal mortality ratio has decreased considerably, but is not parallel to neonatal mortality, which continues to be high [16]. Several initiatives to improve obstetrical and neonatal care in the country, such as advocacy for facility delivery, new infrastructure for delivery and neonatal services, and capacity strengthening for health providers through the Human Resources for Health training program, are ongoing [16]. Between 2010 and 2015, deliveries by skilled health providers improved from 69% to 90% [16]. In Rwanda, 13.0–14.7% of births in 2014 were delivered by cesarean section [16, 17]. More than 60% of the operations performed at rural district hospitals in the country are cesarean sections [18]. Similar to other low-resource settings, Rwandese mothers experience delays in obtaining cesarean section [8]. This study described the delays pregnant women face when a decision for cesarean delivery was made, and assessed the effect of the delays on neonatal outcomes at three rural district hospitals in Rwanda.

Methods

Study design and setting

This retrospective cross sectional study was conducted at three rural district hospitals (Butaro, Kirehe and Rwinkwavu) in Rwanda. These district hospitals are under the management of the Rwandan Ministry of Health (MOH) with technical and operational support provided by an international non-governmental organization, Partners In Health, known locally as Inshuti Mu Buzima (PIH/IMB). These district hospitals receive patients referred from 46 health centers in their catchment area. At each of the district hospitals, there are two operating rooms where cesarean deliveries can be performed and most cesarean deliveries are conducted by general practitioners.

In Rwanda, pregnant women and their families are responsible for their transport from home to the health center in their catchment area. Sometimes community health workers accompany laboring women to the health center. At the health center, registered nurses or midwives manage the woman. In the event of a potential complication for the fetus or the woman, the nurses/midwives will transfer the woman to the nearest district hospital via ambulance or with transport arranged by the woman's family if no ambulance is available. Each district hospital has five ambulances for all emergencies, while only 11 out of the 46 health centers in the districts of study have ambulances. The rest of the health centers depend on ambulances from the district hospital for emergency transport. Most of the roads in these rural settings are unpaved and public transport has limited reliability. In cases where the health center is located in the same compound as the district hospital, an ambulance is not necessary for the transport. On rare occasions, laboring women present directly to the district hospital.

At the district hospital, registered nurses or midwives perform initial obstetrical review and call general practitioners for further laboratory and ultrasound assessments, and decision for cesarean delivery. If cesarean delivery is decided, the pregnant woman is transferred to a delivery room where nurse-anesthetists administer anesthesia and the general practitioner, supported by nurses or midwives, performs cesarean section. Each hospital assists with 10–12 deliveries per day. During the day, one general practitioner is assigned to the delivery room; at night, one general practitioner covers the entirety of the maternity department. At all times, two nurses or midwives are assigned to the delivery room. After delivery, the woman and the neonate are transferred to the post-partum room where midwives closely monitor their progress with daily check-ups by the general practitioners and until discharge. Obstetricians are sometimes but not always available at the district hospitals.

The decision to seek care at a health facility depends on the ability to pay or having a valid health insurance [16]. The majority of Rwandan households (79%) have at least one member with health insurance [16]. For women who have community-based health insurance (97% of households with insurance [16]), the insurance covers 90% of the total cost of care and the woman pays the remaining balance. Women without health insurance cover entirety of the cost out of pocket.

Study population

The study included mothers and their neonates born via emergency cesarean section between 01 January 2015 and 31 December 2015 at the three hospitals. All emergency cesarean sections without intrauterine fetal death prior to the decision for cesarean section were eligible for inclusion. Because of the large population of cesarean deliveries at the district hospitals, we calculated a study sample size that could detect differences in neonatal outcomes by delays. Due to limited data a priori, we assumed that the overall negative neonatal outcome was 50% and that delay categories were binary to calculate the largest sample size possible. To have a 90% power to detect a 20% difference in neonatal outcome (i.e. one group had 40% negative neonatal outcome and the second group had 60% negative neonatal outcome), with $\alpha=0.05$, we calculated a necessary sample of 140 women per group (delayed or not delayed). In anticipation of missing data, we increased the sample size by 30% to 200 per group or 400 women total. We further increased the sample size to 600 women, 200 per hospital, to account for any losses in statistical efficiency due to stratification by hospital and differences in group sizes.

As the majority of cesarean deliveries at these hospitals were due to the referral of emergent and complicated cases from health centers, we originally assumed all cesarean deliveries were emergency and used segmented sampling to sample 200 women in each hospital. However, if a woman's chart did not meet the inclusion criteria, that is if the cesarean delivery was indicated as elective or the infant died before the decision for cesarean section, we removed and replaced the chart with an eligible chart, randomly picked from the same month of admission. Among the sampled cesarean section deliveries, we performed in-depth review of indications for cesarean section. During the data cleaning stage, we excluded any deliveries whose indication for cesarean section was not emergent. These included women whose sole indication for cesarean delivery was previous cesarean delivery, women who were past their due date, or women who were having twins without any other emergent indication. Included emergency cesarean deliveries had at least one of the following indications: cord prolapse, uterine rupture with a previous cesarean section scar, fetal distress, eclampsia, obstructed labor, mal-presentation, cephalopelvic disproportion, prolonged rupture of membranes with a previous cesarean section scar, and pre-eclampsia [19, 20]. Finally, any neonate who did not have record of neonatal outcome, either death within the first 24 h or APGAR at 5 min after delivery was excluded from analysis.

Data collection and definitions

Trained data collectors extracted chart data on women's demographic and clinical characteristics, individual and health facility delays, and neonatal outcomes. We categorized the indication for cesarean delivery as very severe or severe through consultation with a local obstetrician and based on complications to the fetus. Very severe indications included fetal distress, cord prolapse, uterine rupture, eclampsia, abruption placenta, and obstructed labor. Severe indications included prolonged rupture of membranes, pre-eclampsia, placenta previa, cephalopelvic disproportion, and mal-presentation, including breech presentation, transverse presentation, and occiput posterior presentation. If a woman had more than one indication, we prioritized the most severe indication. A neonatal outcome was considered favorable if the neonate was alive and had an APGAR score ≥ 7 at 5 min and unfavorable if there was death within 24 h after delivery or an APGAR score < 7 at 5 min.

We captured four measures of delays in reaching and receiving care that were routinely collected in the charts (Fig. 1). We used two measures for delays in reaching care. First, we looked at the duration of labor prior to district hospital admission, as self-reported by the women. We also used the average ambulance travel time from the health center, where an emergency condition occurred or could have been detected, to the district hospital. The latter was a standardized time based on health center records and did not include the actual time from when the emergency was detected until the ambulance was called or the actual travel time for the mother in case an ambulance was not available. We used three cutoffs for this measure: less than 30 min (indicating that the health center was located on the same compound as the district hospital), 30–60 min, and more than 60 min. Delays in receiving care were measured by the time from admission to the district hospital to surgery start and the time from the decision for a cesarean section by a doctor to surgical incision (decision-to-incision interval).

Data analysis

We assessed the relationship between neonatal outcome and potential confounders using Chi-squared tests. Types of delays were described using frequencies. We assessed the relationship between each of the delays and the neonatal outcome using multivariate logistic regression, controlling for potential confounders. We developed a separate model for each delay predictor. Potential confounders considered for this study were mother's age, gestational age, number of fetuses, woman's heart rate, fetal heart rate, district hospital, history of prior pregnancy, and severity of indication. To determine the appropriate confounders for each delay and neonatal outcome, i.e. the specific factors that were potentially related to the delay and the outcome but were not on the causal pathway, we constructed directed acyclic graphs (DAGs) (Fig. 2). For the duration of labor prior to admission at the district hospital, we controlled for district hospital, gestational age, number of fetuses, history of prior pregnancy, and woman's age as potential confounders. For the travel time from health center to district hospital, we controlled for district hospital as a potential confounder. For the admission to surgical incision and decision to incision intervals, we controlled for district hospital, gestational age, number of fetuses, woman's age, woman's heart rate, fetal heart rate, and severity of cesarean section indication. We reported the resulting odds ratios (OR), adjusted odds ratios (aOR), 95% confidence intervals (95% CIs), and p-values.

For bivariate analyses, we excluded all observations with missing data. We also excluded observations if delay for that individual was not measured; however, if a confounder was included in a multivariate analysis, we created a missing category for that confounder if more than 15% of patients had missing data in order to avoid excluding these patients from the analysis. We used $\alpha = 0.05$ significance level for all analyses and completed all analyses using Stata v14 (College Station, TX: StataCorp LP).

Results

In 2015, there were 2339 emergency cesarean section deliveries in the three district hospitals, of which we

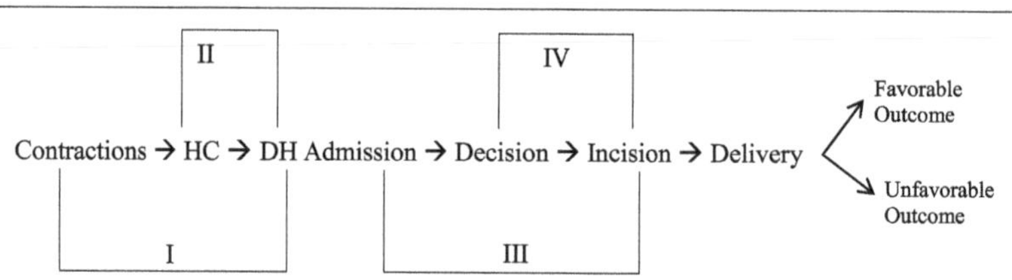

Key:

Delay	Definition	Linking to the "three delays framework"
I.	Time from onset of contractions to district hospital admission.	Delays in seeking and reaching care
II.	Time of travel from health center (HC) to the district hospital (DH).	Delays in reaching care
III.	Time from district hospital admission to surgical incision.	Delays in receiving care
IV.	Time from decision for cesarean delivery to surgical incision.	Delays in receiving care

Fig. 1 Possible delays for emergency cesarean section

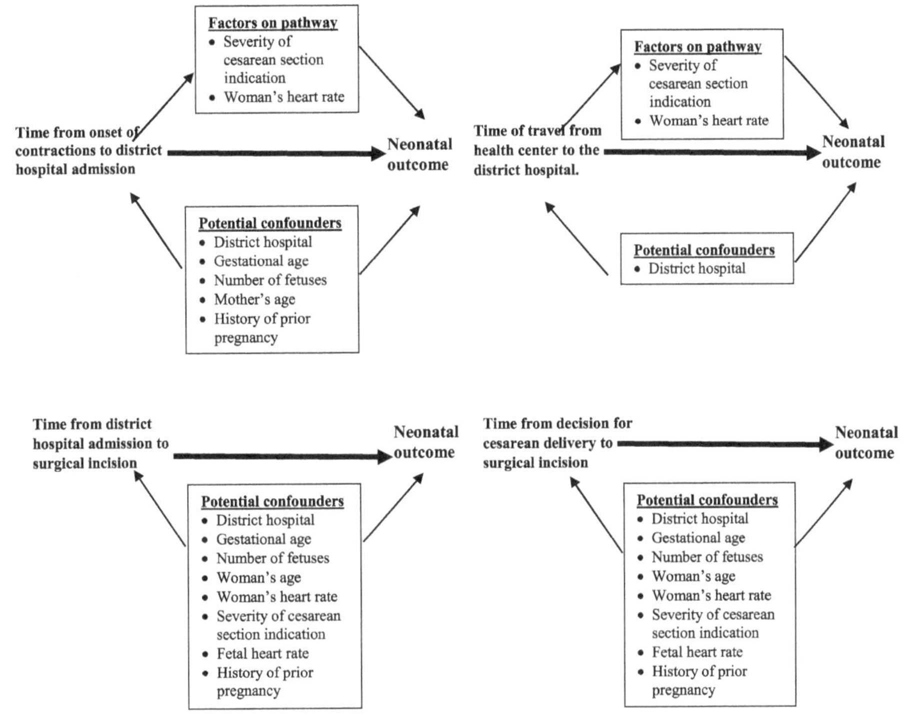

Fig. 2 Directed acyclic graphs (DAGs) mapping the relationship between the four possible delays and neonatal outcomes, noting potential confounders

sampled 597 deliveries corresponding to 622 neonates (Fig. 3). Of the 622 neonates, we confirmed that 455 had emergent indications for their cesarean sections. An additional 14 were excluded due to lack of neonatal outcome records, resulting in 441 neonates included in the analysis. Of these, 401 (90.9%) survived and had APGAR score ≥7 at 5 min while 40 (9.1%) died or had five-minute APGAR score <7 (Table 1). Overall, 13 (2.9%) neonates died, 27 (6.1%) had APGAR scores <7, and 14 (51.9%) of those with APGAR scores <7 were transferred or admitted to neonatology unit. Among the potential confounders, most had no significant association with the neonatal outcome with $p > 0.10$ for district hospital, mother's age, gestational age, number of fetuses, systolic blood pressure, maternal heart rate, and fetal heart rate. However, there was a trend between severity of indication for cesarean section and outcome, as very severe indications had a higher rate of neonatal deaths or low APGAR scores compared to severe indications (12.2% vs. 6.9%, $p = 0.06$).

In assessing rates of delay, among 279 neonates whose mother's duration of labor was recorded, the mothers of 108 (38.7%) neonates were in labor for 12-24 h prior to admission at the district hospital (Table 2). For the 356 neonates whose mother's ambulance travel time from health center to district hospital was calculated, 159 (44.7%) were from health centers located 30-60 min away from the district hospital. Cesarean deliveries were started within 5 h after admission in 178 out of 370 cases (48.1%). In an additional 100 (27%) cases, the operation started more than 15 h after admission. For the majority of cesarean sections ($n = 288$ out of 338, 85.2%), the decision to incision interval was greater than 30 min.

In the unadjusted model, both the duration of labor prior to admission as well as the varying times between admission and surgery start were not significantly linked to neonatal outcome ($p > 0.05$ for all categories). The shorter decision to incision interval had a trend towards a negative neonatal outcome ($p = 0.09$). Longer ambulance travel time from health center to district hospital had a strong association with poor neonatal outcome ($p = 0.07$ for 30–60 min, $p = 0.04$ for 60–90 min and $p = 0.01$ for 90+ minutes compared to the individuals from health centers located on the same compound as the district hospital).

After adjusting for potential confounders, there was no statistically significant association between duration of labor before hospital admission and time from admission to surgery with neonatal outcome. Compared to less than 12 h of labor prior to arrival, the adjusted odds ratio (aOR) for neonatal death or low APGAR score for deliveries within 12-24 h, 24-36 h and 36+ h of labor were ≤1.20 ($p > 0.05$ for all categories) (Table 3). Compared to the time from admission to surgery of <5 h, time from admission to surgery of 5–10 h and 10-15 h both had an aOR ≥1.12 ($p \geq 0.08$) and time from

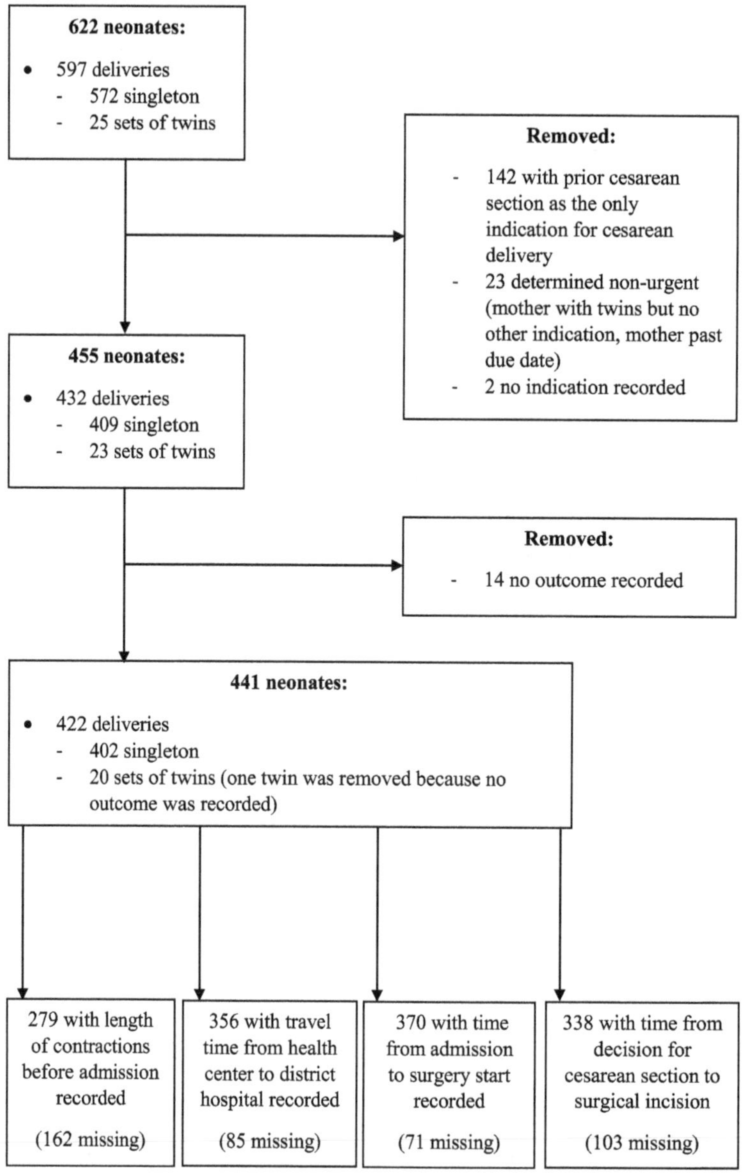

Fig. 3 Study inclusion criteria

admission to surgery >15 h had an aOR of 0.50 (p = 0.35).

However, while adjusting for confounders, a longer travel time from the health center to the district hospital remained significantly associated with death or low APGAR score. Compared to travel time from health centers located on the same compound as the district hospital, travel time of 30–60 min had an aOR of 3.02 (95% CI: 0.84, 10.84), travel time of 60–90 min had an aOR of 4.31 (95% CI: 1.02, 18.29), and travel time of more than 90 min had an aOR of 5.12 (95% CI: 1.30, 20.21). For the decision to incision interval, neonates whose mothers had a decision to incision interval of 30 min or more were significantly less likely to die or have low APGAR scores (aOR = 0.32, 95% CI: 0.11, 0.96). In analysis not shown in the tables, 13 deliveries had intra-operative complications, 11 of which were bleeding. Of the 13 complications, ten occurred with a decision to incision interval of <60 min (three for <30 min and seven for 30–60 min), and three with a decision to incision interval ≥ 60 min.

Discussion

In this study, we found that pregnant women experience diverse and considerable delays from the initiation of labor to the start of an emergency cesarean section. Nearly a third of women had labored for over 24 h

Table 1 The effect of demographic factors on neonatal outcomes post emergency cesarean section in Rwanda ($N = 441$)

	Survived and APGAR ≥7		Died or APGAR <7		
	n	%	*n*	%	*p-value*
Overall	401	90.9	40	9.1	N/A
Neonatal death	-	-	13	3.0	N/A
Neonates with APGAR <7	-	-	27	6.1	N/A
District hospital					
Butaro	147	91.3	14	8.7	0.47
Kirehe	129	92.8	10	7.2	
Rwinkwavu	125	88.7	16	11.3	
Woman's age (years) ($N = 436$)					
15–24	163	92.6	13	7.4	0.41
25–34	171	90.5	18	9.5	
35–44	62	87.3	9	12.7	
Gestational age (weeks) ($N = 366$)					
< 37	35	92.1	3	7.9	0.88
37–41	247	92.5	20	7.5	
> 41	56	91.8	5	8.2	
Number of fetuses					
1	368	91.5	34	8.5	0.15
2	33	84.6	6	15.4	
Indication for cesarean section					
Very severe[a]	158	87.8	22	12.2	0.06
Severe[b]	243	93.1	18	6.9	
Systolic blood pressure ($N = 404$)					
< 90	3	100.0	0.0	0.0	0.85
90–140	354	91.5	33	8.5	
> 140	13	92.9	1	7.1	
Maternal heart rate (beats per minute) ($N = 383$)					
≤ 100	311	92.3	26	7.7	0.46
> 100	41	89.1	5	10.9	
Fetal heart rate (beats per minute) ($N = 429$)					
< 120	54	91.5	5	8.5	0.46
120–160	323	91.8	29	8.2	
>160	15	83.3	3	16.7	

[a]Very severe indication: intrauterine rupture, fetal distress, cord prolapse, abruption placenta
[b]Severe indication: preeclampsia, prolonged rupture of membranes, cephalopelvic disproportion, prolonged labor and mal-presentation

Table 2 Time delays for emergency cesarean section in Rwanda

Type of Delay	*n*	%
Duration of labor before hospital admission (hours) ($N = 279$)		
< 12	83	29.7
12 to <24	108	38.7
24 to <36	46	16.5
≥ 36	42	15.1
Travel time from HC to DH (minutes) ($N = 356$)		
HC located on the same compound as the DH (<30)	91	25.6
30 to <60	159	44.7
60 to <90	45	12.6
≥ 90	61	17.1
Time from admission to surgery (hours) ($N = 370$)		
≤ 5	178	48.1
> 5 to ≤10	55	14.9
> 10 to ≤15	37	10.0
> 15	100	27.0
Decision to delivery interval (minutes) ($N = 338$)		
< 30	50	14.8
≥ 30	288	85.2

HC Health Center
DH District Hospital

before arriving at the district hospital. Of note, most women first go to their catchment health center to seek care and are only referred to the district hospital once an emergency occurs [21]. If they are referred, the travel time from the health center to the district hospital was often 30 min or more. This is likely an underestimation of the actual time since our study did not capture the real-time duration between when an emergency was detected until the woman reached the district hospital. More delays can occur when a woman waits for the ambulance to arrive or when she has to arrange her own transport if an ambulance is not available. These prehospital delays have previously been attributed to delays in deciding to seek healthcare due to limited finances or lack of family support [7–10, 16], underestimation of the severity of complication, previous poor experience with the health care system, lack of or prolonged transport, and seeking care in many health facilities that lack the needed capacity [1, 16, 22].

Additional delays in receiving care occur between a woman's presentation at the health center and her arrival at the district hospital. At the health center, lack of ambulances for emergency transport or insufficient ambulance staff delay referral to the district hospital. After admission to the district hospital, midwives and registered nurses monitor women, while the general practitioner assesses and determines the need for an emergency cesarean section. The majority of women in our study received surgery more than 5 h after admission. Furthermore, most women received surgery more than 30 min after a general practitioner had decided that she needed a cesarean section. This delay, which could be due to too few providers, inadequate medication and equipment, and too few operating rooms [8–10], is consistent with other studies in sub-Saharan Africa, suggesting a 30-min decision to incision interval may not be realistic in low- or middle-income

Table 3 The effect of time delays for emergency cesarean section on neonatal outcomes in Rwanda

	Unadjusted			Adjusted		
	OR	*p*-value	95% CI	aOR	*p*-value	95% CI
Duration of labor before hospital admission (hours)[a]						
< 12	ref	-	-	ref	-	-
12 to <24	0.65	0.42	[0.23, 1.87]	0.81	0.71	[0.26, 2.50]
24 to <36	0.43	0.29	[0.09, 2.10]	0.54	0.38	[0.10, 2.92]
≥ 36	0.99	0.98	[0.27, 3.49]	1.20	0.80	[0.31, 4.65]
Travel time from HC to DH (minutes)[b]						
HC located on the same compound as the DH (<30)	ref	-	-	ref	-	-
30 to <60	3.28	0.07	[0.93, 11.59]	3.02	0.09	[0.84, 10.84]
60 to <90	4.51	0.04	[1.07, 18.98]	4.31	0.05	[1.02, 18.29]
≥ 90	5.75	0.01	[1.51, 21.87]	5.12	0.02	[1.30, 20.21]
Time from admission to surgery (hours)[c]						
≤ 5	ref	-	-	ref	-	-
> 5 to ≤10	1.85	0.22	[0.70, 4.90]	3.00	0.08	[0.89, 10.08]
> 10 to ≤15	0.73	0.68	[0.16, 3.36]	1.12	0.89	[0.20, 6.15]
> 15	0.81	0.68	[0.30, 2.20]	0.50	0.35	[0.12, 2.10]
Decision to incision interval (minutes)[c]						
< 30	ref	-	-	ref	-	-
≥ 30	0.48	0.09	[0.20, 1.13]	0.32	0.04	[0.11, 0.96]

Ref Reference value
HC Health Center
DH District Hospital
OR Odds Ratio
aOR adjusted Odds Ratio
[a]Adjusted for district hospital, gestational age, number of fetuses, and woman's age
[b]Adjusted for district hospital
[c]Adjusted for district hospital, gestational age, number of fetuses, woman's age, woman's heart rate, severity of cesarean section indication, and fetal heart rate

settings [23]. Of note, there could also be a potential unmeasured delay between nurse notification and doctor assessment, which was not captured systematically in the patient files for inclusion in this study but should be assessed in future studies.

While delayed emergency cesarean section is often linked to poor neonatal outcomes [3], two of the delays we considered, the duration of labor prior to admission to the district hospital and the time from admission to surgery start, were not significantly associated with neonatal death or low APGAR scores. However, we found a significant association between ambulance travel time from the health center to the district hospital, with longer travel time associated with higher odds for neonatal death or low APGAR scores. This is consistent with other studies that link poor maternal and neonatal outcomes to distance traveled by the woman before she reaches the hospital [24]. In Rwanda, we believe that this effect is compounded when there are no ambulances available to transport a laboring woman to the district hospital. For the 46 health facilities in the catchment area of the district hospitals included in this study, only 11 have an ambulance available at the facility and the remainder request for an ambulance to be dispatched from another location. Increasing timely access from health centers to the district hospital, either by adding more district hospitals or by increasing the availability of ambulances, will likely result in better neonatal outcomes after emergency cesarean delivery.

While some studies in sub-Saharan Africa have not reported a link between the decision to incision interval and neonatal outcomes [25], the prevailing consensus is that a shorter interval is associated with improved neonatal outcomes [14], with a 30 min target commonly set for the decision to incision interval [23, 26]. To our surprise, we found that neonates born with a longer decision to incision interval had better outcomes. We propose possible hypotheses that could explain this result. First, this may be due to triaging by hospital staff, where patients who were determined to be less emergent and therefore more likely to have better outcomes, are less likely to go to the operating theatre immediately. Such a phenomenon is a noted confounder in a meta-analysis on this topic [27]. However, a second explanation could be that rushing the surgery may lead to less than ideal surgical conditions, for example, due to a lack of optimization of the patient or inadequate materials due to lack of preparation. Complications from emergency cesarean section include sepsis, wound dehiscence, anemia, and others [28]. It is also possible that some indications for cesarean section such as fetal distress were not actually present but were documented to reflect a decision to perform a cesarean section. Further studies related to the quality of care are needed to explore the relationship between decision to incision interval and neonatal outcome in this context.

Our study has several limitations to consider. First, we used routinely collected clinical data, and as a result, some data were incomplete. However, because we expected to have missing data, we accounted for this when calculating our minimum sample size. For all of the women whom we collected data on, the majority (280 patients) had information on major delays, which was adequate to detect a difference in outcomes. Second, given that this study was only conducted at three district hospitals, all of which receive some support from Partners In Health, the results may have limited generalizability, as there may be variations in staffing and supply chain at these hospitals. However, the Rwandan Ministry of Health manages all three public hospitals, with the same standardized structures in place as other district hospitals throughout Rwanda. Therefore, we believe our findings to be representative of the Rwandan rural setting and may be similar to other rural district hospitals in the region. Additionally, since time estimates relied on information existing in the medical charts, we were not able to measure some delays, such as delay in deciding to seek care, the actual travel time from health center to district hospital, or the time between nurse or midwife notification for cesarean section assessment by doctor and doctor assessment and decision for cesarean delivery. Furthermore, some of the time estimates such as duration of labor before hospital admission were self-reported by the women and thus subject to recall bias. The self-reported time data did not capture moments such as when labor began, when decision to seek care was made, and when initial care was sought. We recommend future prospective studies to tease out delays in seeking care and factors leading to these delays, which are important in improving maternal and neonatal outcomes in this setting. Finally, as observed in a previous systematic review [19], the definitions of cesarean section indications such as fetal distress were ambiguous and our classification of cesarean sections as emergency or as severe and very severe were subjective, limiting generalizability. In addition, due to time and resource constrains, we did not report outcomes for neonates admitted to neonatology units. A prospective audit of cesarean section rates in Rwanda should provide more evidence on the categorizations for urgency of cesarean section, and follow neonates admitted to neonatology units to report outcomes.

Conclusions

Our study found that a longer travel time from health centers to the district hospital was associated with adverse neonatal outcomes. This emphasizes the need for strategies to reduce the transfer delay from health centers to district hospitals, including improving detection of maternal/fetal complications and response time, referral systems, improving road networks, increasing the number of ambulances and district hospitals, and subsidizing transport costs. However, longer time lag from a decision to perform an emergency cesarean section to the surgical incision was associated with less risk of poor neonatal outcome possibly due to an opportunity of thorough pre-operative interventions including resuscitation and triage. The achievability of a 30-min decision to incision interval and the relationship between this interval and neonatal outcomes requires further prospective studies to make appropriate recommendations for this context and investigate factors leading to delays that worsen neonatal outcomes.

Abbreviations

95% CI: 95% Confidence Interval; aOR: Adjusted Odds Ratio; APGAR: Appearance, Pulse, Grimace, Activity and Respiration; DAGS: Directed acyclic graphs; OR: Odds Ratio

Acknowledgements

We acknowledge Partners In Health/Inshuti Mu Buzima (PIH/IMB) for their support of this work. This study was developed under the PIH/IMB Intermediate Operational Research Training Program, developed and facilitated by Bethany Hedt-Gauthier and Jackline Odhiambo. We are thankful to all three PIH/IMB-supported district hospital staff for their contributions. We appreciate the Harvard Global Health Initiative Burke Global Health Fellowship grant for their financial support in data collection and training costs. We also thank the Rwandan Human Resources for Health faculty, the Government of Rwanda, the Global Fund to fight AIDS, Tuberculosis and Malaria, and the Centers for Disease Control and Prevention for their financial support for this project.

Funding

All data collection and training costs were covered by the Harvard Global Health Initiative Burke Global Health Fellowship grant. Some training facilitators and mentors are Rwanda Human Resources for Health faculty, funded with the support of the Government of Rwanda, the Global Fund to fight AIDS, Tuberculosis and Malaria and Centers for Disease Control and Prevention.

Authors' contributions

JN and GN led the study design, protocol development, data analysis, results interpretations, and manuscript preparation. AS, BHG, JO, YL and TN provided inputs in study design, data analysis and results interpretation. YL and JO led data collection and BHG and YL led data cleaning. TN, RR, SR, PB, HM, MM and RH supported study design, results interpretation. All authors critically reviewed drafts of the manuscript and approved the final version for publication.

Competing interests
The authors declare that they have no competing interests.

Author details
[1]Department of Anesthesia, Critical Care and Emergency Medicine, School of Medicine and Pharmacy, College of Medicine and Health Sciences, University of Rwanda, P.O. Box 3286, Kigali, Rwanda. [2]Ministry of Health, Kigali, Rwanda. [3]Program in Global Surgery and Social Change, Harvard Medical School, Boston, MA, USA. [4]Miller School of Medicine, University of Miami, Miami, FL, USA. [5]Partners In Health, Boston, MA, USA. [6]Department of Surgery, University of Colorado Hospital, Aurora, CO, USA. [7]Partners In Health / Inshuti Mu Buzima, Kigali, Rwanda. [8]Department of Surgery, Brigham and Women's Hospital, Boston, MA, USA. [9]School of Medicine and Pharmacy, College of Medicine and Health Sciences, University of Rwanda, Kigali, Rwanda. [10]Division of Global Health Equity, Brigham and Women's Hospital, Boston, MA, USA. [11]Division of General Pediatrics, Boston Children's Hospital, Boston, MA, USA. [12]Department of Global Health and Social Medicine, Harvard Medical School, Boston, MA, USA.

References

1. Chan M, Sundby J, Vangen S. Maternal mortality in the rural Gambia, a qualitative study on access to emergency obstetric care. Reprod Health. 2005;2(1):3.
2. Korhonen J, Kariniemi V. Emergency cesarean section: the effect of delay on umbilical arterial gas balance and Apgar scores. Acta Obstet Gynecol Scand. 1994;73(10):782–6.
3. Morris JA, Rosenbower TJ, Jurkovich GJ, Hoyt DB, Harviel JD, Knudson MM, et al. Infant survival after cesarean section for trauma. Annals of Surgery. 1996;223(5):481–91.
4. Pacagnella R, Cecatti J, Osis M, Souza P. The role of delays in severe maternal morbidity and mortality: expanding the conceptual framework. RHM. 2012;20(39):155–63.
5. Meara JG, Leather AJM, Hagander L, Alkire BC, Alonso N, Ameh E, et al. Global Surgery 2030: evidence and solutions for achieving health, welfare, and economic development. Lancet. 2015;386(9993):569–624.
6. McCord C, Mbaruku G, Pereira C, Nzabuhakwa C, Bergstrom S. The quality of emergency obstetrical surgery by assistant medical officers in Tanzanian district hospitals. Health Affairs. 2009;28:5.
7. Rutherford ME, Mulholland K, Hill PC. How access to health care relates to under-five mortality in sub-Saharan Africa : systematic review. Trop Med Int Health. 2010;15(5):508–19.
8. Grimes CE, Bowman KG, Dodgion CM, Lavy CBD. Systematic Review of Barriers to Surgical Care in Low-Income and Middle-Income Countries. World J Surg. 2011;35(5):941–50.
9. Onah H, Okaro J, Umeh U, Chigbu C. Maternal mortality in health institutions with emergency obstetric care facilities in Enugu State, Nigeria. J Obstet Gynaecol. 2005;25(6):569–74.
10. Gulliford M, Figueroa-munoz J, Morgan M, Hughes D, Gibson B, Beech R, et al. What does 'access to health care' mean? J Health Serv Res Pol. 2002;7(3):186–9.
11. Galukande M, von Schreeb J, Wladis A, Mbembati N, Miranda H, Kruk ME, et al. Essential Surery at the District Hospital: A Retrospective Descriptive Analysis in Three African Countries. PLoS Med. 2010;7(3):1–10.
12. Chu K, Cortier H, Maldonado F, Mashant T, Ford N, Trelles M. Cesarean Section Rates and Indications in Sub-Saharan Africa: A Multi-Country Study from Medecins sans Frontieres. PLoS One. 2012;7(9):e44484.
13. Volpe FM. Correlation of Cesarean rates to maternal and infant mortality rates: an ecologic study of official international data. Rev Panam Salud Publica. 2011;29(5):303–8.
14. American Academy of Pediatrics, American College of Obstetricians and Gynecologists. Guidelines for perinatal care. 7th ed. Elk Grove Village (IL): AAP; Washington, DC: American College of Obstetricians and Gynecologists. 2012. p.109-110, 160, 192-194, 248.
15. Liu L, Oza S, Hogan D, Perin J, Rudan I, Lawn J, et al. Global, regional, and national causes of child mortality in 2000–13, with projections to inform post-2015 priorities: an updated systematic analysis. Lancet. 2015;385(9966):430 40.
16. National Institute of Statistics of Rwanda (NISR), Ministry of Health (MOH) Rwanda, and ICF International. Rwanda Demographic and Health Survey 2014-15. 2015. Rockville, Maryland, USA: NISR, MOH, and ICF International. http://www.statistics.gov.rw/publication/demographic-and-health-survey-20142015-final-report. Accessed 25 Nov 2016
17. Rwanda Ministry of Health. Rwanda Annual Health Statistics Booklet. Rwanda Annual Health Statistic. 2014. http://moh.gov.rw/fileadmin/templates/HMIS_Docs/MOH_Statistical_Booklet_2014.pdf. Accessed 28 Dec 2016.
18. Petroze R, Nzayisenga A, Rusanganwa V, Ntakiyiruta G, Calland J. Comprehensive national analysis of emergency and essential surgical capacity in Rwanda. Br J Surg. 2012;99:436–43.
19. Torloni MR, Betran AP, Souza JP, Widmer M, Allen T, Gulmezoglu M, et al. Classifications for Cesarean Section: A Systematic Review. PLoS One. 2011; 6(1):e14566.
20. Nakamura-Pereira M, Leal MC, Esteves-Pereira AP, RMSM D, Torres JA, MAB D, et al. Use of Robson classification to assess cesarean section rate in Brazil: the role of source of payment for childbirth. BMC Reprod Health. 2016;13(Supple 3):128.
21. Rwanda Ministry of Health. Service Packages for Health Facilities at Different levels of Service Delivery. Ministry of Health. 2011. www.moh.gov.rw/fileadmin/templates/Clinical/SERVICE-PACKAGES-FOR-HEALTH-FACILITIES-AT-DIFFERENT-LEVELS-OF-SERVICE-DELIVERY-last-version.pdf . Accessed 23 Nov 2016.
22. Ghebrehiwet M, Morrow RH. Delay in Seeking and Receiving Emergency Obstetric care in Eritrea. J Eritrean Med Assoc. 2007;2(1):8–12.
23. Onuoha O, Ramaswamy R, Srofenyoh EK, Kim SM, Owen MD. The effects of resource improvement on decision-to-delivery times for cesarean deliveries in a Ghanaian regional hospital. Int J Gynecol Obstet. 2015;130(3):274–8.
24. Grzybowski S, Stoll K, Kornelsen J. Distance matters: a population based study examining access to maternity services for rural women. BMC Health Serv Res. 2011;11:1.
25. Bloom S, Leveno K, Spong C, Gilbert S. Decision-to-Incision Times and Maternal and Infant Outcomes. Obstet Gynecol. 2006;108(1):6–11.
26. Royal College of Obtetricians and Gynaecologists. Report of a joint working group:organisational standards for maternity services. London. 2008. https://www.rcog.org.uk/globalassets/documents/guidelines/wprmaternitystandards2008.pdf. Accessed 15 Dec 2016.
27. Tolcher MC, Johnson RL, El-Nashar SA, West CP. Decision-to-Incision Time and Neonatal Outcomes. A Systematic Review and Meta-analysis. Obstet Gynecol. 2014;123:536–48.
28. Daniel CN, Singh S. Cesarean delivery: An experience from a tertiary institution in north western Nigeria. Niger J Clin Pract. 2016;19(1):18–24.

15

Mental health after first childbirth in women requesting a caesarean section

Louise Möller[1], Ann Josefsson[1], Marie Bladh[1], Caroline Lilliecreutz[1], Ellika Andolf[2] and G. Sydsjö[1*]

Abstract

Background: Psychiatric illness before delivery increases the risk of giving birth by caesarean section on maternal request (CSMR) but little is known about these women's mental health after childbirth. In this study we aimed to compare the prevalence of psychiatric disorders five years before and after delivery in primiparae giving birth by CS on maternal request to all other primiparae giving birth, indifferent on their mode of delivery.

Methods: The study population comprised all women born in Sweden 1973–1983 giving birth for the first time in 2002–2004. Psychiatric diagnoses, in- and outpatient care were retrieved from the National Patient Register in Sweden. The risk of psychiatric care after childbirth was estimated using CSMR, previous mental health and sociodemographic variables as covariates.

Results: Psychiatric disorders after childbirth were more common in women giving birth by CSMR compared to the other women (11.2% vs 5.5%, $p < 0.001$). CSMR increased the risk of psychiatric disorders after childbirth (aOR 1. 5, 95% CI 1.2–1.9). The prevalence of psychiatric disorders had increased after compared to before childbirth (mean difference 0.02 ± 0.25, 95% CI 0.018–0.022, $p < 0.001$). Women giving birth by CSMR tended to be diagnosed in the inpatient care more often (54.9% vs. 45.8%, $p = 0.056$) and were more likely to have been diagnosed before childbirth as well (39.8% vs. 24.2%, $p < 0.001$).

Conclusions: Women giving birth by CSMR more often suffer from psychiatric disorders both before and after delivery. This indicates that these women are a vulnerable group requiring special attention from obstetric- and general health-care providers. This vulnerability should be taken into account when deciding on mode of delivery.

Keywords: Psychiatric disorders, Caesarean section, Maternal request

Background

The rate of caesarean sections (CS) is increasing with an average rate of 15% worldwide and 21% in developed countries [1]. One reason for this trend is an increase in the frequency of CS on maternal request (CSMR). In Stockholm, Sweden, CSMR increased from 10.5% of all elective CS in 1992 to 38.5% in 2005, i.e. 4% of all deliveries [2]. Fear of childbirth (FOC) is the most common reason given for CSMR [3–7]. FOC affects approximately 7–15% of all pregnant women [8–11]. The fear may be due to a previous negative birth experience, obstetric complications such as an emergency CS/vacuum extraction [5, 8, 9], lack of trust in the obstetrical staff, loss of control, pain, as well as fear of one's own death and/or the infant's death [12]. Maternal characteristics associated with the preference for a CS are higher maternal age, smoking, lower educational attainment, unemployment [3, 5], living alone [5], personality, and being an immigrant [13].

These women giving birth by CSMR (hereafter CSMR women) suffer more often from psychiatric illness than women giving birth by other modes of delivery. Mood disorders, anxiety [10, 14, 15], and the use of psychotropic medications are more common in women fearing childbirth [11, 14]. We have earlier reported that the presence of psychiatric disorders five years before childbirth increases

* Correspondence: Gunilla.Sydsjo@liu.se
[1]Department of Obstetrics and Gynaecology, and Department of Clinical and Experimental Medicine, Linköping University, SE-581 85 Linköping, Sweden
Full list of author information is available at the end of the article

the risk of giving birth by CSMR (aOR 2.5, 95% CI 2.0–3.2) [16]. The most common disorders were mood-, anxiety disorders and mental and behavioural disorders due to psychoactive substance use [16]. To our knowledge, no one has studied the long-term mental health after childbirth of CSMR women. Because having had psychiatric care before pregnancy and FOC have both been shown to increase the risk of requiring psychiatric care after delivery [14], we hypothesize that CSMR women are more likely to suffer from an increased psychiatric disease burden after delivery than any other group.

Therefore, the aim of this study was to compare the prevalence of psychiatric care five years before and after delivery in primiparae giving birth by CSMR with prevalence in all other primiparae giving birth during the study period. This knowledge is important in order to provide optimal care for these women. By using the identical study population as in our previous study [16], we have been able to compare the prevalence of psychiatric disorders before and after delivery. The study population comprises a nationwide cohort of all women born in Sweden 1973–1983, giving birth for the first time in 2002–2004.

Methods

The study population is identical to the study population in our previous study and the methods for collecting the data have been described before [16].

The material is based on data from several Swedish National registries. By using the women's unique personal identification number, data from several registries were linked. Assigning every woman a new de-identified number anonymised the dataset.

The Swedish Medical Birth Register (MBR) contains information on maternal characteristics, pregnancies, deliveries and birth characteristics. The MBR was begun in 1973 and has high validity, covering approximately 99% of all deliveries [17]. From this register mode of delivery and maternal characteristics at admission to antenatal care (age, BMI, tobacco use and somatic disorders) were gathered. The National Patient registry (NPR) started to record inpatient care in 1987 and from 2001 and onwards it also contains outpatient care except for primary health care. The coverage of the inpatient care is generally high with 90–94% having a main diagnosis recorded during the study period. The data from the outpatient care are less reliable with 34–79% having a main diagnosis registered during the study period [18]. The outcome of interest in this part of the study was psychiatric illness five years after delivery. Psychiatric illness was defined as in- and/or outpatient care registered together with a psychiatric diagnosis according to the International Classification of Diseases (ICD). Psychiatric diagnoses were identified as codes F00-F99 and these codes were divided into 11 categories according to ICD-10 (Table 1) [19, 20]. The time

Table 1 Categories of psychiatric disorders according to ICD-10

F00-F09	Organic, including symptomatic, mental disorders
F10-F19	Mental and behavioural disorders due to psychoactive substance use
F20-F29	Schizophrenia, schizotypal and delusional disorders
F30-F39	Mood (affective) disorders
F40-F48	Neurotic, stress-related and somatoform disorders
F50-F59	Behavioural syndromes associated with physiological disturbances and physical factors
F60-F69	Disorders of adult personality and behaviour
F70-F79	Mental retardation
F80-F89	Disorders of psychological development
F90-F98	Behavioural and emotional disorders with onset usually occurring in childhood and adolescence
F99-F99	Unspecified mental disorder

period was defined as date of first delivery plus five years. Only dates of admission or dates of visit during this timeframe were included. The prevalence of psychiatric illness five years before delivery has been published in our previous study and was retrieved using the same methods [16].

Background data on sociodemographic variables were gathered from the Total Population register (TPR) [21], the Education register [22], and the Multi-generation register [23]. TPR contains data on births, deaths, citizenship, marital status, migration and country of birth for Swedish residents born abroad [21]. The Education register records data on highest educational attainment and the multi-generation register records kinship [22]. By using the multi-generation register we could identify the parents of our study sample [23].

The study population comprised all women born in Sweden 1973–1983 who were alive and still living in Sweden at 13 years of age (n = 500,245). The original dataset was sorted based on data from the Causes of Death registry, which has reported on causes of deaths since 1961 and has a high validity [24]. For the purpose of another study using the same dataset, women with missing values on birthweight, gestational length as well as implausible birthweights compared to length of gestation at their own birth were excluded (n = 5553). From the final cohort we selected women giving birth for the first time in 2002 to 2004 (n = 64,834). Only primiparae were included because we were interested in primary FOC.

The exposure of interest was CSMR. CSMR was defined as the delivery diagnosis O82.8 in ICD-10 [10, 20]. In the Swedish version of ICD-10 it is labelled "Caesarean section on psychosocial indication" and it is the code that should be used for CSMR [19] (labelled as "encounter for caesarean without indication" in the English version of ICD-10) [20]. However, we do not know whether the women actually requested a CS.

CSMR women (n = 1009, 1.6%) were compared to women giving birth by other modes of delivery (n = 63,826) (hereafter referred to as "the reference group") including vaginal delivery (n = 55,012, 84.9%), emergency CS (n = 5826, 9%) and elective CS for all other reasons except maternal request (n = 2859, 4.4%). Vaginal delivery was defined as ICD-10 codes; spontaneous vaginal delivery (O80), single instrumental vaginal delivery by forceps or vacuum extraction (O81), other assisted single delivery (O83) or multiple vaginal delivery (O84.1 and O84.9). Included were also women missing a delivery diagnosis but having the diagnosis "care after vaginal delivery" (Z.39.0A/B) or a notation in MBR that the delivery ended "vaginally", "by forceps" or "by vacuum extraction". Emergency CS was defined as single (O82.1) and multiple delivery (O84.8) by emergency CS or a notation in MBR that the delivery was by "emergency CS", "not an elective CS" or "delivery ended by CS". Elective CS single delivery (O82, O82.0, O82.9) and multiple delivery by elective CS (O84.2 and O84.3) as well as women missing delivery diagnosis but having the diagnosis "care after CS" (Z.39.0C/D) or a notation in MBR saying "delivery by elective CS before contractions started", "delivery by elective CS" or "delivery started by CS". The following background variables were registered in MBR at admission to antenatal care; age, body mass index (BMI), smoking status, the use of snuff, and somatic diseases (recurring urinary tract infection, inflammatory bowel disease, epilepsy, asthma/lung disease, diabetes mellitus, kidney disease, hypertension and systemic lupus erythematosus). Age was categorized into ≤25 or >25 years old. BMI was divided into five categories (<18.5, 18.5–24.9, 25–24.9, 25–29.9, 30–34.9 and ≥35 kg/m^2). Smoking and the use of snuff were collapsed into one variable called "tobacco use" which thus includes the use of snuff and/or smoking. From the other registers, marital status, educational attainment, parents' country of birth and working status were gathered. Marital status was categorized into "married", "unmarried" and "divorced/widowed". Highest educational attainment was assessed in 2004 and divided into three categories; "Elementary", "High School" and "University". Parents' country of birth were categorised as born inside or outside of Scandinavia. Working status was defined as an income >39,300 SEK per year in 2004 according to Statistics Sweden's definition of paid work.

Missing data

Mode of delivery was missing for 128 (0.2%) women. Educational attainment was missing for 193 (0.3%) women. Working status was missing for 92 (0.1%) and BMI was missing for 8765 (13.5%) of women. Missing data were included in the analysis and applied their own category in each variable.

Background data

Comparisons of sociodemographic variables and psychiatric illness five years before delivery between CSMR women and the reference group have been published earlier [16]. CSMR women were older (68.4 vs. 64.7% >25 years, $p < 0.001$), used tobacco more often (18.3 vs. 13.0%, $p < 0.001$), had a lower educational attainment (16.0 vs. 10.1% elementary school, $p < 0.001$), were more often married (36.2 vs 32.8%, p < 0.001), unemployed (13.1 vs 8.6%, p < 0.001), had a higher BMI ($p < 0.001$) and more often parents born outside of Scandinavia (9.1 vs 6.0%, $p < 0.001$) compared to the reference group. They had also more often recurrent urinary tract infection (22.5 vs 16.8%, p < 0.001), asthma/lung disease (13.1 vs 9.2%, p < 0.001) and inflammatory bowel disease (1.4 vs 0.7%, $p = 0.01$). No significant differences were found for kidney disease (0.8 vs 0.5%), diabetes mellitus (0.9 vs 0.5%), epilepsy (1.1 vs 0.6%), SLE (0.1 vs 0.1%) or hypertension (0.3 vs 0.3%) compared to the reference group.

Statistics

CSMR women were compared to the reference group. The outcome of interest was psychiatric illness five years after first childbirth. Each category of psychiatric illness was treated as a binary variable. A binary variable for one or more registered psychiatric diagnosis in the in- and/or outpatient care ("any psychiatric disorder") was constructed. A similar variable was created for outpatient care only and another variable including those diagnosed in the inpatient care only and/or both the in- and outpatient care. The prevalence of each category of psychiatric disorder, the distribution of in- and outpatient care as well as the prevalence of any psychiatric disorder in CSMR women was compared to the reference group five years after delivery using Pearson's Chi square test. Whenever ≥20% of the expected values were below five, Fishers exact test was used instead. The prevalence of psychiatric disorders five years before delivery was compared to five years after delivery in the whole study population as well as within the two groups respectively by paired T-test. A paired T-test was considered appropriate since the sampling distribution of binary variables becomes approximately normally distributed in large samples according to the Central Limit Theorem.

To compare the rate of new cases (i.e. women diagnosed with a psychiatric disorder after first childbirth who had not been diagnosed during the five years before first childbirth), a binary variable was constructed for any psychiatric disorder after delivery that excluded cases diagnosed before delivery. Comparisons between the groups were made by Pearson's Chi Square test in the whole study population as well as only for women diagnosed with a psychiatric disorder after childbirth to compare the proportion of new cases among the cases.

The risk of psychiatric illness after delivery was estimated by multiple logistic regression analysis. Psychiatric disorders five years after delivery was considered the outcome and CSMR the exposure. To adjust for potential confounding, previous psychiatric care and background variables (age, BMI, educational attainment, tobacco use, marital status, parents' country of birth, working status and somatic diseases) were added to the model as covariates. Any psychiatric disorder as well as each of the eleven categories of psychiatric disorders were modelled separately in the logistic regression. CSMR and previous psychiatric care were tested for interaction effect in the logistic regression model. No significant interaction effect was found. A sensitivity analysis excluding all women diagnosed with a psychiatric disorder before first delivery was performed and no significant differences were found. All analyses were carried out in SPSS 22.0 (IBM SPSS Inc., Armonk, NY, USA). A p-value <0.05 was considered significant.

Results

Of all the women in the study, 2316 (3.6%) women had been diagnosed with one or more psychiatric disorder during the five years before first childbirth [16] and 3607 (5.6%) women had been diagnosed during the five years after first childbirth. Eight hundred ninety-two women had been diagnosed both before and after first childbirth. During the five years after the first childbirth, 1946 women were diagnosed only in the outpatient care register and 1661 women were diagnosed in both the in- and outpatient care register or in the inpatient care register only. Women in the reference group tended to more often be diagnosed only in the outpatient care register (54.2% vs. 45.1%, $p = 0.056$) (Table 2). The majority, i.e. 75.3%, of the women with a psychiatric diagnosis after childbirth, had not been diagnosed during the five years before childbirth. In the group of CSMR women 60% ($n = 68$) with a psychiatric diagnosis had not been diagnosed before childbirth compared to 76% ($n = 2647$) of the women in the reference group ($p < 0.001$, data not shown).

Table 2 Distribution of psychiatric in- and outpatient care by mode of delivery in women diagnosed with one or more psychiatric disorder after delivery

Mode of delivery	Outpatient care only n (%)	Inpatient care with/without outpatient care n (%)	P
Caesarean section on maternal request	51 (45.1)	62 (54.9)	0.056
Other mode of delivery	1895 (54.2)	1599 (45.8)	
Total	1946 (54.0)	1661 (46.0)	

The prevalence of psychiatric disorders had increased after childbirth (3.6% vs. 5.6%, mean difference 0.2 ± 0.25, 95% CI 0.018–0.022, $p < 0.001$). There was an increase in the prevalence within both the reference group (3.5% vs. 5.5%, mean difference 0.02 ± 0.25, 95% CI 0.018–0.022, $t = 20.250$, p < 0.001) and in CSMR women (10.0% vs. 11.2%) but the increase was not significant in CSMR women (mean difference 0.01 ± 0.35, 95% CI -0.010: 0.034, $t = 1.078$, $p = 0.281$). There were significant increases in all categories of psychiatric disorders except "Organic, including symptomatic, mental disorders", "Unspecified mental disorder" and "Disorders of psychological development" in the reference group. However the differences were small (<1%) except for "mood disorders" (mean difference 0.015 ± 0.17, 95% CI 0.013–0.016, $t = 21.719$, $p < 0.001$) and "neurotic, stress-related and somatoform disorders" (mean difference 0.016 ± 0.19, 95% CI 0.014–0.017, $t = 20.347$, $p < 0.001$). The prevalence of mood disorders had increased significantly in the group of CSMR women (mean difference 0.027 ± 0.23, 95% CI 0.012–0.041, $t = 3.663$, $p < 0.001$) but no significant differences were found for the other disorders. However new cases, i.e. women with a psychiatric diagnosis registered only after childbirth, were more common in CSMR women (6.7% vs. 4.1%, $p < 0.001$, data not shown). Being diagnosed with one or more psychiatric disorder after childbirth was more common in CSMR women (11.2% vs. 5.5%, $p < 0.001$) (Table 3). The following categories of psychiatric disorders were significantly more common in CSMR women; "Mental and behavioural disorders due to psychoactive substance use" (2.7% vs 0.8%, $p < 0.001$), "Disorders of adult personality and behavior" (1.3% vs 0.5%, p=0.001), "Behavioural syndromes associated with physiological disturbances and physical factors" (1.3% vs 0.6%, $p = 0.003$), "Neurotic, stress-related and somatoform disorders" (6.9% vs 3.1%, $p < 0.001$), "Mood disorders" (6.0% vs 2.5%, p < 0.001) and "Unspecified mental disorder" (0.3% vs 0.0%, $p = 0.013$). No significant differences were found for the other psychiatric disorders in ICD-10 (Table 3).

CSMR increased the risk of one or more psychiatric disorder after delivery (OR 2.2, 95% CI 1.8–2.7) (Table 4). The risk was significant and increased for all categories of psychiatric disorders except "Mental retardation" (OR 2.4, 95% CI 0.3–18.0) and "Schizophrenia, schizotypal, and delusional disorders" (OR 0.5, 95% CI 0.1–3.7) (Table 4). After adjustment for potential confounders (previous psychiatric care, age, BMI, educational attainment, tobacco use, marital status, parents' country of birth, working status and somatic diseases) the risk decreased but remained significant for "Mental and behavioural disorder due to psychoactive substance use" (aOR 2.0, 95% CI 1.3–3.1), "Neurotic, stress-related and somatoform disorders" (aOR 1.6, 95% CI 1.2–2.1), "Mood disorders" (aOR 1.7, 95% CI 1.3–2.2) and "Unspecified

Table 3 Psychiatric disorders five years after childbirth among women in the two study groups

	Mode of delivery		
	Caesarean section on maternal request n (%)	Other delivery [a] n (%)	*P*
Any psychiatric disorder			
Yes	113 (11.2)	3494 (5.5)	<0.001
No	896 (88.8)	60,331 (94.5)	
Mental and behavioural disorders due to psychoactive substance use			
Yes	27 (2.7)	504 (0.8)	<0.001
No	982 (97.3)	63,321 (99.2)	
Disorders of adult personality and behaviour			
Yes	13 (1.3)	297 (0.5)	0.001**
No	996 (98.7)	63,528 (99.5)	
Behavioural syndromes associated with physiological disturbances and physical factors			
Yes	13 (1.3)	367 (0.6)	0.003
No	996 (98.7)	63,458 (99.4)	
Behavioural and emotional disorders with onset usually occurring in childhood and adolescence			
Yes	4 (0.4)	90 (0.1)	0.059 **
No	1005 (99.6)	63,735 (99.9)	
Neurotic, stress-related and somatoform disorders			
Yes	70 (6.9)	1993 (3.1)	<0.001
No	939 (93.1)	61,832 (96.9)	
Mood disorders			
Yes	61 (6.0)	1620 (2.5)	<0.001
No	948 (94.0)	62,205 (97.5)	
Mental retardation			
Yes	1 (0.1)	26 (0.0)	0.345**
No	1008 (99.9)	63,799 (100.0)	
Organic, including symptomatic, mental disorders			
Yes	2 (0.2)	29 (0.0)	0.084**
No	1007 (99.8)	63,796 (100.0)	
Schizophrenia, schizotypal, and delusional disorders			
Yes	1 (0.1)	123 (0.2)	1.0 **
No	1008 (99.9)	63,702 (99.8)	
Disorders of psychological development			
Yes	2 (0.2)	24 (0.0)	0.061**
No	1007 (99.8)	63,801 (100.0)	
Unspecified mental disorder			
Yes	3 (0.3)	29 (0.0)	0.013**
No	1006 (99.7)	63,796 (100.0)	

**Calculated by Fisher's exact test
[a]Other delivery, including: "Vaginal delivery", "Emergency caesarean section", "Elective caesarean section" and "Mode of delivery missing"

mental disorder" (aOR 4.0, 95% CI 1.2–13.8). The adjusted odds ratio for one or more psychiatric disorders was 1.5 (95% CI 1.2–1.9) (Table 4). There was no significant interaction effect between previous psychiatric care and CSMR. To evaluate the robustness of the estimates two different sensitivity analyses were performed. In the first analysis, all women previously diagnosed with psychiatric illness were removed from the analysis and in the second analysis no adjustments for previous psychiatric illness were included. None of these both analyses changed the parameter estimates substantially and no statistical differences in the estimates were detected. The

Table 4 Unadjusted and adjusted odds ratios for psychiatric disorders five years after childbirth by caesarean section on maternal request

Psychiatric disorder five years after childbirth	Caesarean section on maternal request			
	OR	95% CI	aOR [a]	95% CI
Any psychiatric disorder	2.2	1.8–2.7	1.5	1.2–1.9
Mental and behavioural disorder due to psychoactive substance use	3.5	2.3–5.1	2.0	1.3–3.1
Disorders of adult personality and behaviour	2.8	1.6–4.9	1.4	0.8–2.5
Behavioural syndromes associated with physiological disturbances and physical factors	2.3	1.3–3.9	1.5	0.9–2.7
Behavioural and emotional disorders with onset usually occurring in childhood and adolescense	2.8	1.0–7.7	1.5	0.5–4.3
Neurotic, stress-related and somatoform disorders	2.3	1.8–3.0	1.6	1.2–2.1
Mood disorders	2.5	1.9–3.2	1.7	1.3–2.2
Mental retardation	2.4	0.3–18.0	0.2	0.2–3.3
Organic, including symptomatic, mental disorders	4.4	1.0–18.3	2.9	0.7–12.7
Schizophrenia, schizotypal, and delusional disorders	0.5	0.1–3.7	0.3	0.0–1.8
Disorders of psychological development	5.3	1.3–22.4	2.5	0.5–11.5
Unspecified mental disorder	6.6	2.0–21.6	4.0	1.2–13.8

[a]Adjusted for previous psychiatric disorder, age, marital status, BMI, parent's country of birth, working status, tobacco use, educational attainment, urinary tract infection, inflammatory bowel disease, SLE, hypertension, diabetes mellitus, epilepsy, kidney disease and lung disease/asthma

largest risk factor for psychiatric illness five years, after childbirth was previous psychiatric care (aOR 9.9, 95% CI 8.9–10.9).

Discussion

In this study we found that CSMR is an independent risk factor for psychiatric illness after first childbirth. CSMR women more often suffer from psychiatric disorders both before and after first delivery compared to other primiparae. As in the general population, the most common disorders were "Mood disorders", "Neurotic, stress-related and somatoform disorders" and "Mental and behavioural disorders due to psychoactive substance use" [25]. The prevalence of psychiatric disorders had increased after compared to before delivery and the majority of the women were diagnosed with a psychiatric disorder only after childbirth. When comparing within the two groups the increase in the prevalence of psychiatric disorders were significant in the reference group but not in the CSMR group except for "mood disorders". The observed increase in the prevalence of psychiatric disorders may be caused by the fact that many of the most common psychiatric disorders increases with age, e.g. mood disorders with a median age of onset in the 4th decade [26]. The postpartum period is also a well-known risk factor for the first onset of psychiatric disorders [27]. However the increase in the prevalence of psychiatric disorders was only significant in the reference group. For most separate disorders the increase was small and not clinically significant but there was an overall increase as well as a clinically significant increase in both mood disorders and neurotic, stress-related and somatoform disorders. Since the sample size differed in the two groups, the lack of a significant increase in the CSMR group may be caused by a lack of power to detect such a difference. Furthermore the women in the reference group showed a tendency towards more often being diagnosed in the outpatient care system. Because the reporting from the outpatient care started in 2001 [18], the data before delivery (1997–2004) have a lower coverage in the outpatient care. Therefor the observed increase may merely reflect a better coverage of the outpatient care and therefore not a true increase in the prevalence. The outpatient care excludes admissions to hospital but the care is provided by specialists in psychiatry and does not include primary health care. Being diagnosed mainly in the psychiatric outpatient care may indicate that the reference group suffer from a lighter psychiatric disease burden, possible to treat in the outpatient care. These findings are in accordance with a previous study by Rouhe et al. who compared psychiatric care before and after childbirth in women with FOC or without FOC during pregnancy. They found women with FOC had an increased risk of requiring psychiatric care 5–12 years after delivery but the risk was even higher among women without FOC [14]. One speculates that the larger increase in the prevalence of psychiatric disorders after childbirth among women in the reference group may be explained by the fact that CSMR women are diagnosed and treated earlier. In Sweden women cannot choose a CS, they must meet with an obstetrician to discuss the reasons for the request and receive information on risks and benefits of CS. This meeting may lead to consultation with a psychologist/therapist. In this process the woman can be diagnosed and referred to treatment, medication and/or psychotherapy which may have improved these women's mental health. Indeed of those women with psychiatric disorders after delivery, CSMR women were more likely to have been diagnosed before.

This could indicate that CSMR women are diagnosed earlier or suffer from more complex psychiatric disorders that are relapsing in character. However the incidence of new cases with psychiatric disorders after delivery was higher among CSMR women compared to the reference group, indicating that these women still have a higher risk of psychiatric disorders also after delivery even when they were not diagnosed during pregnancy.

The prevalence of psychiatric disorders was lower than reported in previous studies [14, 25], including studies on pregnant women [15]. It is difficult to compare rates because different studies use different methods of diagnosing such as use of registers, diagnostic interviews, self-rating questionnaires and measure prevalence during different lengths of time [14, 15, 25]. The reason for the lower prevalence in our study is unknown but may be because the diagnoses in NPR are made by a physician rather than by self-rated questionnaires for example. Furthermore the coverage of NPR is incomplete [18]; and not all psychiatric disorders are diagnosed and treated in the public psychiatric healthcare system and therefore not all are registered. The coverage of the outpatient care is less valid than the inpatient care and this may have affected our results as the reference group showed a tendency towards more often be diagnosed in the outpatient care. This could make us underestimate the true prevalence of psychiatric disorders in the reference group and is a limitation in our study. However when only comparing inpatient care the prevalence of psychiatric disorders was significantly higher in CSMR women. Our inclusion criteria limited the age distribution and excluded women born outside of Sweden. These are factors associated with CSMR [3, 5, 13], and immigrants may suffer more often from psychiatric illness [28], therefore we might underestimate the frequency of CSMR and psychiatric disorders. We also lack a clear definition for CSMR. In Sweden the diagnostic code O82.8 is referred to as "CS on psychosocial indication" and is the diagnostic code that should be applied for CSMR. However some women may be misclassified as elective CS for example and thereby lower our number of cases. In our previous study we found somatic disorders such as e.g. dyspareunia increases the risk of CSMR [29]. This may be a confounding factor since these women more often report mental ill-health. However, the prevalence of dyspareunia is low and should not alter the results significantly. It is impossible to adjust for all possible somatic diseases, however this should be taken into account when interpreting the results.

Our nationwide sample with access to a range of important variables is a major strength of our study making the results more generalizable. In NPR the diagnoses are set by a physician and probably are more valid than diagnoses resulting from questionnaires that can only detect symptoms of e.g. depression or anxiety. By only including primiparae we avoided the potential confounding of a previous negative birth experience. We adjusted for sociodemographic variables, somatic diseases registered in MBR and previous psychiatric care since these variables could possibly be associated to CSMR as well as psychiatric illness. This was important since these variables were all found to have an impact on the risk of psychiatric disorders, especially previous psychiatric care (OR 13.8, 95% CI 12.6–15.2).

Conclusion

We have previously found CSMR women more often suffer from psychiatric disorders before delivery [16] and we can now confirm that these women have an equally high prevalence of psychiatric disorders after delivery. The tendency towards a higher prevalence of inpatient care indicates these women may suffer from a heavier psychiatric disease burden. This shows that these women are a vulnerable group requiring special attention from both obstetric- and general health care providers, and this vulnerability should be taken into account when deciding on mode of delivery. The higher incidence of psychiatric disorders also indicates that these women may require a more intense follow-up. We hypothesize that these women benefit from the care during pregnancy, the incidence might have been even higher without the care. In conclusion, women giving birth by CSMR share a greater burden of mental illness before and after delivery.

Abbreviations

BMI: Body mass index; CS: Caesarean section; CSMR women: women giving birth by caesarean section on maternal request; CSMR: Caesarean section on maternal request; FOC: Fear of childbirth; MBR: Swedish Medical Birth Registry; NPR: National patient registry; Reference group: All primiparae giving birth by other modes of delivery than caesarean section on maternal request; TPR: Total population register

Funding

This study was supported by grants from The Research Council in the southeast of Sweden, FORSS.

Authors' contributions

GS, EA, CL and AJ had the original idea for the study. All authors planned the study. LM and MB analysed the data and drafted the article. All authors contributed to the interpretation of the data and to the revisions, and gave input at all stages of the study. All authors have approved the final version of the article for publication.

Competing interests

The authors declare that they have no competing interests.

Author details

[1]Department of Obstetrics and Gynaecology, and Department of Clinical and Experimental Medicine, Linköping University, SE-581 85 Linköping, Sweden.

[2]Division of Obstetrics and Gynaecology, Department of Clinical Sciences, Karolinska Institutet, Danderyd Hospital, Stockholm, Sweden.

References

1. Betran AP, et al. Rates of caesarean section: analysis of global, regional and national estimates. Paediatr Perinat Epidemiol. 2007;21:98–113.
2. Stjernholm YV, Petersson K, Eneroth E. Changed indications for cesarean sections. Acta Obstet Gynecol Scand. 2010;89:49–53.
3. Fuglenes D, et al. Why do some pregnant women prefer cesarean? The influence of parity, delivery experiences, and fear. Am J Obstet Gynecol. 2011;205:45.
4. Hildingsson I, et al. Few women wish to be delivered by caesarean section. BJOG. 2002;109:618–23.
5. Kringeland T, Daltveit AK, Moller A. What characterizes women in Norway who wish to have a caesarean section? Scand J Public Health. 2009;37:364–71.
6. Nieminen K, Stephansson O, Ryding EL. Women's fear of childbirth and preference for cesarean section–a cross-sectional study at various stages of pregnancy in Sweden. Acta Obstet Gynecol Scand. 2009;88:807–13.
7. Wiklund I, Edman G, Andolf E. Cesarean section on maternal request: reasons for the request, self-estimated health, expectations, experience of birth and signs of depression among first-time mothers. Acta Obstet Gynecol Scand. 2007;86:451–6.
8. Rouhe H, et al. Fear of childbirth according to parity, gestational age, and obstetric history. BJOG. 2009;116:67–73.
9. Lukasse M, Schei B, Ryding EL. Prevalence and associated factors of fear of childbirth in six European countries. Sex Reprod Healthc. 2014;5:99–106.
10. Storksen HT, et al. Fear of childbirth; the relation to anxiety and depression. Acta Obstet Gynecol Scand. 2012;91:237–42.
11. Nordeng H, et al. Fear of childbirth, mental health, and medication use during pregnancy. Arch Womens Ment Health. 2012;15:203–9.
12. Sjogren B. Reasons for anxiety about childbirth in 100 pregnant women. J Psychosom Obstet Gynaecol. 1997;18:266–72.
13. Wiklund I, et al. Personality and mode of delivery. Acta Obstet Gynecol Scand. 2006;85:1225–30.
14. Rouhe H, et al. Mental health problems common in women with fear of childbirth. BJOG. 2011;118:1104–11.
15. Andersson L, et al. Point prevalence of psychiatric disorders during the second trimester of pregnancy: a population-based study. Am J Obstet Gynecol. 2003;189:148–54.
16. Sydsjo G, et al. Psychiatric illness in women requesting caesarean section. BJOG. 2015;122:351–8.
17. National Board of Health and Welfare, Centre for Epidemiology. The Swedish medical birth register; a summary of contents and quality. 2003; 2003–112-3: http://www.socialstyrelsen.se/Lists/Artikelkatalog/Attachments/10655/2003-112-3_20031123.pdf. Accessed 14 June 2016.
18. National Board of Health and Welfare and Centre for Epidemiology. Kvalitet och innehåll i patientregistret. 2009. http://www.socialstyrelsen.se/publikationer2009/2009-125-15. Accessed 18 June 2016.
19. National Board of Health and Welfare and Centre for Epidemiology. Internationell statistisk klassifikation av sjukdomar och relaterade hälsoproblem – Systematisk förteckning, svensk version 2017 (ICD-10-SE). http://www.socialstyrelsen.se/Lists/Artikelkatalog/Attachments/20574/2017-4-2.pdf. Accessed 26 Sept 2017.
20. World Health Organisation. International Statistical Classification of Diseases and Related Health Problems 10th Revision. Available at: http://apps.who.int/classifications/icd10/browse/2016/en. Accessed 22 Nov 2015.
21. Statistics Sweden. A new total population register system. More possibilities and better quality. Örebro: Statistics Sweden; 2002.
22. Statistics Sweden. Educational attainment of the population 2004. 2005. http://www.scb.se/statistik/UF/UF0506/2005A01/UF0506_2005A01_SM_UF37SM0501.pdf. Accessed 18 June 2016.
23. Statistics Sweden. Multi-generation register 2010. A desciption of contents and quality. 2011. http://www.scb.se/statistik/_publikationer/BE9999_2011A01_BR_BE96BR1102.pdf. Accessed 18 June 2016.
24. National Board of Health and Welfare and Centre for Epidemiology. Causes of death 2011. 2012. http://www.socialstyrelsen.se/Lists/Artikelkatalog/Attachments/19001/2013-2-30.pdf. Accessed 18 June 2016.
25. Wittchen HU, et al. The size and burden of mental disorders and other disorders of the brain in Europe 2010. Eur Neuropsychopharmacol. 2011;21: 655–79.
26. Kessler RC, et al. Lifetime prevalence and age-of-onset distributions of DSM-IV disorders in the National Comorbidity Survey Replication. Arch Gen Psychiatry. 2005;62:593–602.
27. Munk-Olsen T, Laursen TM, Pedersen CB, Mors O, Mortensen PB. New parents and mental disorders: a population-based register study. JAMA. 2006;296:2582–9.
28. Tinghog P, Hemmingsson T, Lundberg I. To what extent may the association between immigrant status and mental illness be explained by socioeconomic factors? Soc Psychiatry Psychiatr Epidemiol. 2007;42:990–6.
29. Möller L, Josefsson A, Bladh M, Lilliecreutz C, Sydsjö G. Reproduction and mode of delivery in women with vaginismus or localised provoked vestibulodynia: a Swedish register-based study. BJOG. 2015;122:329–34.

Cesarean deliveries and maternal weight retention

Kandice A. Kapinos[1], Olga Yakusheva[2*] and Marianne Weiss[3]

Abstract

Background: Cesarean delivery accounts for nearly one-third of all births in the U.S. and contributes to an additional $38 billion in healthcare costs each year. Although Cesarean delivery has a long record of improving maternal and neonatal mortality and morbidity, increased utilization over time has yielded public health concerns and calls for reductions. Observational evidence suggests Cesarean delivery is associated with increased maternal postpartum weight, which may have significant implications for the obesity epidemic. Previous literature, however, typically does not address selection biases stemming from correlations of pre-pregnancy weight and reproductive health with Cesarean delivery.

Methods: We used fetal malpresentation as a natural experiment as it predicts Cesarean delivery but is uncorrelated with pre-pregnancy weight or maternal health. We used hospital administrative data (including fields used in vital birth record) from the state of Wisconsin from 2006 to 2013 to create a sample of mothers with at least two births. Using propensity score methods, we compared maternal weight prior to the second pregnancy of mothers who delivered via Cesarean due to fetal malpresentation to mothers who deliver vaginally.

Results: We found no evidence that Cesarean delivery in the first pregnancy causally leads to greater maternal weight, BMI, or movement to a higher BMI classification prior to the second pregnancy.

Conclusions: After accounting for correlations between pre-pregnancy weight, gestational weight gain, and mode of delivery, there is no evidence of a causal link between Cesarean delivery and maternal weight retention.

Keywords: Cesarean delivery, Post pregnancy weight, Fetal malpresentation

Background

Cesarean delivery is the most common surgery in the U.S. occurring in nearly 33% of all live births [1, 2]. Rates of Cesareans have increased from a low of 21% in 1996 to almost 33% where the rate has remained since 2009 [3, 4]. For nearly 3 decades, the World Health Organization (WHO) has argued that although Cesarean deliveries clearly improve maternal and child health outcomes when medically indicated, a population-level Cesarean section rate of greater than 10–15% is not linked with better health outcomes [5]. Evidence suggests Cesarean delivery when *not* medically indicated leads to negative health outcomes - longer postpartum recovery [6], higher rates of re-hospitalization [7], longer hospital stays [8] and greater risk of maternal morbidity [9]. Beyond the impact on the immediate pregnancy outcomes, there may be longer-term adverse impacts on maternal health outcomes, including cumulative weight retention between pregnancies [10, 11].

Several observational studies have documented evidence of an association between Cesarean delivery and subsequent maternal weight. The odds of Cesarean delivery are 1.46 and 2.05 higher for women who are overweight or obese prior to their first pregnancies, respectively, relative to normal weight women [11]. There is also weak-to-moderate evidence on the positive association between gestational weight gain and Cesarean delivery suggesting that greater gestational weight gain is linked to a higher risk of Cesarean delivery even controlling for comorbidities [7, 12–16]. For example, one study using US vital statistics records reported a nearly 40% increase in the adjusted odds of Cesarean delivery for women who gained more than 40 lb during pregnancy [13].

* Correspondence: yakush@med.umich.edu
[2]University of Michigan, School of Nursing and School of Public Health, 400 North Ingalls Building, Ann Arbor, MI 48109-5482, USA
Full list of author information is available at the end of the article

The challenge in identifying a causal effect of Cesarean delivery on maternal weight is that many of the medical indications for Cesarean delivery are also independently associated with both pregravid and postpartum weight. The most common clinical indications for Cesarean delivery are labor dystocia (slow labor) and non-reassuring fetal tracing (interderminate fetal heart), occurring in 34 and 23% of all Cesarean deliveries, respectively [17]. The likelihood of slower labor progression and fetal distress both increase as the mother's pre-pregnancy body mass index (BMI) increases [15, 18, 19]. Pre-pregnancy weight or BMI is also correlated with both gestational weight gain and postpartum weight [15]. Therefore, we might observe a positive association between Cesarean delivery and maternal postpartum weight simply because heavier women are at a greater risk of having the clinical indications for Cesarean delivery and are more likely to weigh more after birth. Therefore, a positive association of Cesarean delivery with maternal postpartum weight retention may be driven by this confounding and not necessarily by the Cesarean itself.

Improved knowledge on the causal effect of Cesarean delivery may better inform provider practices and maternal choices, which can result in a healthier population and may generate significant healthcare cost savings. If Cesareans causally result in greater weight retention for new mothers, for example, due to slower physical recovery, then intervention efforts could focus on removing post-operative barriers. If, instead, the positive association between Caesareans and maternal post-birth weight is really driven by the fact that women who are heavier prior to pregnancy are more likely to have a Cesarean, then that adds to the argument that broader and more intensive efforts to promote healthier lifestyle and weight habits throughout the life course are needed (irrespective of pregnancy). Maternal post-birth weight retention is of significant concern for the growing obesity problem in the U.S. with studies documenting permanent weight retention of 13 to 22 lb for mothers 10 to 15 years after giving birth, [20, 21] the magnitude of which can easily move a woman from normal weight to overweight, or overweight to obese. Cesarean deliveries in the U.S. also cost about $9500 more than vaginal births, on average, for an added $38 billion in delivery costs in the U.S. per year [22]. With 2.5% of all births in the U.S. delivered via Cesarean upon maternal request without any medical indication, nearly $1 billion in excess delivery costs can be attributed to mothers requesting medically unnecessary Cesarean deliveries [22, 23].

This study aims to establish causal evidence on the role of Cesarean delivery on maternal postpartum weight by relying on a natural experiment using fetal malpresentation – any fetal body part position other than vertex, one of the main indicators for Cesarean delivery in uncomplicated low-risk pregnancies. As we discuss in the methods section below, fetal malpresentation satisfies the natural experiment framework for modeling causal impact of Cesarean delivery, because 1) its natural occurrence is essentially random (not chosen by the mother or her clinician, and unrelated to maternal weight prior to pregnancy or gestational weight gain), and 2) it nearly uniformly involves Cesarean delivery. Therefore, a statistical association of fetal malpresentation at delivery with maternal weight during the postpartum period can be interpreted, with a high degree of plausibility, as the causal effect of Cesarean delivery on maternal weight.

Nearly 19% of all primary Cesarean deliveries are due to fetal malpresentation [2], which occurs in approximately 3% of all term deliveries, with breech presentation (bottom/feet down) being the most common form of fetal malpresentation [24]. Consistent with a large body of evidence documenting inferior health outcomes among malpresenting infants delivered vaginally relative to Cesarean [25–27] and because malpresentation is an indication for Cesarean delivery and thus recommended by the American Congress of Obstetricians and Gynecologists' (ACOG), [28] most term malpresenting fetuses are delivered by Cesarean in the U.S.[1]

Methods

Study design

The study is a secondary retrospective data analysis of multi-hospital administrative data on first-time mothers with two births, using pre-pregnancy weight in the second pregnancy as the measure of maternal postpartum weight.

Our study contributes to the literature by relying on the conditional randomness of fetal malpresentation to isolate the causal impact of Cesarean delivery on maternal postpartum weight. As we point out above, in order for fetal malpresentation to serve as a natural experiment for measuring the effect of Cesarean delivery on postpartum weight, occurrence of fetal malplresentation must be uncorrelated with the mother's weight prior to pregnancy and gestational weight gain, as well as with any other obesity risk factors and maternal characteristics that might have a direct influence on maternal post-pregnancy weight. Statistically, this condition is satisfied for approximately 85 to 91% of breech presentations where no cause or risk factor can be identified [29]. However, malpresentation is significantly more likely in earlier gestational age, and among shorter and older women, which are all factors known to be independently associated with maternal weight [29–32]. Some evidence also suggests potential additional risk factors for fetal malplresentation (altered intrauterine contour or volume, as well altered fetal shape or mobility), all of which could have unknown independent associations with post-partum weight [30, 33–38]. Although most of these confounding associations become statistically insignificant when gestational age at birth is included in the models [31, 37], use of fetal malpresentation as a natural experiment for Cesarean delivery requires adjusting for these potential confounders—so that, after the adjustment, malpresentation is randomly assigned.

To further address potential issues of confounding, we employ a propensity score matching method, matching first-time mothers who delivered by Cesarean where fetal malpresentation is the *only* clinical indicator to first-time mothers who delivered vaginally.

Data and sample

Data

We relied on data previously obtained from PeriData.Net®, a data platform that contains data covering about 92% of hospital births in Wisconsin from 2006 to 2013. Following IRB approval at Marquette University (Weiss, PI) and data use agreements with 31 hospitals, we analyzed a de-identified dataset containing 236,820 birth records (64.78% of the total database) over the study period.

We restricted the sample to women for whom we observe *both* their first and second births with non-missing values on all key measures (see Appendix). We included mothers greater than age 17 at the time of the first birth and whose first birth was a singleton delivered between 28 and 42 weeks of gestation.[2] We excluded women who delivered their first infant by Cesarean due to any clinical indication other than fetal malpresentation. Fetal malpresentation is listed as a clinical indication for Cesarean delivery only (it is not observable in the records for vaginal deliveries). Our analytic sample of first-time mothers with a second birth includes 29,463 women across 31 hospitals: 777 Cesarean deliveries due to fetal malpresentation (2.64% of sample) and 28,686 vaginal deliveries (97.36% of sample).

We examined the following maternal weight outcomes: the mother's weight (in pounds), body mass index (BMI), and whether she was obese (BMI > 30) at the beginning of pregnancy 2; we refer to these measures as post-pregnancy or postpartum (to pregnancy 1). Pre-pregnancy weight for each pregnancy was derived from prenatal records submitted to the hospitals by the obstetrical provider prior to the birth. This measure was either self-reported to the obstetrical provider by the mother or measured at the first prenatal visit, but the method of obtaining the pre-pregnancy weight measure was not submitted. Maternal weight at delivery was recorded by hospital personnel as the weight measured either on admission in labor or at the last prenatal visit.

We included the following measures as matching characteristics in propensity score models: maternal age, maternal height, an indicator for any congenital anomalies of the newborn, perinatal death, or diagnosed fetal anomalies prior to delivery, an indicator for any uterine or placenta anomalies (any uterine or cervical anomaly, inverted uterus, incompetent cervix, placenta previa, polyhydramnios or oligohydramnios, eclampsia, uterine or cervical bleeding during the pregnancy), weeks of gestation at delivery, whether the mother reported alcohol or tobacco use during pregnancy, and whether the mother used the Women's, Infants, and Children (WIC) nutritional assistance program during the pregnancy, length of the interpregnancy interval (months between delivery of pregnancy 1 and pregnancy 2), and a set of maternal socio-demographic measures, including an indicator for advanced maternal age (> 35 years), indicators for white race, Hispanic/Latino ethnicity, college degree, and two sources of payment for the delivery (private health insurance, Medicaid, and other as the reference).

Statistical analysis

We used a propensity score matching (PSM) model in order to restrict the sample to mothers with fetal malpresentation matched one-to-one to statistically similar mothers who delivered vaginally [39]. We did this by using a regression-adjusted nearest-neighbor method for matching without replacement. Specifically, we estimated the propensity score, obtained as the predicted values after estimating a logistic regression of fetal malpresentation on maternal pre-pregnancy weight, weight at delivery, malpresentation risk factors (age, height, weeks of gestation, uterine/cervical abnormalities, and fetal/congenital anomalies) and other health and socio-demographic measures described above. We then selected comparison mothers who had vaginal deliveries that are "nearest," based on the estimated propensity score, to each treatment mother who delivered via Cesarean. We conducted t-tests to compare weight outcomes of treatment (Cesarean delivery due to fetal malpresentation) and comparison (vaginal delivery) mothers. Two-sided p-values of less than 0.05 were considered to indicate statistical significance.

We examined the robustness of our results by allowing multiple comparison mothers per treatment mother (instead of just one-to-one matching) and using propensity scores as weights in multivariate regressions. Additionally, as a final check, we excluded all mothers (both Cesarean due to fetal malpresentation and vaginal delivery) with any uterine, placental, or fetal/congenital anomalies, which reduced our sample by 7%.

Results

Sample characteristics

We present descriptive statistics of our analytic sample of first-time mothers with at least two births in the full unadjusted sample (first set of columns) and among the propensity score matched sample (second set of columns) in Table 1. The full sample included 29,463 women across 31 hospitals: 777 Cesarean deliveries due to fetal malpresentation (2.64% of sample) and 28,686 vaginal deliveries. This rate of Cesarean delivery due to fetal malpresentation is similar to the national rate among all hospital births in the U.S. that ended in a Cesarean section due to malpresentation in 2013.[3]

In the first two columns in Table 1, we compared sample means/percentages across the full sample of mothers. Mothers who delivered by Cesarean due to fetal malpresentation tended to weigh more prior to pregnancy and at delivery, were older, delivered earlier, and had higher rates of any fetal or congenital anomalies and uterine, cervical or placental abnormalities. These differences became statistically insignificant in the propensity score matched sample (last columns in Table 1).

Post-pregnancy maternal weight

The average maternal weight at the beginning of pregnancy 2 was 159.24 lb (95% CI, 156.38 to 162.09) for mothers who delivered by Cesarean due to fetal malpresentation (Panel B of Table 2). This is not statistically different for the matched mothers who delivered vaginally (*p*-value = 0.85). The average BMI at the beginning of pregnancy 2 was 26.54 (95% CI, 26.08 to 26.99) and 26.62 (95% CI, 26.17 to 27.06) for mothers who delivered by Cesarean and vaginally, respectively; these are not statistically different (p-value = 0.80). There was also no significant difference in the percent of mothers who were classified as obese at the beginning of pregnancy 2 by mode of delivery: 22.91% (95% CI, 19.95 to 25.87) of mothers delivering by Cesarean relative to 24.20% (95% CI, 21.17 to 27.21) of mothers delivering vaginally ($p = 0.55$).

Sensitivity analyses

In column 1 of Table 3, we present means and 95% CIs by mode of delivery where we have allowed multiple comparison mothers for each treatment mother in the propensity score matching (instead of just a one-to-one match). In column 2, we present adjusted means and 95% CIs from a multivariate regression model using propensity scores as weights and adjusting for the full set of health and socio-

Table 1 Sample Characteristics, Comparison by Mode of Delivery for Unmatched (full) and Propensity Score Matched Samples

	Cesarean *n* = 777		Full Sample: Vaginal *n* = 28,686		*p*-value	Propensity Score Matched Sample: Vaginal *n* = 777		*p*-value
Maternal Weight Measures	Mean/%	SE	Mean/%	SE		Mean/%	SE	
Prior to Pregnancy 1								
Weight (pounds)	154.81	1.41	151.75	0.22	*0.02*	155.30	1.37	*0.80*
BMI	25.88	0.22	25.43	0.03	*0.03*	26.62	0.23	*0.80*
% Obese (BMI > = 30)	18.92	1.40	18.31	0.23	*0.66*	21.10	1.47	*0.28*
At Pregnancy 1 Delivery								
Weight (pounds)	187.83	1.37	183.65	0.22	*0.00*	187.85	1.33	*0.99*
Malpresentation Risk Factors								
Maternal age	28.79	0.17	26.68	0.03	*0.00*	28.88	0.17	*0.69*
% Maternal age > 35	9.40	1.05	4.92	0.13	*0.00*	9.27	1.04	*0.93*
Maternal height (inches)	64.82	0.11	64.76	0.02	*0.58*	64.86	0.1	*0.75*
Weeks of gestation at delivery	38.33	0.08	39.06	0.01	*0.00*	38.32	0.08	*0.9*
% Any fetal or congenital anomaly or infant death	6.43	0.88	2.86	0.09	*0.00*	6.94	0.91	*0.68*
% Any uterine or placental anomalies	13.51	0.01	4.33	0.12	*0.00*	13.90	1.24	
5-Minute APGAR	8.86	0.03	8.89	0.00	*0.14*	3.85	0.03	*0.92*
Interpregnancy Interval (months)	29.44	0.45	30.06	0.08	*0.24*	29.49	0.51	*0.95*
% Tobacco use during pregnancy	9.91	1.07	13.13	0.20	*0.01*	10.17	1.08	*0.87*
% Alcohol use during pregnancy	0.64	0.29	0.64	0.05	*0.99*	0.51	0.26	*0.74*
% Maternal education = College+	48.39	1.79	33.50	0.28	*0.00*	46.85	1.79	*0.54*
% Maternal race = white	89.57	1.10	7.59	0.26	*0.00*	89.06	1.12	*0.74*
% Mother Hispanic/Latino	6.82	0.91	11.82	0.19	*0.00*	6.82	0.91	*1.00*
%Mother married	79.15	1.46	49.89	0.29	*0.00*	80.44	1.42	*0.53*
% Received WIC during pregnancy	14.16	1.25	19.43	0.23	*0.00*	11.45	1.14	*0.11*
% Payer = Private health insurance	65.00	1.71	38.94	0.29	*0.00*	65.51	1.71	*0.83*
% Payer = Medicaid	16.47	1.33	29.06	0.27	*0.00*	15.06	1.28	*0.44*

Notes: Cesarean delivery refers to births with fetal malpresentation as the only clinical indicator. P-values reflect whether sample means/percentages are statistically different by mode of delivery

Table 2 Predicted Maternal Weight Measures Prior to Pregnancy 2

	Weight (pounds)	BMI	% Obese (BMI > 30)
A. Full Sample, *n* = 29,463			
Cesarean Delivery	157.30	26.32	22.53
	(0.42)	(0.06)	(0.67)
Vaginal Delivery	158.05	26.46	24.03
	(0.22)	(0.04)	(0.24)
P-value (statistically different)	0.07	0.02	0.04
B. Propensity Score Matched Sample, *n* = 1554			
Cesarean Delivery	159.24	26.54	22.91
	(1.46)	(0.23)	(1.51)
Vaginal Delivery	159.61	26.62	24.20
	(1.43)	(0.23)	(1.56)
P-value (statistically different)	0.85	0.80	0.55

Notes: Robust standard errors in parentheses. The p-value listed corresponds to the difference between breech Cesarean and vaginal deliveries in each model (column)

economic covariates listed above (and in Table 1). Finally, in column 3, we present means and 95% CIs by mode of delivery where we have excluded all mothers with one of the following risk factors for fetal malpresentation: any congenital anomalies of the newborn, perinatal death, or diagnosed fetal anomalies prior to delivery, any uterine or cervical anomaly, inverted uterus, incompetent cervix, placenta previa, polyhydramnios or oligohydramnios, eclampsia, uterine or cervical bleeding during the pregnancy. The resulting sample included 651 mothers who delivered via Cesarean due to fetal malpresentation and their one-to-one matches. Results are largely consistent with those presented in Table 2.

Table 3 Sensitivity Checks

	Multiple comparisons	Propensity scores as weights	Restricted Sample
Panel A: Maternal weight (pounds)	(1)	(2)	(3)
Cesarean Delivery (Malpresentation)	159.24	158.88	159.08
	(157.54, 158.46)	(157.13, 160.63)	(157.36, 163.40)
Vaginal Delivery	158.00	159.98	160.38
	(158.46, 162.09)	(159.60, 160.36)	(157.36, 163.40)
P-value (statistically different)	0.39	0.18	0.55
Panel B: Maternal BMI			
Cesarean Delivery (Malpresentation)	26.54	26.42	26.54
	(26.08, 26.99)	(26.15, 26.70)	(26.06, 27.03)
Vaginal Delivery	26.46	26.69	26.81
	(26.39, 26.54)	(26.61, 26.76)	(26.34, 27.29)
P-value (statistically different)	0.75	0.04	0.44
Panel C: Mother Obese			
Cesarean Delivery (Malpresentation)	22.91%	24.04%	22.27%
	(19.95, 25.87)	(21.82, 26.27)	(19.07, 25.48)
Vaginal Delivery	24.02	24.62%	25.19%
	(23.53, 24.51)	(24.11, 25.13)	(21.85, 28.54)
P-value (statistically different)	0.47	0.58	0.22
N	29,463	29,463	1302

Notes: Column 1 compares mean postpartum weight measures of mothers with fetal malpresentation Cesarean and vaginal delivery where we have allowed *multiple* comparison matches per treatment observation. Column 2 contains predicted means obtained after a multivariate regression model using the propensity scores as weights and adjusting for covariates listed in the text. Column 3 compares mean postpartum weight measures using a matched sample that excludes mothers with malpresentation risk factors. The p-values listed correspond to the difference between Cesarean (due to fetal malpresentation) and vaginal deliveries in each model (column). The three panels (A-C) correspond to each weight measure

Discussion

Our findings do not support the notion derived from cross-sectional studies that Cesarean delivery leads to greater maternal weight retention after pregnancy. Using a large dataset from the state of Wisconsin that included hospital administrative records that contain vital records data, we found no evidence that first-time mothers delivering via Cesarean due *only* to fetal malpresentation weighed more at the beginning of their second pregnancies relative to their statistically matched mothers who delivered vaginally.

Our study contributes to both the literature examining the effects of Cesarean deliveries and to the literature endeavoring to explain the obesity epidemic in the U.S. we contribute to the ongoing debate about the risks and benefits of Cesarean delivery. In particular, our study suggests that although there are certainly health risks of Cesarean delivery, contribution to maternal weight retention does not seem to be one of them. Although obesity remains a significant public health concern, our findings do not suggest that mode of delivery contributes to weight gain. Instead, previously documented correlations of maternal weight retention and mode of delivery were likely driven by correlations between pre-pregnancy weight, gestational weight gain, and risk factors for Cesareans. Our finding adds to the knowledge base regarding the evolution of perinatal weight and its link to longer-term weight retention, but more research is needed to determine the extent to which other characteristics of the perinatal period matter in explaining long-term weight.

We point out the following limitation of our study. First, women who deliver a malpresenting infant via Cesarean may be a biased (higher-risk) subset of all women with a malpresenting fetus at delivery, potentially causing a bias toward finding an association between Cesarean delivery and poorer health outcomes. To the extent that poor health outcomes are also associated with being overweight or obese, this bias would likely only strengthen our conclusion that Cesarean delivery does not causally impact weight in the long term. Additionally, due to the clinical recommendation that malpresenting infants be delivered via Cesarean, this bias is likely small. In the 2013 national birth data, only 0.01% of all births to first-time adult mothers delivering between 28 and 42 weeks of gestation were malpresenting fetuses delivered vaginally.[4] An additional limitation of the analysis is the use of linked birth data from a single state, which may limit the generalizability of our findings. Results may be different among mothers who deliver via Cesarean but do not go on to have additional children, mothers in other states or for mothers with interpregnancy intervals longer than those available in the dataset. Finally, we note that excluding women who have Cesareans due to other clinical indications was necessary for the quasi-experimental design, but limits the generalizability of our findings.

Conclusions

In the light of a well-documented pattern of weight increase between pregnancies, our findings have important policy implications. Women and providers should be aware that women's postpartum weight changes are not influenced by the mode of delivery. Recommendations for restriction of exercise in the first weeks after Cesarean do not appear to contribute to additional weight retention between pregnancies; attention to interconceptional weight management is equally important for vaginal and Cesarean mothers. Reversing the pattern of maternal weight gain, through counselling and surveillance about weight management during the childbearing years and between pregnancies, could contribute to a more stable weight trajectory for women over the life course.

Endnotes

[1]Among first-time mothers with a term malpresenting fetus, 92% delivered via Cesarean in 2013 based on the authors' calculations using the 2013 National Vital Statistics Systems births data.

[2]Restricting the sample to mothers who deliver full-term (between 37 and 42 weeks of gestation) yields similar results to those presented here.

[3]Based on authors' calculations using the National Vital Statistics System births data for 2013, 3.34% of all births were delivered via Cesarean due to malpresentation.

[4]Authors' calculations using the 2013 NVSS births data. We note that a few states are missing presentation information for a small fraction of births with the exception of Virginia (missing about 50%) and Wyoming (missing on 100%).

Appendix

Table 4 Sample Construction

Criteria	# of Observations
Starting sample	236,820 births
1.Keep only if MONTHS_SINCE_LAST_ LIVE_BIRTH = 0 or is missing (no prior births) or BIRTH==1	97,171 births
2. Drop Cesarean births where fetal malpresentation is not indicator	75,021 births
3. Keep mothers age 18+ at first birth	69,875 births
4. Keep only births delivered between 28 and 42 weeks of gestation	67,480 births
5. Keep only singleton births	66,674 births
6.Keep mothers for whom we observe both first and second births	58,926 births
7. Final Analytic Sample (mothers with 2 births)	29,463 mothers

Acknowledgments
Not applicable.

Funding
This project was supported in part by the National Center for Advancing Translational Sciences, National Institutes of Health, through Grant Number 8UL1TR000055. Its contents are solely the responsibility of the authors and do not necessarily represent the official views of the NIH.

Authors' contributions
KAK conceived of the study, performed statistical analyses and drafted the manuscript. OY participated in the study design, contributed to the statistical analyses and revising the manuscript. MW participated in the study design and in revising the manuscript. All authors read and approved the final manuscript.

Competing interests
The authors declare that they have no competing interests.

Author details
[1]RAND Corporation, 1200 South Hayes, Arlington, VA 22202, USA. [2]University of Michigan, School of Nursing and School of Public Health, 400 North Ingalls Building, Ann Arbor, MI 48109-5482, USA. [3]Marquette University College of Nursing, 530 N 16th St, Milwaukee, WI 53233, USA.

References
1. Hamilton BE, Martin JA, Osterman MJK, Curtin SC. Births: Preliminary data for 2014. Natl Vital Stat Rep. 2015;64(6):1–19.
2. Boyle A, Reddy UM, Landy HJ, Huang CC, Driggers RW, Laughon SK. Primary cesarean delivery in the United States. Obstet Gynecol. 2013;122(1):33–40.
3. Menacker F, Declercq E, Macdorman MF. Cesarean Delivery: Background, Trends, and Epidemiology. Semin Perinatol. 2006;30(5):235–41.

4. Osterman MJ, Martin JA. Changes in cesarean delivery rates by gestational age: United States. NCHS Data Brief. 1996–2011;2013(124):1–8.
5. Betran AP, Torloni MR, Zhang JJ, Gülmezoglu AM. WHO Statement on caesarean section rates. BJOG. 2016;123:667-70.
6. Thompson JF, Roberts CL, Currie M, Ellwood DA. Prevalence and persistence of health problems after childbirth: associations with parity and method of birth. Birth. 2002;29(2):83–94.
7. Declercq E, Barger M, Cabral HJ, Evans SR, Kotelchuck M, Simon C, Weiss J, Heffner LJ. Maternal outcomes associated with planned primary cesarean births compared with planned vaginal births. Obstet Gynecol. 2007;109(3):669–77.
8. Liu S, Liston RM, Joseph K, Heaman M, Sauve R, Kramer MS. Maternal mortality and severe morbidity associated with low-risk planned cesarean delivery versus planned vaginal delivery at term. Can Med Assoc J. 2007; 176(4):455–60.
9. Sanchez-Ramos L, Wells T, Adair C, Arcelin G, Kaunitz A, Wells D. Route of breech delivery and maternal and neonatal outcomes. Int J Gynecol Obstet. 2001;73(1):7–14.
10. Weiss JL, Malone FD, Emig D, Ball RH, Nyberg DA, Comstock CH, Saade G, Eddleman K, Carter SM, Craigo SD, et al. Obesity, obstetric complications and cesarean delivery rate–a population-based screening study. Am J Obstet Gynecol. 2004;190(4):1091–7.
11. Chu SY, Kim SY, Schmid CH, Dietz PM, Callaghan WM, Lau J, Curtis KM. Maternal obesity and risk of cesarean delivery: a meta-analysis. Obes Rev. 2007;8(5):385–94.
12. Viswanathan M, Siega-Riz AM, Moos MK, Deierlein A, Mumford S, Knaack J, Thieda P, Lux LJ, Lohr KN. Outcomes of maternal weight gain. Evid Rep Technol Assess (Full Rep). 2008;168:1–223.
13. Rosenberg TJ, Garbers S, Lipkind H, Chiasson MA. Maternal obesity and diabetes as risk factors for adverse pregnancy outcomes: differences among 4 racial/ethnic groups. Am J Public Health. 2005;95(9):1545.
14. Hemminki E, Shelley J, Gissler M. Mode of delivery and problems in subsequent births: A register-based study from Finland. Am J Obstet Gynecol. 2005;193(1):169–77.
15. Institute of Medicine: Weight Gain During Pregnancy: Reexamining the Guidelines. In. Edited by Rasmussen KM, Yaktine AL: Institute of Medicine, National Research Council; 2009.
16. Li N, Liu E, Guo J, Pan L, Li B, Wang P, Liu J, Wang Y, Liu G, Baccarelli AA, et al. Maternal prepregnancy body mass index and gestational weight gain on pregnancy outcomes. PLoS One. 2013;8(12):e82310.
17. Barber EL, Lundsberg L, Belanger K, Pettker CM, Funai EF, Illuzzi JL. Contributing indications to the rising cesarean delivery rate. Obstet Gynecol. 2011;118(1):29.
18. Kominiarek MA, Zhang J, VanVeldhuisen P, Troendle J, Beaver J, Hibbard JU. Contemporary labor patterns: the impact of maternal body mass index. Am J Obstet Gynecol. 2011;205(3):244. e241-244.e248
19. Cedergren MI. Maternal morbid obesity and the risk of adverse pregnancy outcome. Obstet Gynecol. 2004;103(2):219–24.
20. Linné Y, Dye L, Barkeling B, Rössner S. Long-Term Weight Development in Women: A 15-Year Follow-up of the Effects of Pregnancy. Obes Res. 2004; 12(7):1166–78.
21. Rooney BL, Schauberger CW. Excess pregnancy weight gain and long-term obesity: One decade later. Obstet Gynecol. 2002;100(2):245–52.
22. Truven Health Analytics. The Cost of Having a Baby in the United States. In: Center for Healthcare Quality and Payment Reform; 2013.
23. American Congress of Obstetricians and Gynecologists. Cesarean Delivery on Maternal Request. In: Committee Opinion; 2013.
24. Arulkumaran S: Malpresentation, malposition, cephalopelvic disproportion and obstetric procedures. Dewhurst's Textbook of Obstetric and Gynaecology Edmonds DK (ed) 8th Edition John Wiley and Sons LTD 2012: 311–325.
25. Hannah ME, Hannah WJ, Hewson SA, Hodnett ED, Saigal S, Willan AR, Collaborative TBT. Planned caesarean section versus planned vaginal birth for breech presentation at term: a randomised multicentre trial. Lancet. 2000;356(9239):1375–83.
26. Berhan Y, Haileamlak A: The risks of planned vaginal breech delivery versus planned Caesarean section for term breech birth: a meta-analysis including observational studies. BJOG 2015:n/a-n/a.
27. Jensen VM, Wüst M. Can Caesarean section improve child and maternal health? The case of breech babies. J Health Econ. 2015;39:289–302.
28. American Congress of Obstetricians and Gynecologists Committee on Obstetric Practice. ACOG Committee Opinion No. 340. Mode of term singleton breech delivery. Obstet Gynecol. 2006;108(1):235.
29. Luterkort M, Persson PH, Weldner BM. Maternal and fetal factors in breech presentation. Obstet Gynecol. 1984;64(1):55–9.
30. Fruscalzo A, Londero AP, Salvador S, Bertozzi S, Biasioli A, Della Martina M, Driul L, Marchesoni D. New and old predictive factors for breech presentation: our experience in 14 433 singleton pregnancies and a literature review. J Mater-Fetal Neonatal Med. 2014;27(2):167–72.
31. Rayl J, Gibson PJ, Hickok DE. A population-based case-control study of risk factors for breech presentation. Am J Obstet Gynecol. 1996;174(1 Pt 1):28–32.
32. Hickok DE, Gordon DC, Milberg JA, Williams MA, Daling JR. The frequency of breech presentation by gestational age at birth: a large population-based study. Am J Obstet Gynecol. 1992;166(3):851–2.
33. Westgren M, Edvall H, Nordstrom L, Svalenius E, Ranstam J. Spontaneous cephalic version of breech presentation in the last trimester. Br J Obstet Gynaecol. 1985;92(1):19–22.
34. Ben-Rafael Z, Seidman DS, Recabi K, Bider D, Mashiach S. Uterine anomalies. A retrospective, matched-control study. J Reprod Med. 1991;36(10):723–7.
35. Michalas SP. Outcome of pregnancy in women with uterine malformation: evaluation of 62 cases. Int J Gynaecol Obstet. 1991;35(3):215–9.
36. Sekulic S, Ilincic M, Radeka G, Novakov-Mikic A, Simic S, Podgorac J, Kekovic G. Breech presentation and the cornual-fundal location of the placenta. Croatian Med J. 2013;54(2):198–202.
37. Mostello D, Chang JJ, Bai F, Wang J, Guild C, Stamps K, Leet TL. Breech presentation at delivery: a marker for congenital anomaly? J Perinatol. 2014; 34(1):11–5.
38. Soernes T, Bakke T. The length of the human umbilical cord in vertex and breech presentations. Am J Obstet Gynecol. 1986;154(5):1086–7.
39. Rosenbaum PR, Rubin DB. The central role of the propensity score in observational studies for causal effects. Biometrika. 1983;70(1):41–55.

Lack of controlled studies investigating the risk of postpartum haemorrhage in cesarean delivery after prior use of oxytocin

Karin Bischoff[1], Monika Nothacker[2], Cornelius Lehane[3], Britta Lang[1], Joerg Meerpohl[1] and Christine Schmucker[1*]

Abstract

Background: Postpartum haemorrhage (PPH) is a major cause of maternal mortality and morbidity worldwide. Experimental and clinical studies indicate that prolonged oxytocin exposure in the first or second stage of labour may be associated with impaired uterine contractility and an increased risk of atonic PPH. Therefore, particularly labouring women requiring cesarean delivery constitute a subset of patients that may exhibit an unpredictable response to oxytocin. We mapped the evidence for comparative studies investigating the hypothesis whether the risk for PPH is increased in women requiring cesarean section after induction or augmentation of labour.

Methods: We performed a systematic literature search for clinical trials in Medline, Embase, Web of Science, and the Cochrane Library (May 2016). Additionally we searched for ongoing or unpublished trials in clinicaltrials.gov and the WHO registry platform. We identified a total of 36 controlled trials investigating the exogenous use of oxytocin in cesarean section. Data were extracted for study key characteristics and the current literature literature was described narratively.

Results: Our evidence map shows that the majority of studies investigating the outcome PPH focused on prophylactic oxytocin use compared to other uterotonic agents in the third stage of labour. Only 2 dose-response studies investigated the required oxytocin dose to prevent uterine atony after cesarean delivery for labour arrest. These studies support the hypotheses that labouring women exposed to exogenous oxytocin require a higher oxytocin dose after delivery than non-labouring women to prevent uterine atony after cesarean section. However, the study findings are flawed by limitations of the study design as well as the outcome selection. No clinical trial was identified that directly compared exogenous oxytocin versus no oxytocin application before intrapartum cesarean delivery.

Conclusion: Despite some evidence from dose-response studies that the use of oxytocin may increase the risk for PPH in intrapartum cesarean delivery, current research has not investigated the prepartal application of oxytocin in well controlled clinical trials. It was striking that most studies on exogenous oxytocin are focused on PPH prophylaxis in the third stage of labour without differing between the indications of cesarean section and hence the prepartal oxytocin status.

Keywords: Oxytocin, Uterotonics, Postpartum haemorrhage, Intrapartum cesarean section

* Correspondence: schmucker@cochrane.de
[1]Cochrane Germany, Medical Center – University of Freiburg, Faculty of Medicine, University of Freiburg, Freiburg, Germany
Full list of author information is available at the end of the article

Background

Postpartum haemorrhage (PPH) is a major cause of maternal mortality and morbidity worldwide [1–4]. Approximately 36% of all lower segment cesarean deliveries and between 6 and 14% of spontaneous deliveries are complicated by PPH, depending on the definition used and the population studied [5–7]. Although global mortality from PPH is falling, its incidence is increasing in several high resource settings [8, 9]. In the United States, between 1994 and 2006, the rate of atonic PPH increased by 160% among women undergoing cesarean section after induction of labour and 130% among women undergoing non-induced cesarean section [10]. This increase may be explained by the increasing rates of cesarean sections and associated complications caused by general anesthesia, operative techniques or complications such as placental abruption leading to an emergency cesarean section [8, 11–14], but also due to an extensive use of uterotonics to induce or augment labour [7, 14].

The most widely used uterotonic drug for augmenting labour or to maintain uterine contractility during labour is oxytocin [15, 16]. Oxytocin, which was first synthetically synthesized in 1953 is also the first choice in the prevention and treatment of uterine atony [17]. When given in low-dose, oxytocin induces rhythmic uterine contractions which are indistinguishable in frequency, duration and strength from contractions observed during spontaneous labour [18, 19]. On the other hand, oxytocin for inducing or augmenting labour may desensitise the oxytocin receptors, thereby impairing oxytocin's post-delivery effects on uterine contractility [18]. For example, Balki et al. showed in different in vitro studies that pretreatment with oxytocin decreases oxytocin-induced myometrial contractions in pregnant humans and animals [20–22]. In addition, Grotegut et al. conducted a retrospective study on women who experienced severe PPH and found that these women received significantly greater amounts of oxytocin during labour compared with women without PPH, suggesting that prolonged pre- or intrapartum exposure to oxytocin might lead to decreased drug efficacy [23]. Similarly, Belghiti et al. investigated in a population-based case-control study the association between the level of oxytocin exposure during labour and the risk of severe atonic PPH [24, 25]. The study showed that oxytocin exposure during labour appears to be an independent risk factor for severe PPH in woman with spontaneous labour who did not receive prophylactic oxytocin after delivery (odds ratio after adjustment for all potential confounders [adjusted OR]: 1.8, 95% CI 1.3 to 2.6). Thereby, the strength of the association increased with the amount of oxytocin infused during labour [24, 25].

Considering that PPH rates are higher in cesarean section compared to spontaneous labour [7], particularly labouring women requiring cesarean delivery may constitute a subset of patients that may exhibit a negative response to exogenous oxytocin [14–16]. Therefore, we mapped the current literature for controlled clinical studies investigating the risk of atonic PPH in labouring women requiring cesarean delivery (intrapartum cesarean section) after oxytocin use for labour induction or augmentation in comparison to no exogenous oxytocin.

Methods

Sources

We adhered to the Preferred Reporting Items for Systematic reviews and Meta-Analyses (PRISMA) protocol for identifying, screening and eligibility of studies to conduct the present research work [see Additional file 1].

We searched for controlled clinical studies investigating exogenous oxytocin in cesarean delivery, irrespective of delivery indication, age, comorbidity or woman's parity. Primary maternal outcomes, we were interested in, included PPH rates, adverse effects or the need for additional uterotonics. In addition we collated any neonatal outcomes reported. A review protocol can be accessed from the corresponding author (CS).

Published studies were identified from searches of electronic databases. We searched Medline (OvidSP), Embase, Web of Science, the Cochrane library from inception until May 2016. The search strategy was based on combinations of medical subject headings (MeSH) and keywords and was not restricted to specific languages. The search strategy used in Medline (OvidSP) is presented in an additional file [see Additional file 2]. Search strategies for other databases were modified to meet the requirements of each database. The searches were supplemented by screening the bibliographies of relevant studies and systematic reviews. Potential ongoing studies were identified in the International Clinical Trials Registry Platform WHO (http://www.who.int/ictrp/en/) and the Register for Clinical Trials (http://clinicaltrials.gov/).

Study selection

One author (KB) screened the titles and abstracts of all reports identified by electronic searches. We obtained full-text copies of all potentially relevant articles and 2 reviewers (KB, CS) assessed them for inclusion. These authors also independently carried out data extraction for key characteristics of the study, participant and intervention.

Data analysis (mapping the evidence)

First, study characteristics such as country, study design, details of the intervention and control intervention, time point of drug application, week of gestation, sample size, age and indication for cesarean section were extracted and tabulated. Second, we looked whether the given PPH rates were stratified after the indication for cesarean delivery and/or when only women with intrapartum cesarean section were included whether the results were stratified after the use of oxytocin versus no oxytocin before surgery. By considering key characteristics of all studies investigating oxytocin in cesarean section, evidence gaps for a subset of women could be identified and a narrative description of the current literature provided.

Results

Published studies

We identified 7866 titles and abstracts; for 432 of these, the full text was evaluated. Figure 1 outlines the screening and selection process of the articles. Table 1 presents the key characteristics of the 36 controlled trials investigating the risk of PPH after the use of exogenous oxytocin in cesarean section: 23 randomized controlled trials (RCTs) (including 4084 patients), 2 comparative dose-response studies (including 100 patients) and 11 non-RCTs (including 3896 patients).

Intrapartum cesarean delivery

From 36 studies identified, 8 studies (1705 patients) included solely women requiring intrapartum cesarean delivery, mainly because of labour arrest [26–33]. However, from these 8 studies, only 2 dose-response studies addressed the hypothesis whether parturients who receive intrapartum exogenous ocytocin are prone to a higher risk of PPH by evaluating uterine contraction after delivery [26, 27]: *(i)* Thereby, the dose-response study from Lavoie et al. investigated whether women who receive intrapartum exogenous oxytocin, and who subsequently undergo cesarean delivery for labour dystocia, need a higher estimated effective dose of oxytocin in 90% of women (ED90) compared with non-labouring parturients [27]. Thirty-two women participated in the labouring and 38 women in the non-labouring group. The reported oxytocin ED90 was significantly greater for the labouring group requiring cesarean delivery compared with that for the non-labouring group (mean difference:

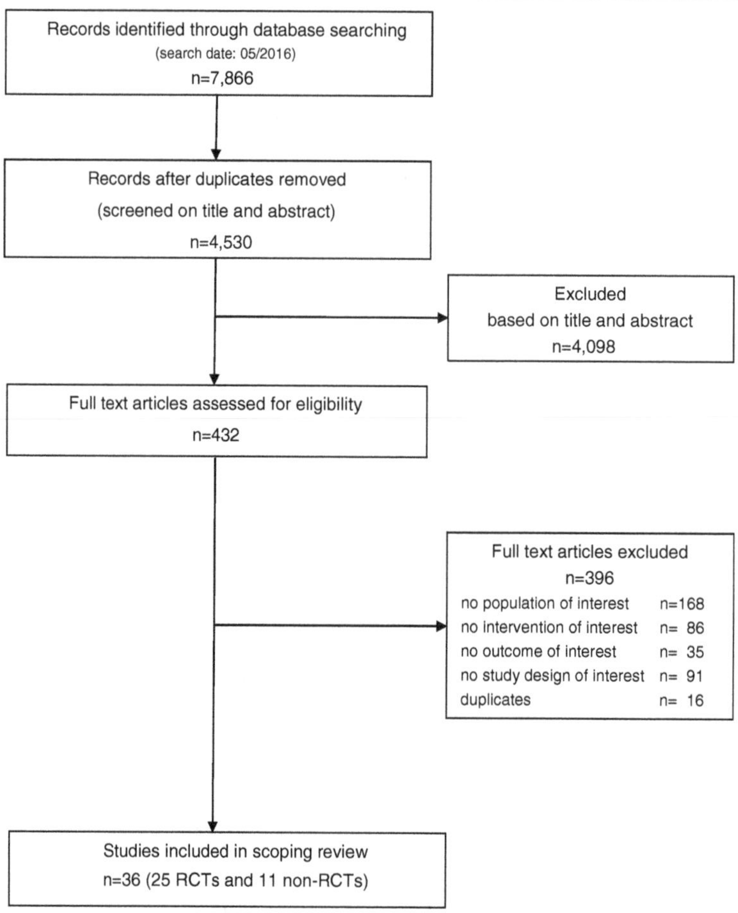

Fig. 1 PRISMA flow diagram: Results of the bibliographic literature search in Medline, Embase, Web of Science, and the Cochrane Library in May 2016 (as published by *Moher D* et al. *in BMJ 2009;339:b2535*). RCT: randomized controlled trial

Table 1 Studies Included in Scoping Review

	Study & Country	Study type	Intervention (I1) & Control (I2)	Time point of drug application	Population				Follow-up & beginning and end of study
					Week of gestation (mean ± SD)	Women (n)	Age (mean ± SD; median [range])	Indication	
Comparative dose-response studies	Balki 2006 [26] Canada	RCT	"the dose of oxytocin for each patient was determined by the response of the previous patient (±0,5 IU) to the drug, according to a biased coin up-and-down sequential allocation scheme to cluster doses close to the minimum effective dose (ED_{90})"[a]	"immediately upon delivery of the anterior shoulder of the infant"	39.9 ± 1.1	total: 30	32.7 ± 4.4	CS for labour arrest "augmentation with iv oxytocin for a minimum of 2 h"	48 h 03/04–12/04
	Lavoie 2015 [27] US	RCT	"dose-response study using a 9:1 biased-coin sequential allocation method to estimate the ED_{90} of an infusion of prophylactic oxytocin in women undergoing CS with neuraxial anesthesia. The starting infusion rate was 18 IU/h, with an incremental dose of 2 IU/h."	"immediately after the umbilical cord was clamped"	I1: 40 (40–41) I2: 39 (39–39)	I1: 32 I2: 38	I1: 33 (28–35) I2: 33 (31–36)	I1:"labouring group: women scheduled for intrapartum CS after prior exposure to exogenous oxytocin"[b] I2:"non-labouring group: women scheduled for CS"	24 h 08/12–06/13
Different Oxytocin doses	Munn 2001 [28] US	RCT	I1: Oxytocin 10 IU, *iv*, 30 min I2: Oxytocin 80 IU, *iv*, 30 min +prn Oxytocin for labour induction;[c] after delivery in the postanesthesia care unit, all patients received oxytocin, 20 IU, *iv*, 8 h	"after cord clamping"	I1: 37 ± 4.3 I2: 37 ± 4.9	I1: 163 I2: 158	I1: 25 ± 6.0 I2: 25 ± 6.1	labour before CS[d]	1 day 01/97–11/99
	Ayedi 2011 [55] Tunisia	RCT	I1: Oxytocin 2 IU (in 5 ml volume), *iv*, single-dose, 5–10 s I2: Oxytocin 5 IU (in 5 ml volume), *iv*, single-dose, 5–10 s +prn uterotonics	"after delivery of the baby and cord clamping"	≥37	total: 60	–	–	–
	Chou 2015 [56] Malaysia	RCT	I1: Oxytocin 40 IU (in 500 ml NaCl), *iv*, over 6 h I2: Oxytocin 80 IU (in 500 ml NaCl), *iv*, over 6 h +all P. were given an oxytocin bolus of 5 IU	"post-delivery"	–	–	–	–	- 11/12–05/13

Table 1 Studies Included in Scoping Review *(Continued)*

	Study & Country	Study type	Intervention (I1) & Control (I2)	Time point of drug application	Population				Follow-up & beginning and end of study
					Week of gestation (mean ± SD)	Women (n)	Age (mean ± SD; median [range])	Indication	
	Khan 2012 [32] India	RCT	I1: Oxytocin 10 IU (in 500 ml NaCl), *iv*, over 1 h I2: Oxytocin 20 IU (in 500 ml NaCl), *iv*, over 1 h +prn uterotonics	–	–	total: 200	–	emergency	24 h study duration: 6 mos
	Kintu 2012 [54] Uganda	RCT	I1: Oxytocin 2.5 IU, no further information I2: Oxytocin 10 IU, no further information +prn uterotonics	"following cord clamping"	–	total: 380	–	emergency and elective	24 h -
	Lee 2014 [48] US	Non-RCT (retrospective)	I1: Oxytocin 10 IU, *iv* Infusion was continued until P. transfer to the recovery room I2: Oxytocin 30 IU, *iv*, over 1 h	"following cord clamping"	–	I1: 483 I2: 418	I1: 32 ± 6 I2: 33 ± 6	–	- I1: 09/08–11/08 I2: 11/08–01/09
	Pursche 2012 [42] Germany	Non-RCT (retrospective)	I1: Oxytocin 3 IU, *iv*, single-dose + continuously 3 IU oxytocin, *iv*, infusion rate 100 ml/h I2: Oxytocin continuously 3 IU oxytocin, *iv*, infusion rate at least 120 ml/h	"postpartum"	I1: 37.9 I2: 37.9	I1: 228 I2: 227	–	elective (n = 71) and during labour (n = 384)[e]	4 h 01/11–12/11
	McClune 2011 [44] UK	Non-RCT (retrospective)	Different doses oxytocin, not administered uniformly[f] + prn uterotonics	"given at cord clamping"	–	total: 50	–	–	- 08/10–09/10
Application schema	Mangla 2012 [59] India	RCT	I1: Oxytocin 20 IU, *iv* I2: Oxytocin 5 IU, *imy* I3: Oxytocin 5 IU, *imy* No information about additional uterotonics	I1 + I2: "after separation of placenta" I3: "before separation of placenta"	–	I1: 50 I2: 50 I3: 50	–	–	1 h -
Oxytocin vs other uterotonics time-dependent	Adefuye 2012 [50] Nigeria	RCT	I1: Oxytocin 20 IU, *iv* I2: Misoprostol 2 × 400 μg, *sublingual* +prn uterotonics intraop	I1: "after delivery" I2: "before delivery"	I1: 38.0 ± 0.2 I2: 38.1 ± 0.3	I1: 50 I2: 50	I1: 28.7 ± 0.7 I2: 29.9 ± 0.8	elective (28%) and emergency (72%)[g]	24 h 04/09–03/11
	Chaudhuri 2010 [60] India	RCT	I1: Oxytocin 8 × 5 IU, *iv* + placebo, *rectal* I2: Misoprostol 4 × 200 μg, *rectal* + 8 placebo, *iv* +prn uterotonics	I1: "after delivery" I2: "before incision"	I1: 39.2 ± 1.4 I2: 39.5 ± 1.7	I1: 100 I2: 100	I1: 24.3 ± 5.0 I2: 24.0 ± 3.4	elective and emergency[h] without risk factors for PPH	24 h 12/07–06/09

Table 1 Studies Included in Scoping Review *(Continued)*

	Study & Country	Study type	Intervention (I1) & Control (I2)	Time point of drug application	Population				Follow-up & beginning and end of study
					Week of gestation (mean ± SD)	Women (n)	Age (mean ± SD; median [range])	Indication	
Oxytocin vs placebo	King 2010 [49] Canada	RCT	I1: Oxytocin 5 IU, *iv*, über 30 s, single-dose I2: Placebo NaCl, *iv*, 30 s, single-dose +routinely oxytocin (40 IU, *iv*, 30 min) followed by oxytocin (20 IU) immediately after study drug +prn uterotonics	"as soon as the umbilical cord was clamped"	I1: 37.0 ± 3.0 I2: 38.0 ± 2.0	I1: 75 I2: 75	I1: 34 ± 5 I2: 34 ± 6	elective (*n* = 76) and non-elective (*n* = 67) at least one risk factor for PPH	24 h 11/05–10/06
Oxytocin vs other uterotonics	Attilakos 2010 [34] UK	RCT	I1: Oxytocin 5 IU, *iv*, 30–60 s I2: Carbetocin 100 μg, *iv*, 30–60 s +prn uterotonics (Oxytocin for PPH prophylaxis or treatment)	"after the birth of the baby"	≥37	I1: 189 I2: 188	I1: 32 (18–44) I2: 32 (18–42)	elective (60%) and emergency (40%) 1/3 showed risk factors for PPH	until discharged 11/06–07/07
	Borruto 2009 [35] Italy	RCT	I1: Oxytocin 10 IU, *iv*, 2 h I2: Carbetocin 100 μg, *iv*, single-dose +prn uterotonics	"immediately following placental delivery"	≥36	I1: 52 I2: 52	32.2 (22–41)	planned and emergency[j] at least one risk factor for PPH	24 h 09/07–01/08
	Catanzarite 1990 [47] US	RCT	I1: Oxytocin 20 IU, *imy* I2: Carboprost tromethamine 125 μg, *imy* +routinely oxytocin (20 IU, *iv*) after placental delivery	"immediately following placental delivery"	–	I1: 21 I2: 25	I1: 24.5 I2: 24.1	planned and emergency[j]	3 days -
	Chaudhuri 2014 [33] India	RCT	I1: Oxytocin 8 × 5 IU, *iv*, 12 h + placebo *rectal* I2: Misoprostol 4 × 200 μg, *rectal* + placebo *iv*, 12 h +routinely oxytocin, not later than 1 min after delivery	"at the end of the operation"	I1: 38.8 ± 1.2 I2: 39.0 ± 1.1	I1: 96 I2: 96	I1: 23.2 ± 3.7 I2: 23.5 ± 4.5	emergency without risk factor for PPH	24 h 05/11–05/12
	Lapaire 2006 [36] Switzerland	RCT	I1: Oxytocin 20 IU, *iv*, 8 h + placebo *oral* I2: Misoprostol 800 μg, *oral* + placebo *iv*, 8 h +routinely oxytocin (5 IU, *iv*) after cord clamping	"immediately after cord clamping"	I1: 38.7 ± 1.3 I2: 38.6 ± 1.3	I1: 28 I2: 28	I1: 31.2 ± 5.1 I2: 32.2 ± 6.5	elective and indicated[k] low risk for PPH	48 h 01/99–02/02
	Lokugamage 2001 [37] UK	RCT	I1: Oxytocin 10 IU, *iv*, single-dose + placebo, *oral* I2: Misoprostol 500 μg, *oral* + placebo *iv*, single-dose +prn uterotonics	"immediately after the delivery of the baby"	I1: 38.3 ± 1.1 I2: 36.7 ± 8.9	I1: 20 I2: 20	I1: 31.4 ± 5.5 I2: 32.3 ± 6.4	elective (n = 38) and emergency (*n* = 2) excluded: previous rupture of the uterus	3 days -

Table 1 Studies Included in Scoping Review *(Continued)*

Study & Country	Study type	Intervention (I1) & Control (I2)	Time point of drug application	Population: Week of gestation (mean ± SD)	Population: Women (n)	Population: Age (mean ± SD; median [range])	Population: Indication	Follow-up & beginning and end of study
Owonikoko 2011 [51] Nigeria	RCT	I1: Oxytocin 20 IU, *iv* I2: Misoprostol 400 µg, *sublingual* +prn Oxytocin *iv*	"immediately after extraction of the baby"	I1: 39.7 ± 1.9 I2: 38.7 ± 2.3	I1: 50 I2: 50	I1: 30.4 ± 4.8 I2: 31.5 ± 4.1	elective (35%)[l] and emergency (65%)[m]	24 h 06/06–04/07
Razali 2016 [30] Malaysia	RCT	I1: Oxytocin 10 IU, *iv*, single-dose I2: Carbetocin 100 µg, *iv*, single-dose +prn uterotonics	"after delivery"	"at term"	I1: 300 I2: 300	I1: 29.7 ± 4.3 I2: 29.5 ± 4.6	emergency[n]	24 h 14/08–09/12
Vimala 2006 [61] India	RCT	I1: Oxytocin 20 IU, *iv*, 6 h I2: Mis +prn uterotonics	"immediatiely after delivery of the neonate"	I1: 38.7 ± 1.1 I2: 38.7 ± 1.2	I1: 50 I2: 50	I1: 26.3 ± 3.7 I2: 25.6 ± 5.1	elective (17%) and emergency (83%)[o] without risk factors for PPH	24 h 08/04–04/05
El Behery 2016 [29] Egypt	RCT	I1: Oxytocin 20 IU, *iv* I2: Carbetocin 100 µg, *iv*, 2 min +prn uterotonics	"after delivery of the infant preferably before placental removal"	I1: 38.2 ± 0.8 I2: 38.2 ± 1.2	I1: 90 I2: 90	I1: *n* = 90 I2: n = 90	emergency	24 h 01/13–06/14
Whigham 2016 [31] Australia	RCT	I1: Oxytocin 5 IU, *iv* I2: Carbetocin 100 µg, *iv* +prn uterotonics	"immediately after birth of the baby"	I1: 40.0 ± 1.4 I2: 39.6 ± 1.5	I1: 53 I2: 59	I1: 28.9 ± 5.8 I2: 28.3 ± 5.9	non-elective and emergency[p]	- 08/12–02/13
Alli 2013 [53] Nigeria	RCT	I1: Oxytocin 10 IU, *iv*, single-dose I2: Misoprostol 600 µg, *sublingual* +prn uterotonics	"immediately after delivery of the baby"	–	total: 100	–	–	–
Begum 2015 [57] Bangladesh	RCT	I1: Oxytocin 20 IU (in 100 ml Dextrose NaCl), *iv* I2: Misoprostol 400 µg, *sublingual* +prn uterotonics	"soon after delivery"	"term pregnancy"	total: 100	–	–	–
Pizzagalli 2015 [41] France	Non-RCT (prospective)	I1: Oxytocin 5 IU *iv*, followed by 10 IU *iv* during surgery, further infusions 10 IU 8 h postop I2: Carbetocin 100 µg *iv* I3: Oxytocin 5 IU *iv*, followed by 10 IU *iv* during surgery, further infusions 10 IU 8 h + Sulprostone	"during cord clamping"	≥37	I1: 282 I2: 262 I3: 258	–	CS before labour (*n* = 283) and unclear indication (*n* = 519)	24 h I1: 07/10–12/10 I2: 02/11–12/11 I3: 08/11–01/12

Table 1 Studies Included in Scoping Review *(Continued)*

	Study & Country	Study type	Intervention (I1) & Control (I2)	Time point of drug application	Population: Week of gestation (mean ± SD)	Population: Women (n)	Population: Age (mean ± SD; median [range])	Population: Indication	Follow-up & beginning and end of study
	Triopon 2010 [62] France	Non-RCT (retrospective)	I1: Carbetocin 100 µg, *iv* I2: Oxytocin 5 IU, *iv*	"after cord clamping"	I1: 38.2 ± 3.0 I2: 37.9 ± 3.2	I1: 155 I2: 155	I1: 30.6 ± 5.3 I2: 30.7 ± 5.4	elective and during labour	24 h I1: 04/09–07/09 I2: 03/07–06/07
	Demetz 2013 [46] France	Non-RCT (retrospective)	I1: Oxytocin 10 IU, *iv*, single-dose[q] +3 h after delivery: 10 IU Oxytocin *iv* over 12 h I2: Carbetocin 100 µg, *iv*, single-dose +3 h after delivery: 10 IU Oxytocin *iv* over 12 h	"at the delivery"	I1: 35.5 ± 2.5 I2: 34.3 ± 3.1	I1: 24 I2: 39	I1: 31.6 ± 4.3 I2: 31.1 ± 5.8	planned (n = 31) and unclear (n = 32)	48 h I1: 08/09–01/10 I2: 02/10–07/10
	Testa 2013 [45] Italy	Non-RCT (retrospective)	I1: Oxytocin 10 IU, *iv*, 2 h I2: Carbetocin 100 µg, *iv*, single-dose	–	–	I1: 14 I2: 14	–	planned and emergency	24 h after drug application -
	Brzozowska 2015 [63] Polska	Non-RCT (retrospective)	I1: Oxytocin 10 IU, *im* I2: Carbetocin 100 µg, *iv* +prn uterotonics	–	I1: 38.3 ± 1.9 I2: 38.1 ± 1.9	I1: 140 I2: 139	I1: 30.5 ± 4.6 I2: 31.5 ± 5.1	–	- 03/14–10/14
Combination therapy	Koen 2016 [52] South Africa	RCT	I1: Oxytocin 2,5 IU, *iv*, single-dose + placebo *im* I2: Oxytocin + Ergometrine Placebo *iv* + Oxytocin 5 IU, *im* + Ergometrine 0.5 mg, *im* +routinely 10 IU Oxytocin	"after delivery of the neonate"	I1: 38.4 ± 2.2 I2: 38.5 ± 1.9	I1: 214 I2: 202	I1: 28.6 ± 6.0 I2: 28.9 ± 5.4	elective (36%) and emergency (64%)[r]	6–24 h 01/4–06/14
	Mahmud 2014 [58] Pakistan	Non-RCT (prospective)	I1: Oxytocin 10 IU *iv* I2: Oxytocin 10 IU *iv* + Ergometrine 0,25 mg *im*	"intraoperatively"	I1: 37.5 ± 2.0 I2: 38.0 ± 1.8	I1: 378 I2: 323	I1: 28.0 ± 3.5 I2: 29.0 ± 3.4	elective and emergency	6 h I1: 11/10–12/10 I2: 01/11–02/11
	Bayoumeu 2003 [38] France	Non-RCT (retrospective)	I1: Oxytocin 5 IU *iv (single dose)*, 10 IU *iv* 30 min, afterwards 25 IU *iv* 24 h I2: Oxytocin 5 IU *iv (single dose)*, 10 IU *iv* 30 min, afterwards 25 IU *iv* 24 h + Dinoprost/Sulprostone	"after clamping the last umbilical cord"	I1: 32.0 ± 2.7 I2: 32.8 ± 1.7	I1: 14 I2: 28	I1: 29.1 ± 3.2 I2: 30.2 ± 3.3	elective and emergency	48 h I1: 01/93–11/96 I2: 12/96–12/00

Table 1 Studies Included in Scoping Review *(Continued)*

Study & Country	Study type	Intervention (I1) & Control (I2)	Time point of drug application	Population				Follow-up & beginning and end of study
				Week of gestation (mean ± SD)	Women (n)	Age (mean ± SD; median [range])	Indication	
Lourens 2007 [40] UK	Non-RCT (prospective)	I1: Oxytocin 5 IU iv, single-dose I2: Oxytocin 5 IU *iv*, single-dose + Ergometrine 0.5 mg *im*	Oxytocin: "after delivery" Ergometrine: "during abdominal closure"	I1: 38.0 ± 1.0 I2: 38.0 ± 1.0	I1: 158 I2: 107	–	elective (n = 120) and emergency (n = 145)	- I1: 02/06–03/06 I2: 04/06–06/06

[a]The dose of oxytocin for each woman was determined by the response of the previous woman to the drug, (…). If a woman did not respond adequately to the initial bolus of oxytocin, the initial dose for the next one was increased by 0.5 IU. If the woman responded to the initial bolus, the dose for the next one was decreased by 0.5 IU with a probability of 1/9; otherwise it remained unchanged. (…) . The starting dose of oxytocin was arbitrarily chosen as 0.5 IU

[b]CS due to labour dystocia, defined as arrest of dilation in first stage of labour or arrest of descent in second stage of labour

[c]Results were not reported separately for women with or without prepartal oxytocin administration

[d]Labour was defined as at least two contractions in 10 min and either an initial cervical dilation of at least 2 cm or progressive cervical change. Indications: non-reassuring FHR tracing (58%), arrest of labour (75%), abnormal lie (44%), other reasons (24%)

[e]Cardiotocography abnormalities (92), breech presentation (67), macrosomia (19), preeclampsie/HELLP (14), state after recesarean (22), twins/triplets (24/2), obstructed labour (29), fetal abnormalities/disease (22), maternale disease (54), placenta praevia/ bleeding (21)

[f]Initial bolus dose of oxytocin given at cord clamping and any subsequent bolus doses were recorded along with the concentration and rate of the maintenance oxytocin infusion if used and any other uterotonic drugs

[g]Indications: severe pregnancy induced hypertension/hypertensive disorders (20), uncontrolled diabetes mellitus (1), precious baby (bad obstetric history/pregnancy after infertility treatment) (2), fetal distress (33), abnormal lie (transverse/oblique lie) (3), malpresentation (face/brow) (5), dystocia (foeto-pelvic disproportion/occipito-posterior/transverse arrest) (23), macrosomia (3), breech (6), prolonged pregnancy (4)

[h]Indications: previous cs (51), prolonged pregnancy (failed induction) (23), malpresentation (10), preeclampsie (11), PROM (9), cephalopelvic disproportion (14), fetal distress (27), non-progress of labour (19), poor obstetric history (6), IUGR/oligohydramnios (7), elderly primigravida/infertility treated (13)

[i]Indications: previous cs (28), abnormal presentation (24), dystocia (18), FHR anomalies (16), umbilical cord prolapse (2), feto-pelvic disproportion (2), IUGR (2), fetal megalosomy (2), abruptio placentae (2), placenta previa (2), maternal disease (2), failed induction of labour (2), maternal request (2)

[j]Indications: elective, prior to labour (35), early labour (7), cephalopelvic disproportion (4)

[k]Indications: elective cs or breech presentation (31), malposition (1), twin pregnancy (1), repeated cs (5), ineffective induction of labour (2), ineffective induction of labour and infection (1), failure of labour to progress (1), hip dysplasia (1), IUGR (2), ankylosing spondylitis (1), macrosomia (2), placenta previa (2), Increased pressure not indicated (retinal disease, colposuspension) (3)

[l]Indication for elective cs: maternal, medical condition (HIV, herpes) (4), two previous cs (9), malpresentation (transverse lie, breech in primigravidae etc.) (6), maternal request for cs (4), fetal macrosomia (12)

[m]Indication for emergency: fetal distress (14), cephalopelvic disproportion (9), malpresentation in labour (9), failed vaginal birth after cs (20), failed induction of labour (4), severe oligohydramnios (9)

[n]Indication for emergency: defined as an unplanned procedure performed after the start of labour and labour as regular contractions at least every 10 min and cervical dilatation >3 cm; non reassuring fetal status (267), failure to progress in labour (189), malpresentation (34), prolonged second stage (15), other reasons (42)

[o]Indication: fetal breech presentation (14), cephalopelvic disproportion (10), nonprogress of labour (16), meconium stained liquor (25), fetal variable decelerations (20), scar tenderness (2), transverse lie (3), Type II decelerations (5), prolonged latent phase (2), previous lower segment cs with unfavorable cervix(3)

[p]Women with planned labour induction, were in early labour or were in active labour but had an epidural anaesthetic. Results were not reported separately for women with or without prepartal oxytocin administration

[q]In case of PPH, French national guidelines were applied

[r]Indications: previous CS (188), fetal distress (87), cephalopelvic disproportion (41), poor progress (30), failed induction of labour (14), breech (14), twins (11), other reasons (24)

CS: cesarean section; dl: decilitre; ED: effective dose; FHR: fetal heart rate; g: gram; GA: gestational age; h: hours; I1: intervention; I2: control intervention; im: intramuscular; imy: intramyometrial; intraop: intraoperatively; IUGR: intrauterine growth retardation; IU: international units; iv: intravenous; mg: milligram; min: minutes; ml: milliliter; mU: milliunit; n: number; NaCl: saline; non-RCT: non-randomized controlled trial; P: participants; postop: postoperatively; PPH: postpartum hemorrhage; prn: pro re nata; PROM: premature rupture of membranes; RCT: randomized controlled trial; s: seconds; SE: standard error; UK: United Kingdom; US: United States; µg: microgram; vs: versus

28 Units/h [95% CI 26–29 Units/h, $P < 0.001$]). Furthermore, significantly more women in the labouring group compared to the non-labouring group required additional uterotonic agents (mean difference: 26% [95% CI 7–44%, $P = 0.008$]). *(ii)* The other dose-response study from Balki et al. estimated the minimum effective intravenous dose of oxytocin required for adequate uterine contraction after cesarean delivery for labour arrest, however, without using an active control group [26]. In this study, all 30 patients received oxytocin infusion at a mean of 9.8 ± 6.3 h before cesarean delivery. After delivery, oxytocin was administered as a slow intravenous bolus according to a coin up-down sequential allocation scheme. The minimum oxytocin ED90 required to produce adequate uterine response was estimated to be 3.0 U (95% CI 2.3–3.7 U). The authors concluded that women with intrapartum cesarean section for labour arrest require an oxytocin dose that is 9 times higher than previously reported after elective cesarean section in non-labouring women at term. However, the results of these dose-response studies are limited by comparing different patient populations without controlling for potential confounders such as women with increased risk of uterine atony, age, anticoagulant medication, general anaesthesia or multiple pregnancy. In addition, the authors used 'satisfactory uterine contraction' assessed by palpating the uterus as main outcome. Beside the fact that this outcome is subjective and not validated to estimate the effect of oxytocin on the uterus, it can not be excluded that due to a lack of blinding of the obstetricians, different thresholds for satisfactory uterine tone in women with prior labour compared with non-labouring women were used. Therefore, theses study results need to be interpreted with caution. The remaining 6 studies including women with intrapartum cesarean sections investigated different doses or application schedules of exogenous oxytocin or compared oxytocin to other uteronotics after cesarean delivery for PPH prophylaxis [28–32]. Whether the prepartal oxytocin status is a risk factor for atonic PPH could not be derived from these studies.

Intrapartum and prelabour cesarean delivery

Our mapping also revealed that the majority of studies investigating PPH rates for different treatment groups are focused on prophylactic uterogenics and included women with different types of cesarean delivery (intrapartum and prelabour cesarean section). However, the PPH rates given in these studies were not stratified according to the indications for cesarean section. In addition, the prepartal oxytocin status was not considered as confounding factor by conducting subgroup analyses [34–63].

Ongoing studies

The search for ongoing and unpublished studies identified 2 RCTs which may provide subgroup data estimating the blood loss and risk for PPH after cesarean section for labour arrest (ClinicalTrials.gov Identifier: NCT01869556 and NCT02794779). The estimated completion date for both studies is by the end of 2017. In addition, we identified HOLDS, a multicentre, double-blind randomised controlled trial to compare standard and high dose regimens of oxytocin for women with confirmed delay in the first stage of labour (http://www.isrctn.com/ISRCTN99841044). This trial randomises 1500 women and measure differences in rates and complications associated with cesarean section. If this study provides a subgroup analysis of PPH rates in those women requiring cesarean sections, important insights addressing the present research question will be given.

Discussion

Current clinical practice guidelines for third stage oxytocin administration do not distinguish between women with prior oxytocin exposure and those without [64, 65]. This practice is also reflected by the current research in cesarean delivery, which showed that the majority of studies investigating oxytocin focus on prophylactic administration in the third stage of labour, without differing between the indications for cesarean section and, hence the prepartal oxytocin status (particularly when labour was induced or augmented). However, taking into account that labouring women requiring cesarean delivery constitute a relevant subset of patients - for whom originally spontaneous labour was anticipated - the lack of studies solely investigating this patient population is not surprising.

In total, our evidence map revealed that only 2 studies investigated the required oxytocin dose to prevent uterine atony after cesarean delivery for labour arrest. These dose-response studies support the hypothesis that labouring women exposed to exogenous oxytocin require a higher oxytocin dose after delivery than non-labouring women to prevent uterine atony after cesarean section. This finding is in accordance with the observations during spontaneous labour [24, 25]. However, the studies investigating this hypothesis in intrapartum cesarean delivery are all flawed by limitations of the study design as well as the outcome selection. Thus, the estimated oxytocin ED90 may be lower in labouring women than actually reported.

A limitation of our research work is that data could not be formally synthesized due to a lack of controlled studies evaluating the impact of ante partum oxytocin use on the risk of PPH in exogenous cesarean delivery. Nevertheless, the current scoping review describes key data of published studies investigating the routine use of oxytocin in caesarean delivery in their quantity, but also reveals major research gaps in this important but under-represented obstetric area. It is obvious that research on this topic is mainly restricted to augmentation or induction of vaginal delivery [16, 66, 67] or the prophylactic use in the third stage of labour to prevent PPH [15, 68]. But such data would have been only relevant to address our research question, if they had allowed us to derive PPH rates for those women who required intrapartum cesarean delivery (e.g., data from subgroup analyses). A Cochrane Review from 2013 investigated oxytocin augmentation of labour in women with epidural analgesia for reducing operative deliveries [69]. This review provides rates for cesarean sections after oxytocin exposure in comparison to placebo, but whether there is a difference in PPH rates for women requiring cesarean section were also not provided. Taking into account that the current research does not provide us with rigorous controlled data to address our research question, access to individual and/or unpublished study data may be desirable [70]. Although overall progress has been made to obtain such study data, there are still major issues related to unrestricted data access. For example, released data may be incomplete, selective or not in compliance with the results reported in the corresponding publications. Facing these issues, we did not undertake efforts to include such data in our research work.

We believe that the current scoping review is important because it reveals that published research on oxytocin is restricted to the use for inducing or augmenting labour or for PPH prophylaxis, without considering women requiring intrapartum cesarean section – not even in subgroup analyses. Given the increasing rates in cesarean sections and labour inductions in many developed countries [71], well controlled studies are needed focusing on these parturient. Taking into account that different studies suggest that induction of labour increases the risk of postpartum hemorrhage and blood transfusion [24, 71], caution is needed when intrapartum cesarean section is performed, particularly when labour is induced or augmented, as it may result in increased maternal morbidity.

Conclusions

Considering that research on the risk of PPH after oxytocin exposure is generally restricted to the use of PPH prophylaxis and vaginal births, future controlled studies should evaluate whether administration of oxytocin in cesarean delivery is associated with a higher risk of PPH taking into account that labouring and non-labouring women may show a difference response to exogenous oxytocin. In addition, these studies should control for known confounding factors associated with a higher risk of PPH such as multiple pregnancy, assisted reproductive technologies, general anaesthesia, type of uterine incision or advanced maternal age [6, 13, 14, 72]. As long as there is no evidence-based guideline available for labouring women requiring cesarean delivery, obstetricans and anaesthesiologists should always be aware of an increased risk of PPH due to prior oxytocin exposure in this patient population.

Abbreviations

CI: Confidence Interval; ED: Effective Dose; IU: International Unit; OR: Odds Ratio; PPH: Postpartum Haemorrhage; PRISMA: Prefered Reporting Items for Systematic Reviews and Meta-Analyses; RCT: Randomized Controlled Trial; WHO: World Health Organization

Acknowledgements

This project was initiated by the German Society for Gynecology and Obstetrics to answer a clinical question for the multidisciplinary expert group of the German evidence- and consensus-based guideline project "Sectio Cesarea" (AWMF-Registry number 015-084, coordinator: Prof. Dr. med. F. Louwen). The authors also thank Edith Motschall from the University of Freiburg for conducting the comprehensive systematic literature search and Katharina Kunzweiler (Cochrane Germany) for conducting the search for ongoing studies in the study registries.

Funding

This project was funded by the German Federal Ministry of Health, #GE20160425. The funders had no role in the conduct or reporting of the scoping review.

Authors' contributions

CS and MN are responsible for the coordination, conception and design of the review. KB reviewed titles and abstracts. Screening of full-texts and data extraction were undertaken by CS and KB. CS wrote a first draft and JM, CL, MN and BL revised the manuscript critically for important intellectual content. All authors have read and approved the final version of the publication.

Competing interests

The authors declare that they have no competing interests.

Author details

[1]Cochrane Germany, Medical Center – University of Freiburg, Faculty of Medicine, University of Freiburg, Freiburg, Germany. [2]AWMF-Institute for Medical Knowledge Management (IMWi), Karl-von-Frisch-Street 1, 35043 Marburg, Germany. [3]Department of Anesthesiology and Critical Care, University Heart Center Freiburg-Bad Krozingen, Medical Center - University of Freiburg, Freiburg, Germany.

References

1. Khan KS, Wojdyla D, Say L, Gulmezoglu AM, Van Look PF. Who analysis of causes of maternal death: a systematic review. Lancet. 2006; 367(9516):1066–74.
2. Zwart JJ, Richters JM, Ory F, de Vries JI, Bloemenkamp KW, van Roosmalen J. Severe maternal morbidity during pregnancy, delivery and puerperium in the netherlands: a nationwide population-based study of 371,000 pregnancies. BJOG. 2008;115(7):842–50.
3. Baskett TF, O'Connell CM. Severe obstetric maternal morbidity: a 15-year population-based study. J Obstet Gynaecol Can. 2005;25(1):7–9.
4. Magann EF, Evans S, Hutchinson M, Collins R, Howard BC, Morrison JC. Postpartum hemorrhage after vaginal birth: an analysis of risk factors. South Med J. 2005;98(4):419–22.
5. Gizzo S, Patrelli TS, Gangi SD, Carrozzini M, Saccardi C, Zambon A, Bertocco A, Fagherazzi S, D'Antona D, Nardelli GB. Which uterotonic is better to prevent the postpartum hemorrhage? Latest news in terms of clinical efficacy, side effects, and contraindications: a systematic review. Reprod Sci. 2013;20(9):1011–9.
6. Weeks AD, Neilson JP. Rethinking our approach to postpartum haemorrhage and uterotonics. BMJ. 2015;351:h3251.
7. Bateman BT, Berman MF, Riley LE, Leffert LR. The epidemiology of postpartum hemorrhage in a large, nationwide sample of deliveries. Anesth Analg. 2010;110(5):1368–73.
8. Knight M, Callaghan WM, Berg C, Alexander S, Bouvier-Colle MH, Ford JB, Joseph KS, Lewis G, Liston RM, Roberts CL, et al. Trends in postpartum hemorrhage in high resource countries: a review and recommendations from the international postpartum hemorrhage collaborative group. BMC Pregnancy Childbirth. 2009;9:55.
9. Menard MK, Main EK, Currigan SM. Executive summary of the revitalize initiative: standardizing obstetric data definitions. Obstet Gynecol. 2014; 124(1):150–3.
10. Callaghan WM, Mackay AP, Berg CJ. Identification of severe maternal morbidity during delivery hospitalizations, united states, 1991–2003. Am J Obstet Gynecol. 2008;199(2):133.e1–8.
11. Briley A, Seed PT, Tydeman G, Ballard H, Waterstone M, Sandall J, Poston L, Tribe RM, Bewley S. Reporting errors, incidence and risk factors for postpartum haemorrhage and progression to severe pph: a prospective observational study. BJOG. 2014;121(7):876–88.
12. Mathai M, Hofmeyr GJ. Abdominal surgical incisions for caesarean section. Cochrane Database Syst Rev. 2007;(1):Cd004453.
13. Butwick AJ, Ramachandran B, Hegde P, Riley ET, El-Sayed YY, Nelson LM. Risk factors for severe postpartum hemorrhage after cesarean delivery: case-control studies. Anesth Analg. 2017;125(2):523–32.
14. Combs CA, Murphy EL, Laros RK, Jr. Factors associated with hemorrhage in cesarean deliveries. Obstet Gynecol 1991;77(1):77–82.
15. Westhoff G, Cotter AM, Tolosa JE. Prophylactic oxytocin for the third stage of labour to prevent postpartum haemorrhage. Cochrane Database Syst Rev. 2013;10:CD001808.
16. Bugg GJ, Siddiqui F, Thornton JG. Oxytocin versus no treatment or delayed treatment for slow progress in the first stage of spontaneous labour. Cochrane Database Syst Rev. 2013;6:CD007123.
17. Arthur P, Taggart MJ, Mitchell BF. Oxytocin and parturition: a role for increased myometrial calcium and calcium sensitization? Front Biosci. 2007; 12:619–33.
18. Phaneuf S, Rodriguez Linares B, TambyRaja RL, MacKenzie IZ, Lopez Bernal A. Loss of myometrial oxytocin receptors during oxytocin-induced and oxytocin-augmented labour. J Reprod Fertil. 2000;120(1):91–7.
19. Fraser W, Vendittelli F, Krauss I, Breart G. Effects of early augmentation of labour with amniotomy and oxytocin in nulliparous women: a meta-analysis. BJOG. 1998;105(2):189–94.
20. Balki M, Erik-Soussi M, Kingdom J, Carvalho JC. Oxytocin pretreatment attenuates oxytocin-induced contractions in human myometrium in vitro. Anesthesiology. 2013;119(3):552–61.
21. Balki M, Cristian AL, Kingdom J, Carvalho JC. Oxytocin pretreatment of pregnant rat myometrium reduces the efficacy of oxytocin but not of ergonovine maleate or prostaglandin f 2 alpha. Reprod Sci. 2010;17(3): 269–77.
22. Magalhaes JK, Carvalho JC, Parkes RK, Kingdom J, Li Y, Balki M. Oxytocin pretreatment decreases oxytocin-induced myometrial contractions in pregnant rats in a concentration-dependent but not time-dependent manner. Reprod Sci. 2009;16(5):501–8.
23. Grotegut CA, Paglia MJ, Johnson LN, Thames B, James AH. Oxytocin exposure during labor among women with postpartum hemorrhage secondary to uterine atony. Am J Obstet Gynecol. 2011;204(1):56.e1–6.
24. Belghiti J, Kayem G, Dupont C, Rudigoz RC, Bouvier-Colle MH, Deneux-Tharaux C. Oxytocin during labour and risk of severe postpartum haemorrhage: a population-based, cohort-nested case-control study. BMJ Open. 2011;1(2):e000514.
25. Belghiti J, Coulm B, Kayem G, Blondel B, Deneux-Tharaux C. Oxytocin administration during labor. Results from the 2010 french national perinatal survey. J Gynecol Obstet Biol Reprod. 2013;42(7):662–70.
26. Balki M, Ronayne M, Davies S, Fallah S, Kingdom J, Windrim R, Carvalho JCA. Minimum oxytocin dose requirement after cesarean delivery for labor arrest. Obstet Gynecol. 2006;107(1):45–50.
27. Lavoie A, McCarthy RJ, Wong CA. The ed90 of prophylactic oxytocin infusion after delivery of the placenta during cesarean delivery in laboring compared with nonlaboring women: an up-down sequential allocation dose-response study. Anesth Analg. 2015;121(1):159–64.
28. Munn MB, Owen J, Vincent R, Wakefield M, Chestnut DH, Hauth JC. Comparison of two oxytocin regimens to prevent uterine atony at cesarean delivery: a randomized controlled trial. Obstet Gynecol. 2001;98(3):386–90.
29. El Behery MM, El Sayed GA, Abd El Hameed AA, Soliman BS, Abdelsalam WA, Bahaa A. Carbetocin versus oxytocin for prevention of postpartum hemorrhage in obese nulliparous women undergoing emergency cesarean delivery. J Matern-Fetal Neonatal Med. 2016;29(8):1257–60.
30. Razali N, Latar ILM, Chan YK, Omar SZ, Tan PC. Carbetocin compared to oxytocin in emergency cesarean section: a randomized trial. Eur J Obstet Gynecol Reprod Biol. 2016;198:35–9.
31. Whigham CA, Gorelik A, Loughnan TE, Trivedi A. Carbetocin versus oxytocin to reduce additional uterotonic use at non-elective caesarean section: a double-blind, randomised trial. J Matern Fetal Neonatal Med. 2016:1–4.
32. Khan MS, Sinha SK, Sultana T, Singhal S. Comparison of two oxytocin infusions in patients undergoing emergency cesarean sections: a double blind study. Int J Gynecol Obstet. 2012;119:S389.
33. Chaudhuri P, Mandi S, Mazumdar A. Rectally administrated misoprostol as an alternative to intravenous oxytocin infusion for preventing post-partum hemorrhage after cesarean delivery. J Obstet Gynaecol Res. 2014;40(9):2023–30.
34. Attilakos G, Psaroudakis D, Ash J, Buchanan R, Winter C, Donald F, Hunt LP, Draycott T. Carbetocin versus oxytocin for the prevention of postpartum haemorrhage following caesarean section: the results of a double-blind randomised trial. BJOG. 2010;117(8):929–36.
35. Borruto F, Treisser A, Comparetto C. Utilization of carbetocin for prevention of postpartum hemorrhage after cesarean section: a randomized clinical trial. Arch Gynecol Obstet. 2009;280(5):707–12.
36. Lapaire O, Schneider MC, Stotz M, Surbek DV, Holzgreve W, Hoesli IM. Oral misoprostol vs. intravenous oxytocin in reducing blood loss after emergency cesarean delivery. Int J Gynecol Obstet. 2006;95(1):2–7.
37. Lokugamage AU, Paine M, Bassaw-Balroop K, Sullivan KR, El Refaey H, Rodeck CH. Active management of the third stage at caesarean section: a randomised controlled trial of misoprostol versus syntocinon. Aust N Z J Obstet Gynaecol. 2001;41(4):411–4.
38. Bayoumeu F, Baka NE, Fresson J, Monnier-Barbarino P. Do prophylactic prostaglandins reduce the transfusion rate at cesarean section in high-order multiple pregnancies? Eur J Obstet Gynecol Reprod Biol 2003;111(1):38–42.
39. Brzozowska M, Lisiecki D, Kowalska-Koprek U, Karowicz-Bilinska A. Comparison of carbetocin and oxytocin effectiveness for prevention of postpartum hemorrhage after caesarean delivery. Ginekol Polska. 2015; 86(2):107–12.
40. Lourens R, Paterson-Brown S. Ergometrine given during caesarean section and incidence of delayed postpartum haemorrhage due to uterine atony. J Obstet Gynaecol. 2007;27(8):795–7.
41. Pizzagalli F, Agasse J, Marpeau L. Comparison between carbetocin and oxytocin during cesarean section in the prevention of postpartum haemorrhage. Gynecol Obstet Fertil. 2015;43(5):356–60.
42. Pursche T, Diedrich K, Banz-Jansen C. Blood loss after caesarean section: depending on the management of oxytocin application? Arch Gynecol Obstet. 2012;286(3):633–6.

43. Triopon G, Goron A, Agenor J, Aya GA, Chaillou AL, Begler-Fonnier J, Bousquet PJ, Mares P. Use of carbetocin in prevention of uterine atony during cesarean section. Comparison with oxytocin. Gynecol Obstet Fertil. 2010;38(12):729–34.
44. McClune G, Laird R. Oxytocin doses for caesarean section: a standardised approach. Anaesthesia. 2011;66:20.
45. Testa S, Paoletti O, Dellanoce C, Bassi L, Stramezzi M, Spotti E, Mammoliti D, Riccardi A. Carbetocin increase thrombin generation after cesarean section. JTH. 2013;11(Suppl. 2):738.
46. Demetz J, Clouqueur E, D'Haveloose A, Staelen P, Ducloy AS, Subtil D. Systematic use of carbetocin during cesarean delivery of multiple pregnancies: a before-and-after study. Arch Gynecol Obstet. 2013;287(5): 875–80.
47. Catanzarite VA. Prophylactic intramyometrial carboprost tromethamine does not substantially reduce blood-loss relative to intramyometrial oxytocin at routine cesarean-section. Am J Perinatol. 1990;7(1):39–42.
48. Lee AI, Wong CA, Healy L, Toledo P. Impact of a third stage of labor oxytocin protocol on cesarean delivery outcomes. Int J Obstet Anesth. 2014; 23(1):18–22.
49. King KJ, Douglas MJ, Unger W, Wong A, King RAR. Five unit bolus oxytocin at cesarean delivery in women at risk of atony: a randomized, double-blind, controlled trial. Anesth Analg. 2010;111(6):1460–6.
50. Adefuye PO, Akindele RA, Adefuye BO, Durojaiye BO, Adeiyi TO. Effect of pre-operative sub-lingual misoprostol versus intravenous oxytocin on caesarean operation blood loss. East Afr Med J. 2012;89(9):294–300.
51. Owonikoko KM, Arowojolu AO, Okunlola MA. Effect of sublingual misoprostol versus intravenous oxytocin on reducing blood loss at cesarean section in nigeria: a randomized controlled trial. J Obstet Gynaecol Res. 2011;37(7):715–21.
52. Koen S, Snyman LC, Pattinson RC, Makin JA. A randomised controlled trial comparing oxytocin and oxytocin + ergometrine for prevention of postpartum haemorrhage at caesarean section. SAMJ. 2016;106(4):399–402.
53. Alli QO. Comparing effectiveness of sublingual misoprostol with oxytocin infusion to reduce blood loss at caesarean section: double blind, randomised study. BJOG. 2013;120:77–8.
54. Kintu A, Nakubulwa S, Mijumbi C, Kwizera A, Tindimwebwa J. Uterotonic efficacy of oxytocin 2.5 versus 10 units during caesarean section at mulago hospital: a double blinded placebo controlled randomised clinical trial. Br J Anaesth. 2012;108:197–8.
55. Ayedi M, Zouche I, Smaoui L, Bouaziz I, Smaoui M, Kolsi K. Comparison of 2 versus 5 units of oxytocin in caesarean section. Eur J Anaesthesiol. 2011;28: 159–60.
56. Chou LT, Da AL, Murizah MZ, Rushdan MMN, Rashid ZMRA. Randomised controlled trial on low dose versus high dose oxytocin infusion in prevention of uterine atony at caesarean delivery. J Obstet Gynaecol Res. 2015;41:44–5.
57. Begum T, Yeasmin S, Chakma S. Sublingual misoprostol versus oxitocin infusion to reduce blood loss in caesarean section. BJOG. 2015;122:258.
58. Mahmud G, Javaid K, Tasnim N, Tabassum A, Bangash KT. Where does ergometrine stand in prevention of postpartum haemorrhage in caesarean section? J Pak Med Assoc. 2014;64(8):911–4.
59. Mangla D, Goel JK, Goel R. Prophylactic intramyometrial oxytocin before placenta delivery during cesarean section prevents postpartum hemorrhage: a prospective randomized study of 150 women. J SAFOG. 2012;4(2):93–6.
60. Chaudhuri P, Banerjee GB, Mandal A. Rectally administered misoprostol versus intravenous oxytocin infusion during cesarean delivery to reduce intraoperative and postoperative blood loss. Int J Gynecol Obstet. 2010; 109(1):25–9.
61. Vimala N, Mittal S, Kumar S. Sublingual misoprostol versus oxytocin infusion to reduce blood loss at cesarean section. Int J Gynecol Obstet. 2006;92(2): 106–10.
62. Triopon G, Goron A, Agenor J, Aya GA, Chaillou AL, Begler-Fonnier J, Bousquet PJ, Mares P. Use of carbetocin in prevention of uterine atony during cesarean section. Gynecol Obstet Fertil. 2010;38(12):729–34.
63. Brzozowska M, Lisiecki D, Kowalska-Koprek U, Karowicz-Bilinska A. Comparison of carbetocin and oxytocin effectiveness for prevention of postpartum hemorrhage after caesarean delivery. Ginekol Pol. 2015;86(2):107–12.
64. Acog ACOG. Practice bulletin: clinical management guidelines for obstetrician-gynecologists number 76, october 2006: postpartum hemorrhage. Obstet Gynecol. 2006;108(4):1039–47.
65. Leduc D, Senikas V, Lalonde AB, Ballerman C, Biringer A, Delaney M, Duperron L, Girard I, Jones D, Lee LS, et al. Active management of the third stage of labour: prevention and treatment of postpartum hemorrhage. J Obstet Gynaecol Can. 2009;31(10):980–93.
66. Budden A, Chen LJ, Henry A. High-dose versus low-dose oxytocin infusion regimens for induction of labour at term. Cochrane Database Syst Rev. 2014;10:CD009701.
67. Kenyon S, Tokumasu H, Dowswell T, Pledge D, Mori R. High-dose versus low-dose oxytocin for augmentation of delayed labour. Cochrane Database Syst Rev. 2013;7:CD007201.
68. Oladapo OT, Okusanya BO, Abalos E. Intramuscular versus intravenous prophylactic oxytocin for the third stage of labour. Cochrane Database Syst Rev. 2012;2:CD009332.
69. Costley PL, East CE. Oxytocin augmentation of labour in women with epidural analgesia for reducing operative deliveries. Cochrane Database Syst Rev. 2013;7:CD009241.
70. Schmucker CM, Blumle A, Schell LK, Schwarzer G, Oeller P, Cabrera L, von Elm E, Briel M, Meerpohl JJ. Systematic review finds that study data not published in full text articles have unclear impact on meta-analyses results in medical research. PLoS One. 2017;12(4):e0176210.
71. Grobman WA. Elective induction: when? Ever? Clin Obstet Gynecol. 2007; 50(2):537–46.
72. Nyflot LT, Sandven I, Stray-Pedersen B, Pettersen S, Al-Zirqi I, Rosenberg M, Jacobsen AF, Vangen S. Risk factors for severe postpartum hemorrhage: a case-control study. BMC Pregnancy Childbirth. 2017;17(1):17.

18

Large reductions in cesarean delivery rates in China: a qualitative study on delivery decision-making in the era of the two-child policy

Eileen Wang[1] and Therese Hesketh[1,2*]

Abstract

Background: In 2010, China's cesarean delivery (CD) rates increased to one of the highest in the world, a significant proportion of which were without medical indication. However, recent studies have indicated some declines, coinciding with national and local efforts to promote vaginal birth, as well as the relaxation of the one-child policy. Considering these trends, we aimed to qualitatively explore attitudes towards childbirth and experiences of delivery decision-making among women and physicians.

Methods: Semi-structured interviews were conducted with 45 postpartum women and 7 healthcare providers at one county-level and one provincial-level maternity hospital in Zhejiang Province. We also collected routine data from 2007 to 2016 and observed doctor-patient interactions and hospital facilities as context for the interviews. Interviews were recorded, translated and transcribed into English, and then analyzed using a framework approach.

Results: From 2007 to 2016, cesarean delivery rates at the county-level and provincial-level hospital decreased from 46% to 32% and 68% to 44%, respectively. For low-risk women, vaginal birth was the primary choice of delivery method, encouraged by doctors and nurse-midwives. Elective CD was not as widely accepted, in contrast to previous years. Women were aware of and took into consideration the consequences of CD for future pregnancies. Among those who delivered vaginally, women viewed the existing pain relief methods, epidurals and transcutaneous electrical nerve stimulation, with caution or uncertainty. Even when requested, epidurals were only given under certain circumstances. For multiparas with previous CD, repeat CD remains the norm. Both women and professionals were cautious about vaginal birth after cesarean delivery (VBAC) given the associated risks.

Conclusion: In China, changes in family planning policy and efforts to promote vaginal birth have greatly changed the culture of delivery decision-making, leading to decreased CD rates. This demonstrates the powerful role social factors and public policy can play, and provides a model for other countries with high CD rates. Further research should explore changes in other reproductive decisions during this new multiparous era, particularly across provinces.

Keywords: Cesarean delivery, Two-child policy, Delivery decision-making, China

* Correspondence: t.hesketh@ucl.ac.uk
[1]Institute for Global Health, School of Public Health, Zhejiang University, 866 Yuhangtang Lu, Hangzhou 310058, China
[2]Institute for Global Health, University College London, 30 Guilford St., London, UK

Background

In 1993 the overall rate of cesarean delivery (CD) in China was 5%. By 2010 it had increased to national estimates of 40 to 50%, and rates as high as 70% in some urban areas [1–3]. This steep increase was driven by a host of structural and provider factors, including rapid economic development and urbanization, increasing hospitalization of births, large volume of care with limited resources, and financial incentives to perform CD [1, 4–7]. High rates of CDs without medical indication have also been driven by "social factors" or cesarean deliveries on maternal request (CDMR), which comprised 10% to 28% of all CDs in 2011 [5, 8, 9]. Studies demonstrated that women's reasons for choosing cesarean included anxiety about labor, fear of pain, choice of an auspicious delivery date, and demand for a "perfect" child or birth outcome [4, 10, 11]. Still, there has been increasing concern about the rise in these unnecessary cesarean deliveries. In cases where CDs are non-medically indicated, maternal morbidity and mortality increases compared to cases of women delivering vaginally [2]. Furthermore, a CD for primiparous women increases the risk of uterine rupture, spontaneous miscarriage, abnormal placentation, and other complications in subsequent pregnancies [12].

Given these concerns, China began national and local public health efforts to decrease the CD rate through health promotion, practitioner training and tightening of hospital regulations [13–15]. More recent statistics have shown CD rates in some areas, particularly cities, have since declined by as much as 30% between 2008 and 2014 [16]. This decrease also coincided with the gradual relaxation of the one-child policy, which had been implemented in 1979, and restricted many families to one child [17]. In 2007, all provinces began to permit couples who were both only children to have two children, and in 2013, if one of the partners was an only child. From January 2016 all couples have been allowed two children [18]. The implications of the new policy include increased burden on maternity services, increases in deliveries to older women and women with previous CDs, and changes in reproductive counseling and decision-making [19].

While studies have documented these changes in CD rates, none have explored the changes in delivery decision-making in the context of both the two-child policy and efforts to limit unnecessary CDs. Therefore, the aim of this study was to understand how decisions about delivery method are made, from the perspectives of women and their healthcare providers. The specific objective was to explore attitudes of women and practitioners towards vaginal birth versus cesarean birth, including vaginal birth after cesarean (VBAC), in the era of the two-child policy. We additionally intended to explore women's attitudes towards pain relief during labor and the role it plays in delivery decision-making, particularly as studies have shown how the fear of pain has been a significant contributor to CDMR [5, 11, 20]. We wished to understand changes in CD decision-making in conjunction with the childbirth experience, of which the relief of pain is an integral component.

Methods

Study sample

We conducted the study from November 2016 to April 2017 in Zhejiang, a relatively wealthy coastal province in Eastern China. Study sites were a provincial-level teaching hospital in Hangzhou, and a county-level hospital in Jiangshan. In China, hospitals are classified according to a three-tier system: a primary hospital is usually located in a township and contains less than 100 beds; a secondary hospital contains between 100 and 500 beds; and a tertiary hospital provides the most comprehensive healthcare services with a bed capacity of 500 or more [21]. In this case, the Hangzhou hospital is tertiary-level and a referral unit for high-risk pregnancies, serving a mainly urban population; the Jiangshan hospital is a secondary-level center, serving a mainly rural population. We chose the former because it has been shown in previous studies that tertiary-level hospitals serving an urban population were more likely to have had high rates of CDs and subsequent declines in recent years [3, 16]. We also selected a smaller hospital with a rural patient population to provide comparison and assess differences in rural versus urban attitudes.

Study design

We conducted in-depth, semi-structured interviews with 45 postpartum women, 24 from Hangzhou and 21 from Jiangshan, which allowed us to reach saturation of themes. Nurses and physicians non-randomly identified women who were two to five days postpartum and who were of different parities and birth outcomes. Interviews were conducted on the wards, sometimes with family members present, using a previously-developed interview guide that included questions about the woman's birth experience and views on vaginal versus cesarean birth. We also interviewed four nurse-midwives and three obstetricians about their experience working as health practitioners, and their views of the delivery decision-making process, particularly over time. Interview guides developed and used for this study can be viewed as a Additional files 1 and 2. Prior to each interview, we explained the purpose of the study and obtained participants' verbal consent to be interviewed and recorded.

In addition to interviews, the researcher (EW) spent a month at each hospital observing and taking fieldnotes on doctor-patient relationships and the general environment of maternity care. During that time, the researcher informally interviewed health practitioners and key informants, observed outpatient clinics, inpatient wards and labor and delivery rooms, and attended prenatal classes. Hospitals' routine data from 2007 to 2016, including numbers of births, cesarean deliveries, cesarean indication, maternal age and, if available, parity, were also collected. This provided context for participants' responses.

Analysis

Audio recordings of the interviews were translated and transcribed directly into English by the bilingual researcher (EW). We used previously-identified conceptual codes, guided by preset interview topics, such as their present and past childbirth experiences as well as attitudes towards delivery method, to analyze the data. Responses were extracted, sorted by parity and birth outcome, and then analyzed for patterns. Findings were summarized and organized into a larger explanatory framework based on similarities and differences in responses depending on parity, previous delivery method or hospital. These were compared to and integrated with fieldnotes. The study was approved by the Ethics Committee of Zhejiang University.

Results

Hospital settings

The Jiangshan maternity hospital has one obstetric ward with 72 beds, two operating rooms and one labor-delivery room. There are 15 obstetricians and 26 nurses across all maternity services. The number of births increased from around 2000 in 2007 to 2531 and 2703 in 2012 and 2016, respectively (Table 1). The CD rate was around 46% in 2007, which decreased to 32% in 2016. The percentage of repeat CD out of all CDs increased from 32% to 49% from 2012 to 2016 (data from before 2012 were not obtained). Although daytime epidural services have been available since 2011, only 7% of women delivering vaginally use them. Around 43% instead choose to use transcutaneous electrical nerve stimulation (TENS) on Traditional Chinese Medicine acupoints, available since 2015. Instrumental deliveries account for less than 1% of all vaginal births. Episiotomy rates decreased from 70% in 2007 to 30% in 2016. Women generally enter the labor-delivery room at around 3 cm dilated; family members are not allowed. VBAC is generally not allowed because of the lack of resources in case of emergency surgery.

The Hangzhou maternity hospital has five obstetric wards with a total of 500 beds. There are two large labor rooms, each with ten beds, and six delivery rooms, each with two beds, as well as 40 obstetricians and 60 nurse-midwives. The number of births increased from 10,106 in 2007 to 14,801 and 20,534 in 2012 and 2016, respectively (Table 1). The CD rate was 68% in 2007, and 44% in 2016. The percentage of repeat CD out of all CDs increased from 6% to 51% from 2007 to 2016. Around 40% of women use doula services. In 2016 26% of women delivering vaginally used epidurals, and 8% TENS, available since 2009. Around 5% of eligible women undergo VBAC, but only with an epidural and doula monitoring. In 2016, instrumental delivery rates

Table 1 Collected Hospital Data, 2007–2016

Jiangshan Maternity Hospital[a]										
	2007	2008	2009	2010	2011	2012	2013	2014	2015	2016
Number of births						2531	2372	2649	2116	2703
Cesarean deliveries (% of births)						40%	40%	39%	37%	32%
Age > 35 years (% of births)						16%	20%	15%	11%	22%
Repeat CD (% of all CDs)						32%	35%	32%	40%	49%
Pain relief[b] (% of all vaginal deliveries)						3%	15%	15%	29%	50%
Zhejiang Women's Hospital										
	2007	2008	2009	2010	2011	2012	2013	2014	2015	2016
Number of births	10,106	10,271	10,961	11,414	12,090	14,801	14,332	18,115	14,598	20,534
Cesarean deliveries (% of births)	68%	67%	60%	54%	50%	51%	51%	46%	46%	44%
Age > 35 years (% of births)	7%	7%	8%	8%	8%	7%	10%	10%	16%	18%
Repeat CD (% of all CDs)	6%	7%	10%	12%	15%	18%	21%	30%	43%	51%
Epidurals[b] (% of all vaginal deliveries)						39%	39%	31%	30%	26%
VBAC (% of eligible CDs)						2%	1%	1%	3%	5%

[a]Data from before 2012 from Jiangshan Maternity Hospital were unable to be collected. The approximate number of births and percentage of cesarean deliveries before 2012 were revealed anecdotally in interviews

[b]The pain relief data marked for Jiangshan includes the Traditional Chinese Medicine transcutaneous electrical nerve stimulation (TENS) after its implementation in 2015. Daytime epidural services have been available since 2011. For Zhejiang Women's Hospital, only consecutive data for epidurals were reported, although they also offer other methods of pain relief and social support, such as doulas. Data from before 2012 were unavailable

were around 6%; episiotomy rates were 15%, down from 65% in 2012. Women enter the labor ward from the patient wards at around 3 cm dilated and are then transferred to the delivery room for second stage. Family members are sometimes allowed into the labor ward, depending on volume and time of day. Women are encouraged to move around and choose their position while laboring, but not for delivery. In addition to the wards, there are 20 "VIP," private labor and delivery rooms for women and their families, which cost an average of 6300 RMB (1000 USD) per night.

Table 2 Sociodemographic characteristics of postpartum women interviewed

	Hangzhou	Jiangshan
Delivery Method		
Cesarean	13	11
Vaginal	11	10
Pain Relief Use/Support During Labor		
Epidural	3	1
Transcutaneous Electrical Nerve Stimulation (TENS)	0	8
Doula	3	0
Parity		
Primiparous	10	6
Multiparous	14	15
Mean age of first child ± SD (range)	7 ± 5.1 (2–21)	8.3 ± 5.2 (2–17)
Previous vaginal delivery	6	8
Previous cesarean delivery	8	7
VBAC	1	0
Age		
Mean ± SD (range)	32.5 ± 0.90 (25–44)	32.2 ± 1.28 (23–45)
20–24	0	2
25–29	6	6
30–34	10	6
35–39	7	5
40–45	1	2
Highest Educational Qualification		
Middle School	2	3
High School	1	9
Vocational college	1	6
Bachelor's	17	3
Master's and up	3	0
Currently Employed		
Yes	19	10
No	5	11

Interviews

Of the 45 postpartum women interviewed, 16 were primiparas, 29 multiparas, 24 delivered by cesarean and 21 vaginally. Table 2 lists the characteristics of women interviewed. In general, the women in Hangzhou had higher socio-economic status, in terms of education and employment, than those in Jiangshan, reflecting urban-rural differences. In addition, there was a substantial proportion of women older than 35; this reflects the unusual timeframe in which the study was conducted, in which older women were giving birth to second children immediately after the relaxation of the one-child policy. We note, however, that there has also been a gradual increase in births to older women over time given changes in family planning policy (see Table 1). In this paper, interviewees are referred to by reference initials: H for Hangzhou and J for Jiangshan; V for vaginal and C for cesarean; and F for first birth and S for second birth. We have also included their highest level of education attained.

Attitudes of primiparas

Vaginal birth as the primary choice

In both Hangzhou and Jiangshan, most low-risk primiparas stated that unless there were medical contraindications, they preferred vaginal births. The general remark for their stated preference was that vaginal birth was "better both for the baby and mother." Some mentioned the benefits for the baby, including "fewer respiratory problems," "better immunity" and "stimulation by squeezing through the vaginal canal." However, more women emphasized the disadvantages of surgery: that recovery is slower and more painful, and surgery is harmful to the mother's body. In addition, some explicitly mentioned the effects a cesarean delivery would have on future reproduction, including the spacing of future births and risk for further pregnancies:

> "With vaginal birth, you only have to wait one or two years before having another. But if you had a C-section, you have to wait at the very least three years. That's what I heard from my friend... Also, [with a previous C-section], you have an incision. What if you're older? What if your first was small, and your second is bigger? Your belly is going to be stretched out even larger. It might rupture. So then there's more risk, dangerous both to the mother and child." (JVF3, vocational high school).

> "The doctor will say, if you want to have a second child, you have wait at least five or six years. If you delivered vaginally, you can have another in one to two years, because you recover more quickly if you deliver vaginally. It's better for the woman's body and physique." (HVF1, master's).

One obstetrician at Jiangshan remarked that after the one-child policy was relaxed,

> "It seems that more women at the hospital want natural birth because with a uterine scar, the second child is usually a cesarean birth. [A previous C-section] restricts the choice of delivery method and also adds some risks."

Social norms and hospital promotion

Still, when asked why they decided to try for vaginal birth instead of elective cesarean delivery, most primiparas drew upon the fact that it was commonsense that women would do so. Their responses indicated that their decision was influenced by social norms—that it was what everyone else was saying and doing:

> "They say that recovery is faster, and it's better for the baby. So I wanted a vaginal delivery." (JCF1, high school).

> "With a cesarean, recovery is slower, and it might have more complications than vaginal birth. Usually women will all choose to have a vaginal birth." (HVF4, vocational college).

> "Everyone, at first, wants a vaginal birth. It's only if something happens during labor that you get a C-section. Like my sister, when they told her she needed a C-section [before labor], she ran to the bathroom and cried...she wasn't mentally prepared for a cesarean surgery—the news came so suddenly." (JVF3, vocational high school).

Most received their information about childbirth from friends, family, the internet, and most importantly, the doctor or hospital. A 35-year-old Hangzhou primipara attributed the push for vaginal birth to widespread health promotion in hospitals, whether through doctor recommendations, pamphlets or prenatal classes:

> "They've [the hospital] done health promotion pretty well. They really push natural birth. They constantly recommend natural birth, especially for the first child." (HCF1, bachelor's).

Role of the health care providers

While most women were motivated to try for vaginal delivery, many still worried about their mental and physical ability to give birth. Three primiparas, all of whom Jiangshan women, said they had thought about getting a C-section during labor because of the pain, but the nurse-midwives convinced them that they could persist with it:

> "I did consider a cesarean birth [during labor] because it hurt so much. But the doctor said the baby was very small. They encouraged me to deliver vaginally, because there are more benefits to vaginal birth. If you are already hurting to that point, and you had the C-section, would you not suffer twice?" (JVF1, high school).

> "During labor, I could not handle it. I was anxious, and I was afraid. I just wanted to get the baby out. When I requested a C-section, [the nurse-midwife] said 'right now, there's no problem so you should keep on going.' She said that a C-section is not good for your recovery." (JVF2, middle school).

On the other hand, only one college-educated primipara in Hangzhou specifically wanted and requested an elective cesarean delivery before labor, but was told she was not allowed to get it. She commented:

> "I actually wanted a cesarean, because I feel like it isn't as difficult or painful as vaginal birth. But, now if you are suitable for vaginal birth, you can't get a cesarean section." (HVF5, bachelor's).

Attitudes of multiparas with prior vaginal delivery

Many multiparas with prior vaginal delivery also preferred and tried for vaginal delivery for their second child, giving many of the same reasons as primiparas, with the added comment that there was no point to getting a surgery—and harming the body—if the first child was born vaginally. Only a few expressed a desire for a cesarean delivery pre-labor, either because they were afraid of the pain after having experienced it once, or because they were older and had been waiting for the change in policy to give birth to their second child. Still, like with the primiparas, doctors encouraged vaginal birth, telling them that labor was usually faster the second time and that CDs were not performed at the hospital without a medical indication. For example, one 44-year-old multipara with a previous vaginal birth wanted a CD:

> "The problem is that for those who are older, everything has hardened. We don't have any elasticity down there, so we can't give birth. I fear that the child would get stuck and suffocate. My physique is not good—I'm too fat, too old." (HVS4, middle school).

Another Jiangshan multiparas had previously delivered vaginally, but was overdue and anxious about the labor pain. She said that when she asked the doctor for a CD:

> "The doctor recommended I give birth myself and give it a try. She also said that the second child might

be faster and that it would be a pity if I had a C-section for the second child." (JVS3, vocational college).

Attitudes of multiparas with prior cesarean delivery

Previous culture of cesarean births

These pro-vaginal birth attitudes stand in sharp contrast to previously high rates of CD and previous birth experiences of multiparas who gave birth 5–10 years ago. According to both practitioners and these women, CDs were very common and widely accepted. As one Hangzhou nurse-midwife of 16 years put it,

"[The cesarean rate] was higher before because of 'social factors.' Women would get a cesarean just because their family members wanted one, they feared the pain, or for the slightest problem, like if the amniotic fluid was a bit low. Even women who had severe myopia would get cesareans. Now all these will try for vaginal birth."

This culture resulted from practitioners' encouragement of CDs and willingness to perform it for any reason, without consideration for medical indications, as well as women's apparent low tolerance for risk and labor pain. CDs were perceived as a way to bypass the experience of labor. One 39-year-old college-educated multipara commented on the previous boom in CDs:

"People are finicky. We all knew that labor pain was very painful, and a lot of people did not want to bear it...And during that time everyone was only having one child, so they figured, they would just do the C-section and it would be fine. It also had to do with how people could bear hardship. Before [the widespread availability of CDs] there was no other way—you had to give birth yourself. Now, with this choice, of course people hoped that birth would go more smoothly." (JCS7, bachelor's).

The preference for CD was often justified by the one-child policy, since many women believed they would give birth just once. One multipara regretted requesting a cesarean nine years ago. She said recovering from her second cesarean surgery was much harder, and more painful, compared to the first:

"I thought I would only have one child! And I thought I might as well just get it over with with a cesarean..." (JCS1, bachelor's).

Her husband added,

"The first time around I was worried she could not stand the pain. At the time, we were not allowed a second child so we never considered the risks. Right now, we regret that decision to get a C-section."

Another woman in Jiangshan who requested a CD in 2013 said,

"During that time, I did not even consider [vaginal birth] an option because my belly was so big, and I did not think I would have another baby. [If I had known I would be able to have a second child,] I would have considered vaginal birth, because I heard that then having the second child is easier, and not as painful." (JCS3, high school).

Doctors also admitted that CD indications are much stricter now. Strong messages discouraging CD and extolling the benefits of vaginal birth are consistently promoted through physician recommendations and prenatal classes. This has been reinforced by the relaxation of the two-child policy. Physicians have also become more pressured to manage reproductive complications related to previous CDs. One Hangzhou obstetrician remarked on the need to restrict unnecessary cesareans:

"Now we've realized that we did too many unnecessary cesarean deliveries. As OB/GYNs, we can see that these cesareans have consequences now. There are a lot of women who have cesarean scar ectopic pregnancies or placenta previa. Before there were not that many. There's definitely a relationship there."

Vaginal birth after cesarean (VBAC) as the safer option

While vaginal birth is the primary choice of primiparas or multiparas who have delivered vaginally, CD is the default delivery method for multiparas with previous CD. The Jiangshan hospital did not allow VBACs due to the lack of resources to handle possible uterine rupture, and accordingly, many women at Jiangshan did not know about the possibility of VBAC. Even if they did, they stated that no one else they knew attempted VBAC, and that risks of uterine rupture were high. Only one woman who adamantly wanted a VBAC was pressured by doctors not to:

"The doctors told my family that the rate of success [of a VBAC] is only 25%! They want to scare you. So then my family members said: 'oh, C-section, C-section, let's just do that.'" (JCS8, high school).

The Jiangshan physicians admitted that even though the risk of uterine rupture was comparatively low at 1%, they did not have the resources to monitor whether the uterus is ruptured, or respond appropriately, given that the operating room was on another floor of the hospital. One doctor said:

> "You have to look at the conditions of the hospital. You have to ensure the patients' safety. Only once this prerequisite is fulfilled, and only if they want to try vaginal birth, then we will let them try it. But how can we control these risks?"

She further said she did not feel comfortable with VBAC, because she had not handled many cases:

> "A lot of it depends on the doctors' skills. You have to assess all of the woman's conditions, plus the details of the previous C-section. To tell you the truth, [the circumstances of the previous CD are] not easy to understand, because it might have been five to six years ago, or maybe it wasn't done at our hospital. So I haven't attempted to handle many VBACs."

On the other hand, the Hangzhou hospital did allow VBACs under certain circumstances. Multiparas with previous CDs in Hangzhou were more aware of VBAC, largely from the internet, although some heard of it from their prenatal doctors. Many expressed hope to deliver by vaginal birth. However, almost all had a repeat CD; after doctors' assessment of the thickness of the uterine scar and fetal size, they would be deterred by the risk or their likelihood of "success." A multipara said,

> "Originally I also wanted to try for vaginal birth. But the doctor did an assessment and saw [my scar] was too thin, like 0.7 millimeters thick. She said that a C-section was safer." (HCS5, bachelor's).

One 39-year-old multipara did not consider it at all:

> "I had a uterine scar, which is risky. Also, I felt like I did not have any self-confidence to deliver vaginally. Add to that my age, I felt like the possibility of me giving birth vaginally was practically zero." (HCS6, bachelor's).

Only one woman interviewed gave birth by VBAC because she felt like a cesarean surgery was too painful, despite doctors' comments that they themselves would choose a repeat C-section. But she had made her decision carefully:

> "When they examined my scar, they saw that it was rather thick. I also had gotten pregnant two years after my first which is when the scar's elasticity is the best. I did my own assessment and figured I could possibly deliver vaginally. If I had had any doubt I probably would not have considered it, because after all, safety comes first." (HVS5, bachelor's).

Doctors in Hangzhou were open to VBAC but were relatively conservative about it. Although they acknowledged that they had 24/7 anesthesia services, emergency surgery resources and on-site pediatrics teams to respond to uterine rupture, they believed cesarean birth was a much safer option. Therefore, though they offered VBAC to eligible women, they often recommended repeat CDs. One nurse-midwife in Hangzhou spoke of a patient who insisted on a VBAC, but had an emergency CD anyway:

> "When I heard how tall she was, I felt like she would not be able to do it. She was only 1.5 meters. Her first was a C-section, [the baby was] around 3.5 kg. I did not recommend [VBAC], but her family members wanted her to try...but she ended up with a CD."

One doctor in Hangzhou said that given the difficulty of labor and the added risk of uterine rupture, she could not face the responsibility of an adverse event occurring during VBAC:

> "In China, the doctor-patient relationship is rather tense. If the patient does not have the desire to, we won't force them to a vaginal birth...after all, there's certain risks."

Use of and attitudes towards pain relief

Given that in previous literature fear of pain has been a significant factor in women's decision to have a cesarean, we also inquired about their views of social support and pain relief during labor. In particular, we wanted to understand what role pain relief plays in women's birth experience and how it affects or is tied to their perceptions of vaginal versus cesarean delivery. These experiences differed by hospital. In Hangzhou, most women knew about epidurals prior to labor. Of the 11 interviewees, three chose an epidural, while five felt like they could handle the pain without one. Three requested one, but were refused, mainly because certain standards were not met—either their cervix dilated too quickly or they were multiparous and doctors told them labor would be short. One primipara said:

> "I adamantly wanted an epidural. But then my cervix dilated too quickly, so I could not use it in time... There are not many anesthesiologists here, and many women request epidurals. Even when you call for one, the time it takes the doctor to get there can't match the speed of your cervix dilation. I was already sent to

> "...the delivery room before the anaesthesiologist got to me. I could only brace myself to give birth without it." (HVF5, bachelor's).

Still, when asked about their views towards epidurals, most women—even those that requested it—indicated that they were not too familiar with how it worked, that it might be ineffective, that it could have side effects, or that it would hurt to insert the epidural needle. As two women who opted not to use it remarked:

> "I have heard of epidurals, but some people say it's effective, others say it only slightly relieves the pain, and some say it doesn't work, because everyone's physique and ability to handle labor is different." (HVS1, bachelor's).

> "I feared [the epidural] would be painful. They said they would insert the needle into the spine, and when I heard that, I thought: forget about it. In any case, I'll go with labor pain—and there's medical consequences to [the epidural]. I hear that people's backs will hurt." (HVS2, bachelor's).

Of the three who did get an epidural, two remarked that the pain medication could only be used for a certain period before it ran out, and that it was only a temporary measure of relief:

> "At 3cm they gave me an epidural. The epidural only works for two hours. Then they would add some more for a total of 3.5 hours. During that 3.5 hours, I had only opened from 3cm to 4cm. It wasn't really effective. 4cm until 10cm, I had to depend on myself." (HVF1, master's).

On the other hand, more women were favorable and open to doula services, although this was also dependent on the availability of doulas.

> "To be honest, I think that having someone with you [during labor] is more effective than [the epidural]. You'll feel more calm, especially for your first child because you don't know what it's like." (HVS1, bachelor's).

> "This time I did not ask for a doula, so I just lay on the bed. At that time, the doctor had inserted a drip. When it was all used up, I called for the doctor, but no one came over. Because no family members are allowed in, if there's a person next to you, you'll feel a little better. I think that doulas are great, if you have the money to get one." (HVS2, bachelor's).

In Jiangshan, women did not know about or decide to use any form of pain relief until nurses offered it in the labor-delivery room. Eight opted for transcutaneous electric nerve stimulation (TENS) which involved sticking pads on traditional Chinese medicine acupoints on the back and hand. TENS was the default form of pain relief offered, because it could be easily applied by the nurse-midwives. These women believed TENS worked, but only in the sense that it made labor shorter, not that it reduced pain.

> "I used the stick-on pads, on the hands and back (TENS). The 1000 RMB one. They say it helps open the cervix. But as for the pain...it was still painful." (JVS2, vocational college).

> "Well, the nurses just asked me if I wanted [TENS], and I said I did. She explained to me the benefits, that I would give birth more quickly. I had already labored for a long time, so I decided to use it. I'm not too sure [if it was effective]. They say it is. I think that I gave birth more quickly. Labor was shorter." (JVS5, middle school).

On the other hand, epidurals were available but not consistently offered in the labor-delivery room; as a result, not many women knew it was an option, and only one interviewee used it. When asked if she was offered an epidural, one primipara said,

> "For vaginal birth? They don't have that for vaginal birth, right? It seems like in the delivery room everyone used the electrode pads (TENS)." (JCF3, high school).

Of those who did know about or were offered epidurals, they, like the Hangzhou women, seemed to have a negative impression of it, or heavily depended on their doctors' recommendation and guidance about pain relief options.

> "[The nurses] don't really promote the epidural, just the pads...They say that if you do the shot in the back, it will harm the back. If you stick the pads on, it's like massage, it will be like electric stimulation. It was like a massaging sensation...But usually whatever the doctor says and we'll listen." (JVS1, college).

> "The stick-on ones don't have any side effects. But if you have an injection, then it might affect your body. This is my impression. At the very least you have a needle stuck into you." (JVF3, vocational high school).

> "If they did a shot, then, that might as well be a C-section—that's anesthesia. They only give anesthesia

with a C-section. In any case, no matter C-section or vaginal birth, it's all painful." (JVF2, middle school).

"I was afraid there could be side effects [to the epidural]. I did not trust it. My family is very traditional. They definitely won't agree to using *wutong*." (JVS4, vocational college).

Physicians and nurse-midwives looked favorably upon the introduction of pain relief methods within the past few years, although they viewed it as the woman's choice, except when contraindicated. One nurse-midwife at the Hangzhou hospital said:

"With an epidural, it depends on whether they know about it or their ability to accept it. Some people feel like epidurals are great because it can relieve the pain. If they fear the pain, of course they hope to use it. Some think that because it's a drug, they don't want to use it. Most people who have understood that it's a widely-recognized, safe method would accept it."

However, non-epidural methods were more widely accepted and promoted, because of the epidural-related issues of both anesthesiologist availability and potential side effects, such as its association with lengthening labor and increasing risk of instrumental delivery.

"We promote natural birth... there are also other [non-pharmacological] methods of pain relief to ease the pain [referring to also doulas, massage, water showers, and Lamaze breathing]. The end goal is that they can give birth vaginally." (Hangzhou Nurse-Midwife).

"[The use of epidurals] depends on the doctors' assessment. We also have to see if we can do it—like if the anesthesiologist is very busy, if it's nighttime, or if they're in surgery, then we won't do the epidural. Most people will choose [TENS] because you just need a nurse to put it on and that's it. But for some patients, if they did not sleep the entire night, we'll do an epidural for them so they can rest." (Jiangshan OB/GYN).

Discussion

In 2008, China was purported to have one of the highest rates of cesarean delivery in the world [2]. In the span of just 10 years, rates in urban centers decreased substantially, and the rate of increase in other areas slowed [16]. Such rapid change is unprecedented. The new culture is in sharp contrast to previous encouragement by doctors to undergo CD, and the frequency of maternal requests [5, 22, 23]. In addition, in 2016 China officially ended the one-child policy, creating significant implications for maternity care. This study is the first to examine delivery decision-making at the intersection of these two phenomena. Given the unusual period in which this research was conducted, our interviewees included a disproportionate number of older women with previous CDs. While this unusual situation may not persist, the cohort interviewed does give us some insight into how the culture of delivery decision-making has changed over time.

From our interviews, we found a strong preference and willingness to try for vaginal births among primiparas in both urban and rural settings, representing a huge shift from previous years. Past studies showed that up to 25% of CDs were CDMR, often requested by urban, educated women [5, 9, 22, 24]. In this study, no woman purportedly had CDMR, and in fact, most women of higher socioeconomic status supported vaginal birth. Given that the proportion of CDs had started to drop before changes to the family planning policy were announced, we believe that government policy and promotion have influenced physician suggestions affecting women's choices, as well as women's beliefs about delivery. The relaxation of the one-child policy has further reinforced this change in mindset. The two-child policy has increased awareness of the risk of CD for future pregnancies [25–28]. Previously the impossibility of future births gave women the impetus to request CD, a decision some came to regret for their second pregnancy [1, 5, 29]. This highlights the unintended consequences China's family planning policy has had on delivery decision-making.

We found that regardless of setting, hospitals and practitioners have been key to driving change in delivery method preferences and decision-making. CDs had been encouraged by doctors for convenience, financial and defensive reasons [15, 30, 31]. Moreover, past studies have shown that physicians themselves preferred CD, which can influence maternal preference [29, 31, 32]. However, this is changing. Physicians, at least in Jiangshan and Hangzhou, have become more adherent to medical indications for CD, and they themselves now promote vaginal delivery in most circumstances. They also no longer consider CD as an elective choice for low-risk women, which may also raise questions of maternal autonomy in delivery decision-making.

While the norms for low-risk primiparous women are similar across rural and urban settings, differences in childbirth knowledge, attitudes and experience emerged specifically in two areas: repeat CD and pain relief during labor, which often stemmed from variations in availability of resources and information. In China, repeat CD is the default delivery method for women with previous CD, which suggests the decrease in CD rates has been mainly driven by prevention of the primary CD.

Potential risks of uterine rupture mean that VBACs, like in other countries, are not offered, as in Jiangshan, or are advised against, as in Hangzhou [33–37]. The availability of VBAC and the childbirth environment thus shaped women's perceptions about their childbirth options after CD. As more women are having second children, Chinese hospitals will need to carefully consider the integration of VBAC as a viable delivery method for women with previous CD. As in other contexts, particular attention will have to be paid to childbirth environment, management of labor and perceptions of risk [38–41].

While interviewees' responses demonstrate how delivery preference and decision-making have changed, we also observe that the environment of birth has become more patient-centered, particularly at tertiary-level hospitals. Previous studies have shown how lack of pain relief and social support can drive requests for non-medically-indicated CD [20, 42, 43]. While women did not explicitly connect their birth environment to their decision for vaginal birth, they are becoming aware of and choosing options to ease labor. In Hangzhou, and to a lesser extent Jiangshan, hospitals are promoting freedom of movement during labor, limiting interventions such as episiotomies, and offering private labor and delivery rooms (although at a higher cost)—all options that promote vaginal over cesarean birth. Still, women continue to express anxiety about birth, and certain barriers continue to exist particularly at secondary-level, more rural hospitals: most women still labor alone in open wards, and volume of care continues to be high with limited availability of staff [15, 42, 44]. Moreover, while awareness of pain relief is spreading, the majority of women, particularly in Jiangshan, continue to express negative views of or mistrust towards pharmacological or anesthetic forms of pain relief. This may be because pain relief options are limited, and services are not necessarily guaranteed or widely promoted. Women's responses also indicate that social support and one-on-one encouragement may be seen as a better option to relieve the suffering of labor; however, in China, this is also constrained by the scarcity of resources, particularly at public hospitals [20, 42]. While women's delivery preferences may be influenced by doctors' suggestions or government promotion, they are not enough to ensure the most comfortable childbirth experience or environment.

In a context where many other countries' CD rates are increasing, China provides an example of how top-down efforts can not only reduce CD rates, but also change the perception of childbirth and culture of delivery decision-making. After the release of a 2007–2008 WHO report indicating high rates of CD in China and associating unnecessary CDs with higher rates of maternal mortality and morbidity, the Ministry of Health and the Chinese Maternal-Child Health Association launched a campaign to "Promote Natural Birth and Ensure Maternal-Child Health" [2, 45, 46]. This campaign consisted of various efforts: assessing and adjusting hospital standards, training physicians to follow a less-interventionist approach to childbirth, and disseminating material promoting natural birth [47, 48]. In addition, CD rates became an indicator of hospital quality, providing hospitals' an impetus to reduce CD rates. Provincial governments began offering financial incentives or disincentives to hospitals to decrease their CD rates, which, in turn, filtered down to the doctors to reduce CDs performed [49]. As can be seen from our interviews, such efforts have had an enormous effect on delivery decision-making, maternal preference, and physician behavior. This success emphasizes the social, cultural and economic nature of CD rates, and how they can be addressed. They also provide a lesson for many other countries with high CD rates.

This study has a few limitations. First, the sample was non-randomly drawn from only two hospitals in Zhejiang Province, and is clearly not generalizable to the rest of China, particularly less-developed areas. However, evidence shows that CD rates are decreasing in many cities where they had previously reached 50–70%, so the situation described in this study is probably mirrored elsewhere [16]. Another limitation was that our interviews focused on the woman and healthcare provider; in China, the husband and the family are also important participants in the decision-making process. Selection bias and response bias could have also been a factor; because interviews were conducted in a hospital setting, interviewees may have been more likely to respond according to doctors' wishes. However, given the researcher was not affiliated with the hospital, they seemed to talk candidly about their experiences. Finally, we only interviewed postpartum women, whose responses might have been affected by ex-post rationalization; further research should follow and interview women throughout their pregnancy and after delivery to better describe the process of childbirth decision-making.

Conclusion

In China, changes in family planning policy and efforts to promote vaginal birth have greatly changed the culture of delivery decision-making, leading to decreased CD rates. This demonstrates the powerful role social factors and public policy can play in CD rates, and might provide suggestions for other countries wishing to lower CD rates. At the same time, it also exemplifies the unintended effects of family planning policies on delivery decision-making. Research should further examine changes in CD and other reproductive decisions during this new multiparous era.

Abbreviations
CD: Cesarean delivery; OB/GYN: Obstetrician-gynecologist;
TENS: Transcutaneous electrical nerve stimulation; VBAC: Vaginal birth after cesarean

Acknowledgements
We would like to thank Zhejiang University Women's Hospital and Jiangshan Maternity Hospital for providing hospital statistics as well as supporting the fieldwork and interviews. Special thanks should be given to Dr. Susan Hellerstein, Professor Xudong Zhou, Dr. Xiaoming Zhu, Dr. Lili Huang, Dr. Danqing Chen, Dr. Qiong Luo, Nurses Junqin Li and Fang Wang, Dr. Jinhua Ye and numerous others for their enormous help during this research.

Funding
This research was carried out on a fellowship grant generously sponsored by the U.S. Fulbright Program.

Authors' contributions
EW and TH were both involved in the conception and planning of the study. EW carried out the fieldwork and interviews, analyzed the data, and drafted the article. Both EW and TH revised and edited the paper. Both authors read and approved the final manuscript.

Competing interests
The authors declare that they have no competing interests.

References

1. Hellerstein S, Feldman S, Duan T. China's 50% caesarean delivery rate: is it too high? BJOG. 2014;122:160–4.
2. Lumbiganon P, Laopaiboon M, Gülmezoglu AM, Souza JP, Taneepanichskul S, Ruyan P, et al. Method of delivery and pregnancy outcomes in Asia: the WHO global survey on maternal and perinatal health 2007–08. Lancet. 2010; 375:490–9.
3. Feng XL, Xu L, Guo Y, Ronsmans C. Factors influencing rising caesarean section rates in China between 1988 and 2008. Bull World Health Organ. 2012;90:30–9A.
4. Klemetti R, Che X, Gao Y, Raven J, Wu Z, Tang S, et al. Cesarean section delivery among primiparous women in rural China: an emerging epidemic. Am J Obstet Gynecol. 2010;202:65.e1–6.
5. Zhang J, Liu Y, Meikle S, Zheng J, Sun W, Li Z. Cesarean delivery on maternal request in Southeast China. Obstet Gynecol. 2008;111:1077–82.
6. Sufang G, Padmadas SS, Fengmin Z, Brown JJ, Stones RW. Delivery settings and caesarean section rates in China. Bull World Health Organ. 2007;85:755–62.
7. Bogg L, Huang K, Long Q, Shen Y, Hemminki E. Dramatic increase of cesarean deliveries in the midst of health reforms in rural China. Soc Sci Med. 2010;70:1544–9.
8. Liu Y, Li G, Chen Y, Wang X, Ruan Y, Zou L, et al. A descriptive analysis of the indications for caesarean section in mainland China. BMC Pregnancy Childbirth. 2014;14:410.
9. Liu X, Landon M, Cheng W, Chen Y. Cesarean delivery on maternal request in China: what are the risks and benefits? Am J Obstet Gynecol. 2015; Available from: http://www.sciencedirect.com/science/article/pii/S000293781500099X
10. Tang S, Li X, Wu Z. Rising cesarean delivery rate in primiparous women in urban China: evidence from three nationwide household health surveys. Am J Obstet Gynecol. 2006;195:1527–32.
11. Lee LYK, Holroyd E, Ng CY. Exploring factors influencing Chinese women's decision to have elective caesarean surgery. Midwifery. 2001;17:314–22.
12. D'Souza R, Arulkumaran S. To "C" or not to "C"? Caesarean delivery upon maternal request: a review of facts, figures and guidelines. J Perinat Med. 2013 [cited 2015 Feb 1];41. Available from: http://proxy.library.upenn.edu:2517/view/j/jpme.2013.41.issue-1/jpm-2012-0049/jpm-2012-0049.xml
13. Development of Chinese Women and Children's Development Programme in China [Internet]. Chinese State Council; 2011. Available from: http://www.gov.cn/gongbao/content/2011/content_1927200.htm
14. National Health and Family Planning Commission Notice on the review of the Baby Friendly Hospital Initiative [Internet]. People's Republic of China National Health and Family Planning; 2014. Available from: http://www.nhfpc.gov.cn/fys/s3585/201406/556c0b7673e8470f9641c28d119a9f31.shtml
15. Hellerstein S, Feldman S, Duan T. Survey of obstetric care and cesarean delivery rates in shanghai, China. Birth. 2016;43:193–9.
16. Li H-T, Luo S, Trasande L, Hellerstein S, Kang C, Li J-X, et al. Geographic variations and temporal trends in cesarean delivery rates in China, 2008-2014. JAMA. 2017;317:69–76.
17. Hesketh T, Lu L, Xing ZW. The effect of China's one-child family policy after 25 years. N Engl J Med. 2005;353:1171–6.
18. Zeng Y, Hesketh T. The effects of China's universal two-child policy. Lancet. 2016;388:1930–8.
19. Cheng P, Duan T. China's new two-child policy: maternity care in the new multiparous era. BJOG. 2016;123:7–9.
20. Wang E. Requests for cesarean deliveries: the politics of labor pain and pain relief in Shanghai, China. Soc Sci Med. 2017;173:1–8.
21. Statistical Bulletin of Public Health and Family Planning Development in China [Internet]. National Department of Health Planning and Information; 2014 [cited 2017 Oct 14]. Available from: http://www.moh.gov.cn/guihuaxxs/s10742/201405/886f82dafa344c3097f1d16581a1bea2.shtml
22. Zhu Y, Li H, Zhang Y, Li Z, Zhang L, Liu J. Secular trends of cesarean delivery and cesarean delivery on maternal request among primiparous women with singleton pregnancy in Southern and Northern China during 1993–2010. National Med J China. 2012;92:1734–7.
23. Long Q, Klemetti R, Wang Y, Tao F, Yan H, Hemminki E. High caesarean section rate in rural China: is it related to health insurance (new co-operative medical scheme)? Soc Sci Med. 2012;75:733–7.
24. Qian J. China's national cesarean rate. Analysis and suggestions. J Popul Dev. 2012:39–42.
25. Gilliam M. Cesarean delivery on request: reproductive consequences. Semin Perinatol. 2006;30:257–60.
26. Grobman W, Caughey A, Hahn K. 177: reproductive consequences of elective cesarean: a decision analysis. Am J Obstet Gynecol. 2008;199:S61.
27. Miller ES, Hahn K, Grobman WA, Society for Maternal-Fetal Medicine Health Policy Committee. Consequences of a primary elective cesarean delivery across the reproductive life. Obstet Gynecol. 2013;121:789–97.
28. Ecker J, Frigoletto F. Cesarean delivery and the risk–benefit calculus. N Engl J Med. 2007;356:885–8.
29. Ouyang YQ, Zhang Q. A study on personal mode of delivery among Chinese obstetrician-gynecologists, midwives and nurses. Arch Gynecol Obstet. 2012;287:37–41.
30. Gao Y, Xue Q, Chen G, Stone P, Zhao M, Chen Q. An analysis of the indications for cesarean section in a teaching hospital in China. Eur J Obstet Gynecol Reprod Biol. 2013;170:414–8.
31. Ji H, Jiang H, Yang L, Qian X, Tang S. Factors contributing to the rapid rise of caesarean section: a prospective study of primiparous Chinese women in shanghai. BMJ Open. 2015;5:e008994.
32. Deng W, Klemetti R, Long Q, Wu Z, Duan C, Zhang W-H, et al. Cesarean section in shanghai: women's or healthcare provider's preferences? BMC Pregnancy Childbirth. 2014;14:285.
33. Cheng YW, Eden KB, Marshall N, Pereira L, Caughey AB, Guise J-M. Delivery after prior cesarean: maternal morbidity and mortality. Clin Perinatol. 2011; 38:297–309.
34. Menacker F. Trends in cesarean rates for first births and repeat cesarean rates for low-risk women: United States, 1990–2003. National Vital Statistics Reports. 2005;54:1–8.
35. Black M, Entwistle VA, Bhattacharya S, Gillies K. Vaginal birth after caesarean section: why is uptake so low? Insights from a meta-ethnographic synthesis of women's accounts of their birth choices. BMJ Open. 2016;6:e008881.
36. Dexter S, Windsor S, Watkinson S. Meeting the challenge of maternal choice in mode of delivery with vaginal birth after caesarean section: a medical, legal and ethical commentary. BJOG. 2014;121:133–40.
37. Wanyonyi S, Ngichabe S. Safety concerns for planned vaginal birth after caesarean section in sub-Saharan Africa. BJOG. 2014;121:141–4.

38. Kamal P, Dixon-Woods M, Kurinczuk JJ, Oppenheimer C, Squire P, Waugh J. Factors influencing repeat caesarean section: qualitative exploratory study of obstetricians' and midwives' accounts. BJOG. 2005;112:1054–60.
39. Cox KJ. Providers' perspectives on the vaginal birth after cesarean guidelines in Florida, United States: a qualitative study. BMC Pregnancy Childbirth. 2011;11:72.
40. Lundgren I, van Limbeek E, Vehvilainen-Julkunen K, Nilsson C. Clinicians' views of factors of importance for improving the rate of VBAC (vaginal birth after caesarean section): a qualitative study from countries with high VBAC rates. BMC Pregnancy Childbirth. 2015 [cited 2016 Nov 3];15. Available from: http://bmcpregnancychildbirth.biomedcentral.com/articles/10.1186/s12884-015-0629-6
41. Moffat M, Bell J, Porter M, Lawton S, Hundley V, Danielian P, et al. Decision making about mode of delivery among pregnant women who have previously had a caesarean section: a qualitative study. BJOG. 2007;114:86–93.
42. Raven J, van den Broek N, Tao F, Kun H, Tolhurst R. The quality of childbirth care in China: women's voices: a qualitative study. BMC Pregnancy Childbirth. 2015;15:113.
43. Fenwick J, Staff L, Gamble J, Creedy DK, Bayes S. Why do women request caesarean section in a normal, healthy first pregnancy? Midwifery. 2010;26: 394–400.
44. Qian X, Smith H, Zhou L, Liang J, Garner P. Evidence-based obstetrics in four hospitals in China: an observational study to explore clinical practice, women's preferences and provider's views. BMC Pregnancy Childbirth. 2001;1:1.
45. Chinese Ministry of Health. Ministry of Health on the Issuance of Maternal Health Care Management and Standards [Internet]. 2011 [cited 2017 Apr 30]. Available from: http://www.gov.cn/gzdt/2011-07/08/content_1902348.htm
46. Chinese Ministry of Health. Ministry of Health on the Issuance of the "2011 Health Working Points". 2011.
47. Chinese Maternal and Child Health Association. "Promoting natural childbirth to protect maternal and child health" Hospital Demonstration Project [Internet]. 2012. Available from: http://www.cmcha.org/detail/14582647523257290006.html
48. Li C. China to take measures to reduce high cesarean section rates. Xinhua News Agency [Internet]. Wuhan; 2011 Jun 2 [cited 2017 May 12]; Available from: http://health.sina.com.cn/2011-06-02/095422575131.shtml
49. Mao H, Wang H, Rong H, Wang H, Cao M, Zhang J, et al. Grassroots Intervention to Reduce Cesarean Delivery Rate. China Maternal Child Health [Internet]. 2015;19. Available from: http://www.cnki.com.cn/Article/CJFDTotal-ZFYB201519001.htm

19

The decision delivery interval in emergency caesarean section and its associated maternal and fetal outcomes at a referral hospital in northern Tanzania

Birjna A. Hirani[3], Bariki L. Mchome[1,3], Nicholaus S. Mazuguni[1,3] and Michael J. Mahande[2,3*]

Abstract

Background: Decision delivery interval (DDI) is the time line between a decision to conduct an emergency caesarean section and actual delivery of the baby. Prolong DDI constitute a third phase delay in provision of emergency obstetric care. Intervention designed to minimize DDI are vital, in attempt to prevent maternal morbidity and neonatal morbidity and mortality. The feasibility and practicability of the recommended DDI in recent studies have been questioned especially in limited resource setting and therefore the objective of our study was to determine the DDI and its associated fetalmaternal outcomes at a tertiary referral hospital in Tanzania.

Methods: This was a retrospectivecross-sectional study of inpatient cases who underwent emergency caesarean section from January to September 2014. Data were collected from birth registry and case files of patients. Data analysis was performed using statistical package for social science (SPSS) version 22.0. Odds ratio (ORs) and 95% confidence interval for maternal and fetal outcomes associated with DDI were estimated using Logistic regression models. A *p*-value of less than 5% was considered statistically significant.

Results: A total of 598 women who underwent emergency caesarean section were recruited. The median Decision Delivery Interval was 60 min [IQR 40–120]. Only 12% were operated within 30 min from decision time. Shortest DDI was seen in patients with Cephalopelvic Disproportion (CPD) and uterine rupture (40 min and 45.5 min) as compared to other conditions. Cases with impending uterine rupture, cord prolapse, APH and fetal distress showed to have shorter DDI. There was no significant association between DDI and neonatal transfer,1st and 5thminute Apgar score, maternal blood loss (OR: 5.79; 95% CI 0.63–1.64) and hospital stay (OR: 1.02; 95% 0.63–1.64).

Conclusions: Contrary to the recommended DDI by ACOG & AAP of 30 min is not feasible in our setting, time frame of 75 min could be acceptable but clinical judgment is required to assess on the urgency of caesarean section in order to prevent maternal and neonatal morbidity and mortality.

Keywords: Emergency caesarean section, Decision delivery interval (DDI), Pregnancy outcomes

* Correspondence: jmmahande@gmail.com
[2]Department of Epidemiology & Biostatistics, Institute of Public Health, Kilimanjaro Christian Medical University College, Moshi, Tanzania
[3]Kilimanjaro Christian Medical University College, Moshi, Tanzania
Full list of author information is available at the end of the article

Background

Emergency caesarean section is a type of surgical procedure which is performed when there is an immediate threat to the life of fetus or woman during delivery [1]. According to the American College of Obstetrics and Gynecology (ACOG)& American Academy of Pediatrics (AAP) recommendation, the emergency caesarean section should be performed in a time phase of 30 min from the decision to conduct it [2]. Therefore Decision to Delivery interval (DDI) is the time interval from decision made to perform an emergency caesarean section till the delivery of the baby [1].

Due to overburdened and weak health systems that characterize low income countries often mean the DDI is stretched to 75 min without any significant morbidities [3]. However if the DDI is pushed over 75 min a significant maternal and neonatal morbidities and mortalities are likely to occur [4]. A recent study in Nigeria by Bello and colleagues [4] reported 5.1% perinatal mortality that was statistically significant with increase in DDI beyond 75 min. Other composite outcomes that have been attributed to increased DDI by previous authors include 1% of both fresh and macerated still births,5%.

Apgar score less than 7 in the fifth minute and 3% died in neonatal ICU [5].

Previous investigators also have shown that the standard DDI is not met in many emergency obstetric units and longer duration of DDI of more than 75 min have shown an impact on maternal and neonatal outcomes [3]. In addition, various controversies have risen for the optimal duration of DDI [6]. Since this important duration is being proposed by international professional organization as a benchmark for the standard duration to conduct emergency caesarean section, it therefore becomes important to validate its usage in different clinical setup before it's universally accepted.

Therefore, this study aimed to determine the decision delivery interval and its associated fetal and maternal outcome at Kilimanjaro Christian Medical Centre tertiary hospital in Tanzania.

Methods

Study design and setting

This was a retrospective cross sectional study conducted at Kilimanjaro Christian Medical Centre (KCMC), Moshi, Tanzania. KCMC is one of the four consultant referral hospitals in Tanzania which is located in Kilimanjaro region in the Northern zone of Tanzania. The hospital has an obstetric unit with a labor ward in the same floor with one operating theatre for elective and emergency cesarean section. The unit has around 4000 deliveries annually including inpatient and referrals.

Study subjects

Study subjects consisted of inpatient women who underwent emergency caesarean section from 1st January to 30th September 2014. These were pregnant women who were admitted in the antenatal ward for obstetric care and later underwent emergency caesarean section. Women with incomplete records on delivery model and those referred from other health facility for emergency obstetric care were excluded. Those referred from other health facilities for emergency obstetric care including emergency caesarean section were excluded to reduce first and second delay as potential confounding factors.

Data source

Participant s records were obtained from KCMC medical birth registry and patient case files from medical records. The KCMC medical birth registry contains data for all women who delivered at KCMC from 2000 to date. These include their social, demographic and obstetric information with their neonates. Patient case files were

Table 1 Characteristics of the study participants ($N = 598$)

Characteristics	DDI	
	≤75 min	> 75 min
Age (years)[a]	29.25(5.63)	
Age group (years)		
< 20	13 (3.59)	7 (2.97)
20–24	66 (18.23)	44 (18.64)
25–29	111 (30.66)	79 (33.47)
30–34	98 (27.07)	58 (24.58)
35–39	61 (16.85)	42 (17.80)
≥ 40	13 (3.59)	6 (2.54)
Residence		
Rural	130 (35.91)	77 (32.63)
Urban	232 (64.09)	159 (67.37)
Marital Status*		
Married	314 (86.74)	197 (83.83)
Not Married	48 (13.26)	38 (16.17)
Level of Education*		
No formal education	7 (1.94)	1 (0.43)
Primary	118 (32.69)	88 (37.45)
Secondary	155 (42.94)	86 (36.6)
College/ University	81 (22.44)	60 (25.53)
Occupation*		
Unemployed	55 (15.19)	36 (15.45)
Employed	307 (84.81)	197 (84.55)
Gestational Age (weeks)		
< 32	13 (3.59)	3 (1.27)
32–36	48 (13.26)	24 (10.17)
37–40	237 (65.47)	172 (72.88)
> 41	64 (17.68)	37 (15.68)

[a]Mean (Standard Deviation), *Missing value

Table 2 DDI by indication of emergency caesarean section (*N* = 598)

Indication	n	DDI (minutes) Median (IQ)
Imminent Threat		
Fetal Distress	100	56.5 (37–83.5)
NRFS	38	67.0 (45–172)
APH	29	68.0 (45–139)
Cord Prolapse	2	55.0 (40–70)
Impending Uterine Rupture	2	45.5 (44–47)
Non Imminent Threat		
≥ 2Previous Scar in labour	171	66.0 (43–127)
Poor progress of labor	102	50.0 (38–102)
Hypertensive disorder	88	69.0 (33–159)
PROM	42	61.5 (40–126)
Undiagnosed Breech in labour	22	114.0 (40–172)
Failed Induction	22	59.0 (48–152)
BOH	17	56.0 (30–90)
Big baby	17	70.0 (39–219)
Cervical Dystocia	10	98.0 (45–200)
Prolong Labor	8	214.0 (120–245)
Failure of trial of scar	7	122.0 (61–145)
CPD	3	40.0 (37–100)
Face presentation	2	72.0 (54–90)

used to abstract information to estimate time when the decision to conduct emergency caesarean section was done, anesthesia charts were used to determine the time when induction of anesthesia was initiated and time when the delivery of baby occurred. We used times to compute the DDI (as shown in the formula below).

DDI was defined as the time between decisions to conduct a cesarean section to the actual time when the baby was delivered.

The computed DDI that was recorded in minutes as a continuous variable, then it was categorized into two categories (≤75 & > 75 min, respectively).

Statistical analysis

Data analysis was performed using statistical package for social science (SPSS) version 22. Descriptive statistics were summarized using frequency and proportions for categorical variables. Median and interquartile range was used to calculate the DDI for each diagnosis. A Chi square test was used to determine the associations between a set of variables and DDI, during bivariate analysis Odds ratio (OR) and 95% confidence interval for maternal and fetal outcome associated with DDI were estimated using Logistic regression models. A *P*-value <0.05 was considered statistically significant.

Table 3 Factors influencing DDI (*N* = 598)

Factors	DDI		*P*-value
	≤75 min	> 75 min	
Gestational Age (weeks)			
< 32	13(3.59)	3(1.27)	
32–36	48(13.26)	24(10.17)	0.504
37–40	237(65.47)	172(72.88)	
> 40	64(17.68)	37(15.68)	
Fetal Distress			
No	276(76.24)	184(77.97)	
Yes	86(23.76)	52(22.03)	0.408
APH			
No	344(95.03)	223(94.49)	
Yes	18(4.97)	13(5.51)	0.745
Previous Scar			
No	262(72.38)	164(69.49)	
Yes	100(27.62)	72(30.51)	0.201
Hypertension Disorders			
No	315(87.02)	195(82.63)	
Yes	47(12.98)	41(17.37)	0.037
Prolong labor			
No	360(99.45)	230(97.46)	
Yes	2(0.55)	6(2.54)	0.032
Decision to anesthesia time			
≤ 30	208(57.46)	3(1.27)	
> 30	154(42.54)	233(98.73)	0.000
Anesthesia to delivery of baby			
≤ 10	129(35.64)	71(30.08)	
> 10	233(64.36)	165(69.92)	0.035

Table 4 Association between DDI and Fetal outcome (*N* = 598)

Variables	Transfer to neonatal unit		COR(95% CI)	AOR(95% CI)
	No	Yes		
DDI				
< 30	56(76.7)	17 (23.3)	1	1
30–75	207(71.6)	82(28.4)	1.30(0.72–2.37)	1.29(0.60–2.79)
> 75	170(72.0)	66(28.0)	1.28(0.69–2.36)	0.96(0.39–2.37)
30 min				
≤ 30	56(76.7)	17 (23.3)	1	1
> 30	377(71.8)	148(28.2)	1.29(0.73–2.30)	1.29 (0.60–2.78)
75 min				
≤ 75	262 (72.6)	99(27.4)	1	1
> 75	170(72.0)	66(28.0)	1.03(0.72–1.49)	0.74(0.46–1.20)

AOR: Adjusted for Fetal Distress, APH, Hypertension Disorders, PROM, Decision to anesthesia time and Anesthesia to delivery of baby and weight of child

Table 5 Association between DDI and Fetal outcome ($N = 598$)

DDI, minutes	Apgar Score (1st minutes)				Apgar Score (5th minutes)			
	<7	≥7	COR(95% CI)	AOR(95% CI)	<7	≥7	COR(95% CI)	AOR(95% CI)
DDI								
< 30	3(4.1)	70(95.9)	1	1	1(4.8)	72(12.5)	1	1
30–75	20(6.9)	269(93.1)	1.73[0.5–6.0]	2.47[0.50–6.00]	11(52.4)	278(48.2)	2.85[0.36–22.4]	6.19[0.43–88.9]
> 75	19(72.0)	217(28.0)	2.04[0.59–7.11]	2.04[0.59–7.11]	9(42.8)	227(39.3)	2.85[0.35–22.9]	7.72[0.43–138.7]
30 min								
≤ 30	3(4.1)	70(95.9)	1	1	1(4.8)	72(12.5)	1	1
> 30	39(7.4)	486(92.6)	1.29[0.69–2.43]	1.56[0.68–3.59]	20(95.2)	505(87.5)	1.16[0.48–2.79]	1.25[0.41–3.78]
75 min								
≤ 75	23(6.4)	339(93.6)	1	1	12(57.1)	350(60.7)	1	1
> 75	19(8.1)	217(91.9)	1.87[0.56–6.22]	2.29[0.61–8.58]	9(42.9)	227(39.3)	2.85[0.37–21.6]	3.44[0.39–29.9]

AOR: Adjusted for Fetal Distress, APH, Hypertension Disorders, PROM, Decision to anesthesia time and Anesthesia to delivery of baby

Results

Characteristics of the study participants

A total of 598 women who underwent emergency caesarean section during the 9 months study period were legible for the study. Women with previous scar constituted 27.6% (172) of all the participants. Among these, women 9.7% (58) had two previous scars or above and 114(19%) had only one previous scar. Emergency c/sections were conducted for women with 2 or more previous scars who were scheduled for elective c/sections but started labouring while in the ward.

The mean age was 29.25 years (SD 5.63). There was no difference in age, residence, marital status and occupation distribution between those operated within 75 min or those who were operated beyond 75 min (Table 1).

DDI by indication of emergency caesarean section

Previous scar was the leading cause for emergency caesarean section. Others were poor progress of labor, fetal distress, and hypertensive disorders of pregnancy. The median DDI was 60 min (IQR 40–120 min). CPD has the lowest DDI and patients with imminent threat had DDI between 45 and 60 min (Table 2).

Factors influencing DDI

Hypertensive disorders in pregnancy and prolonged labor had statistically significant influence on prolonged DDI of more than 75 min(*P*-value 0.037 vs. 0.032, respectively).The decision to anesthetic time of more than 30 min and anesthesia to delivery of the baby having more than 10 min significantly influenced prolonged DDI (Table 3).

Association between DDI and fetal outcomes

The fetal outcomes that were observed in this study were Apgar score in first and fifth minute, birth weight, transfer to neonate care unit, early neonatal deaths and still births. Since the facility is not capacitated with destructive delivery equipments, cases with stillbirths were operated for obstetric obstructive indication. These outcomes were analyzed in different cut offs of DDI (Tables 4 and 5). A total of 165

Table 6 Association between DDI and Maternal outcome ($N = 598$)

DDI, min.	Blood Loss (mls)				Hospital Stay (days)			
	<1000	>1000	COR(95% CI)	AOR(95% CI)	≤4	>4	COR(95% CI)	AOR(95% CI)
DDI								
< 30	72(98.6)	1(1.4)	1	1	59(12.6)	14(10.9)	1	
30–75	288(99.7)	1(0.3)	0.25[0.02–4.05]	0.55[0.03–10.3]	231(49.3)	58(44.9)	1.06[0.55–2.03]	0.76[0.36–1.61]
> 75	235(99.6)	1(0.4)	0.31[0.0–4.96]	3.21[0.02–653.9]	179(38.1)	57(44.2)	1.34[0.7–2.58]	0.78[0.32–1.81]
30 min								
≤ 30	72(98.6)	1(1.4)	1	1	59(12.6)	14(10.9)	1	1
> 30	523(99.6)	2(0.4)	0.28[0.02–3.07]	0.55[0.03–10.3]	410(87.4)	115(89.1)	1.18[0.64–2.19]	0.76[0.36–1.62]
75 min								
≤ 75	360(99.4)	2(0.6)	1	1	290(61.8)	72(55.8)	1	1
> 75	235(99.6)	1(0.4)	0.77[0.07–8.49]	5.79[0.05–7.18]	179(38.2)	57(44.2)	1.28[0.86–1.9]	1.02[0.63–1.64]

AOR: Adjusted for Hypertension Disorders, Fetal Distress, APH,Decision to anesthesia time and Anesthesia to delivery of baby

babies (28%) were transferred to neonatal unit department. Only 10.3% babies were delivered within 30 min. Half (50%) of the babies who were born between 30 and 75 min were transferred to neonatal unit (Table 4). Neonates born after 75 min, had higher odds of getting Apgar score of less than 7 in the first and fifth minute when compared to other cut off times.

(OR: 2.29; 95% CI: 0.61–8.85, vs. OR: 3.44; 95% CI 0.39–29.9) (Table 5) but this were not statistically significant. There were 8 still births, of whom 7 were fresh and one was macerated. There was one early neonatal death due to low score and prematurity. Five stillbirths were operated after 75 min and this was not statistically significant ($P = 0.45$).

Association between DDI and maternal outcomes

Women operated more than 75 min had 6 times higher odds of losing blood more than 1000mls (OR: 5.79; 95% CI: 0.05–7.18) and 2% higher odds of staying in hospital for more than 4 days compared to those who were operated within 75 min but this was not statistically significant (OR: 1.02; 95% CI: 0.63–1.64), (Table 6).

Discussion

This study found that only 12.3% of the women were operated within 30 min with a median DDI of 60 min. We also found that less time was used to conduct emergency caesarean section compared to other studies which took more 120 min [5–7].Women with imminent threat had shorter DDI. This was consistent with previous study in Ghana [7]. This could be explained by the fact that immediate action was taken to such cases without any form of delay because these patients were within the ward.

The prolonged decision to anesthetic time influenced DDI but factors that caused the delay were not determined as it was a retrospective study. Previous studies conducted elsewhere have reported factors that influenced delay in decision to anesthetic time [4–6, 8, 9].

In the present study, the anesthesia to delivery of the baby was also prolonged. This may be explained by the fact that many patients had previous scars and adhesions can cause delay before extracting the baby. KCMC is also a teaching hospital whereby anaesthetic students get trained for induction of anesthesia which could also prolong the anesthesia to delivery of the baby time.

In the current study, babies with weight of more than 4 kg and risk of infection from premature rupture of membranes (PROM), were more likely to be sent to neonatal unit for observation as per requirements of the hospital protocol. Neonates with difficulty in breathing, low Apgar score and birth asphyxia and still births had DDI more than 75 min. Similarly observations have been reported in England, India, and Nigeria [3, 4, 6, 10].

Our findings also suggest a significant influence on prolonged DDI for hypertensive disease and prolonged labour cases. For hypertensive cases, initial attempts to stabilize blood pressure prior to delivery may contribute to this delay. For prolonged labour cases without imminent threat clinicians may resort to attend indications with imminent threats first due to presence of a single operational theatre.

In this study only blood loss and hospital stay were observed and that may be because most of the patients were clinically stable in the ward and those even who had longer stay of more than 4 days were on antibiotics or anti-hypertensive drugs. However, some previous studies by Chow [8] and Hussein [5] reviewed many other maternal outcomes which were not present in our study.

This study encountered a number of limitations. Detailed information on the intrapartum care of these patients couldn't be ascertained due to a retrospective nature of the study. Specific type of anesthesia and the other detailed aspects of anaesthetic care couldn't be retrieved from our database. Moreover, this study didn't seek to identify specific factors that contributed to the described delays.

Conclusions

The delivery decision interval for caesarean section at KCMC is 60 min, which is longer than the recommended standard interval. The DDI was influenced by decision to anesthesia time, anesthesia to delivery of baby, prolonged labor and hypertension disorders. A time frame of 75 min can be acceptable after triage and need for urgency have been evaluated.

Abbreviations

ACOG: American College of Obstetrics and Gynecology; AOR: Adjusted odds ratio; APH: Antepartum Hemorrhage; BOH: Bad obstetrics history; COR: Crude odds ratio; CPD: Cephalopelvic Disproportion; DDI: Decision Delivery Interval; KCMC: Kilimanjaro Christian Medical College; LW: Labor Ward; NRFS: None Reassuring Fetal Status; OBGYN: Obstetrics and Gynecology; p3: Pediatrics III i.e. intensive care unit; PPH: Postpartum Hemorrhage

Acknowledgements

The authors express their sincere appreciation to all those who made this work possible and special gratitude to Festo Mazuguni for the statistical analysis.

Funding

This work was supported by the Norwegian government through theNorwegian Council for Higher education program and Development Research (NUFU) which supported the establishment of the medical birth registry at KCMC. The funding agent has no competing interest in this research.

Authors' contributions

BAH and BLM designed the study, participated in data collection, performed the statistical analysis and participated in the writing of the manuscript. BLM and NSM contributed in reviewing the manuscript for intellectual content; MJM reviewed the manuscript for intellectual content and provided technical guidance in the statistical analysis. All authors read and approved the final manuscript.

Competing interests

The authors declare that they have no competing interest. All authors of the manuscript have read and agreed its content.

Author details

[1]Department of Obstetrics and Gynecology, Kilimanjaro Christian Medical Centre, Moshi, Tanzania. [2]Department of Epidemiology & Biostatistics, Institute of Public Health, Kilimanjaro Christian Medical University College, Moshi, Tanzania. [3]Kilimanjaro Christian Medical University College, Moshi, Tanzania.

References

1. Rashid N, Nalliah S. Understanding the Decision-Delivery Interval in Cesarean Birth. IeJSME. 2007;1(2):61–8.
2. Nasrallah FK, Harirah HM, Vadhera R, Jain V, Franklin LT, Hankins GD. The 30-minute decision-to-incision interval for emergency cesarean delivery: fact or fiction? Am J Perinatol. 2004;21(2):63–8.
3. Thomas J. National cross sectional survey to determine whether the decision to delivery interval is critical in emergency caesarean section. BMJ, 2004;328(7441):665–0.
4. Bello FA, Tsele TA, Oluwasola TO. Decision-to-delivery intervals and perinatal outcomes following emergency cesarean delivery in a Nigerian tertiary hospital. Int J Gynaecol Obstet. 2015;130(3):279–83.
5. Hussein AH. Emergency Caesarean Section Turnaround Time and Its Effect on Maternal and Newborn Health Outcomes At University of Nairobi Teaching Hospitals. 2012. Available at http://erepository.uonbi.ac.ke:8080/xmlui/handle/123456789/13758. (Accessed 20 June 2016).
6. Radhakrishnan G, Yadav G, Vaid NB, Ali H. Factors affecting " decision to delivery interval " in emergency caesarean sections in a tertiary care hospital : a cross sectional observational study. Int J Reprod Contracept Obs Gynecol. 2013;2(4):651–6.
7. Oppong SA, Tuuli MG, Seffah JD, Adanu RMK. Is there a safe limit of delay for emergency caesarean section in Ghana? Results of analysis of early perinatal outcome. Ghana Med J. 2014;48(1):24–30.
8. Chow KM, Mak SL. Maternal and fetal outcomes in extremely urgent caesarean delivery in relation to the decision-to- delivery interval. Hong Kong J Gynaecol Obstet Midwifery. 2015;15(1):16–22.
9. Cerbinskaite A, Malone S, McDermott J, Loughney AD. Emergency caesarean section: influences on the decision-to-delivery interval. Journal of Pregnancy, vol. 2011, Article ID 640379, 6 pages, 2011. doi:https://doi.org/10.1155/2011/640379.
10. Roy KK, Baruah J, Kumar S, Deorari AK, Sharma JB, Karmakar D. Cesarean section for suspected fetal distress, continuous fetal heart monitoring and decision to delivery time. Indian J Pediatr. 2008;75(12):1249–52.

Measuring the course of anxiety in women giving birth by caesarean section

Philip Hepp[1,4*], Carsten Hagenbeck[1], Bettina Burghardt[1], Bernadette Jaeger[1], Oliver T. Wolf[2], Tanja Fehm[1], Nora K. Schaal[3] and The MAGIC Group

Abstract

Background: Women undergoing elective caesarean section experience anxiety. However, course, extent and duration of anxiety have not been investigated yet. This study aimed to explore anxiety levels during the course of the day of surgery by employing and comparing subjective as well as objective measures. By examining their correlation it is intended to give methodological support for interventional studies.

Methods: This is a monocentric, prospectively planned study in which 47 women with an indication for primary caesarean section took part. Anxiety levels were evaluated using the State-Trait Anxiety Inventory (STAI-trait and STAI-state), the visual analogue scale for anxiety (VASA) as well as saliva cortisol at three time points on the day of the caesarean section (at admission, at skin closure and 2 h post surgery).

Results: Peak anxiety levels for the STAI-state and VASA were highest at admission and showed significant decreases to skin closure ($p < .001$). The subjective measures correlated significantly at all time points (p-values $< .001$). For cortisol levels the peak level of anxiety was shown at skin closure with a significant increase from admission to skin closure and a significant decrease from skin closure to 2 h post operation (p-values $< .001$). Additionally women with STAI-trait scores above the median showed significantly higher levels at the peaks of anxiety.

Conclusion: The study reveals the course of anxiety on the day of the caesarean section. A strong correlation of STAI-state and VASA was demonstrated. Cortisol showed a different course, which fits into its known biological kinetics. Taking into account all measures, anxiety seems to be most bothersome before surgery until skin closure. In a differentiated approach using STAI-trait scores as a discriminator we showed that the group with STAI-trait levels above the median is particularly prone to develop anxiety in the setting of the caesarean section and might therefore mostly be in need of an intervention against anxiety.

Keywords: Caesarean section, Anxiety, STAI questionnaire, Visual analog scale, Saliva cortisol, Saliva

Background

In 2014, 31.8 % of all births in Germany were by caesarean section (CS) [1]. Throughout the world, it is one of the most common surgeries in obstetrics and gynaecology. In contrast to most other surgeries, CS is usually performed in healthy, pregnant women. With regard to a minimized exposition of the newborn to anesthetics and the parents' desire to witness the birth, the majority of women undergo the operation with regional anesthesia without anxiolytic or sedating medication.

Even though data about consequences for the mother and the newborn in terms of physical detriments are vastly available and part of every informed consent, only few studies have elucidated the impact of CS on psychological parameters [2]. Mostly, women see CS as a routine procedure and may be neglecting the potential psychological side

* Correspondence: philip.hepp@helios-kliniken.de
[1]Clinic for Gynecology and Obstetrics, Heinrich-Heine-University, Düsseldorf, Germany
[4]Clinic for Gynecology and Obstetrics, HELIOS Universitätsklinikum Wuppertal, University Witten/Herdecke, Vogelsangstr. 109, 42109 Wuppertal, Germany
Full list of author information is available at the end of the article

effects and the discomfort it may cause [3]. Sparse measurements already showed that preoperative anxiety is associated with reduced satisfaction and worse recovery from CS [4].

A study by Wyatt et al. reported high preoperative anxiety levels in women before an elective CS under regional anaesthesia [5]. To the best of our knowledge, no data exist so far reporting the course of anxiety from before CS until thereafter taking into account subjective (i.e. questionnaires) as well as objective (i.e. anxiety related hormones) parameters. Nevertheless, tools for the quantification of anxiety are at hand, one of the most frequently used being the "State-Trait Anxiety Inventory" (STAI), an introspective inventory comprising 40 self-report items pertaining to anxiety [6]. It distinguishes between two questionnaires with 20 items each, one measuring anxiety perceived in the current situation (STAI-state) and the other evaluating a general tendency towards anxiety (STAI-trait). The STAI-trait questionnaire is not included that often in clinical studies even though it has been shown that it can potentially be used to identify patients who are prone to high levels of anxiety in surgical settings [7] as well as who could benefit most from additional interventions reducing anxiety in medical settings [8]. On the other hand, the STAI-state questionnaire has been used frequently in order to evaluate anxiety levels in clinical settings [9–12]. However, in a surgery setting like CS the repeated evaluation of the 20 items test (STAI-state) is not practicable. Therefore effort has been made to establish a more easily repeatable tool. There is evidence that a simple visual analogue scale depicting anxiety (VASA) predicts STAI-state results reliably [13, 14]. Nevertheless, a correlation of VASA and STAI-state has not been shown in the context of CS.

Looking at objective measures to evaluate anxiety, cortisol levels are often referred to [15]. Its relation to the activation of the hypothalamus-pituitary-adrenal axis (HPAA) is well understood [16]. Although it can be obtained from all kinds of specimens like blood, urine or hair, the sampling in saliva is the most common way inanxiety research as it reflects the activation of the HPAA within the last half hour before the specimen was obtained [17, 18]. Data about the correlation of cortisol and subjective measurements of anxiety are contradictory [19].

Therefore, we aimed to quantify anxiety in women having a CS by repeated measurements at three time points in order to assess the potential psychological impact of CS in regard to anxiety. Furthermore we intended to clarify the correlation of different subjective and objective measurements of anxiety in the context of CS. Finally, we explored whether STAI-trait scores could serve as a predictor to identify those patients who could benefit the most from an intervention in order to reduce anxiety or could be in need of postoperative psychological treatment.

Methods

Study design

The analysis is based on a monocentric, prospectively planned study at the Clinic for Gynecology and Obstetrics at the University Hospital in Duesseldorf, Germany. Patients scheduled for a planned, primary caesarean section with sufficient command of German language to complete the questionnaires were invited to participate. Data were collected from March through June 2015. In this period 47 women were enrolled in the study. The indications for the CS were previous caesarean sections ($N = 23$), breech presentation ($N = 13$), upon patient's request ($N = 6$) and preexisting conditions of the mother (e.g. fracture of the pelvis, fibroids; $N = 5$). Two women did not undergo cesarean section because of spontaneous cephalic version from breech presentation and were therefore excluded from further analysis.

Figure 1 shows a flow chart of the study. During preoperative visitation one to two weeks prior to scheduled surgery, participants were asked to fill in the STAI-trait questionnaire [6].

Each of the following measurements comprised a STAI-state questionnaire (measuring anxiety levels at the moment of evaluation), a visual analog scale depicting anxiety (VASA) and a saliva specimen for cortisol analysis. For the saliva sample patients were asked to thoroughly insalivate a cotton swab.

The first measurement took place at admission on the day of the surgery. The second measurement was taken during skin closure while the child already had left the surgery theater. Two hours after completion of surgery a third and last measurement was conducted before the patient was transferred to the postnatal ward according to the standard procedure in Germany.

Ethics, consent and permissions

Written informed consent was obtained from all included patients. The study was approved by the ethics committee of the Heinrich-Heine-University Duesseldorf, Germany (protocol number 3625).

Statistics

Sample size was calculated using the software G*power [20] with an estimated medium effect size, a power of 0.9 and with an alpha error probability of 0.05.

The analysis was performed using IBM SPSS Statistics® Ver. 22. The scores of the STAI-trait as well as STAI-state at the three time points were compared to the standard normative data of the German Version of the STAI [21] using one sample t-tests. Repeated measures ANOVAs were conducted independently for the three dependent variables (STAI-state, VASA and cortisol) with *time point* (admission vs. Skin closure vs. 2 h post caesarean) as the within-subject variable. Additionally planned post-hoc

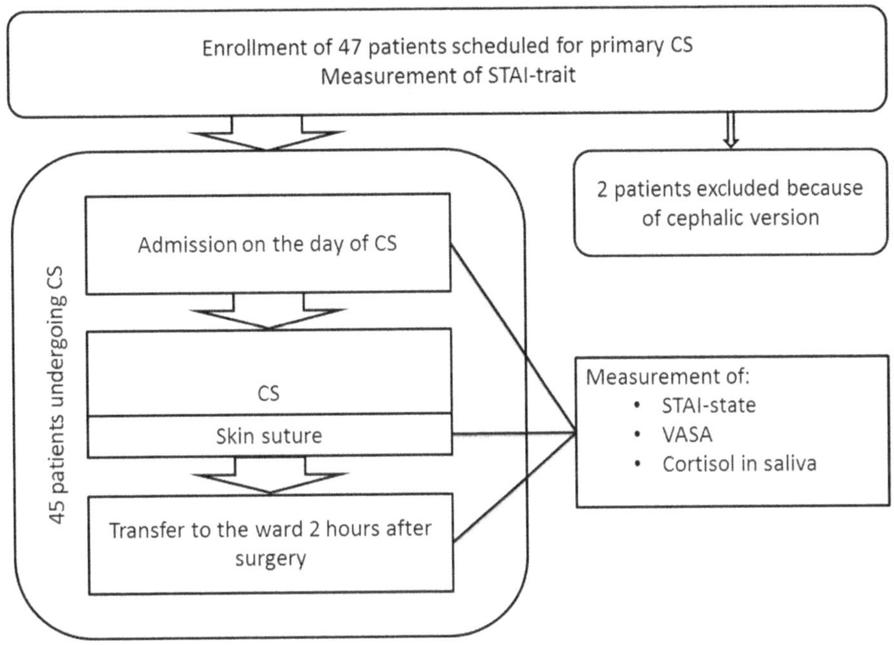

Fig. 1 Flow chart of the study

paired-sample t-tests were applied in order to disentangle significant main effects. Furthermore for a more detailed analysis the between-subject variable *STAI-trait group* (splitting the sample above/below the median = 36 of the STAI-trait score of our sample which is comparable to the mean value of 36.85 of the normative data [21]) was added to the ANOVAs. Here, planned post-hoc independent sample t-tests were conducted to disentangle the interactions.

In order to disclose possible correlations between the dependent variables Pearson product–moment bivariate correlations were calculated.

Greenhouse-Geisser corrections are reported when sphericity was violated. Bonferroni corrections were applied adequately throughout the analysis in order to avoid alpha I error associated with multiple testing.

Additionally, we ran the whole analysis using non-parametric tests (e.g. Friedman's ANOVAs and Wilcoxon tests) as normality was not met for all of the dependent variables. But as the results were comparable to the parametric tests, we only report the results of the parametric tests, as they are more robust.

Results

Data are available from 45 women with an average age of 35.5 years (SD = 5.1). For the analysis including the factor *STAI-trait group,* 40 women are included as data were missing from five participants.

Comparison with normative data

No significant difference ($t(39) = -.827$, $p = .414$) was observed between STAI-trait scores of our sample (M = 35.9, SD = 8.5) and the standard normative value for females (M = 36.85) [21]. The STAI-state at admission (M = 47.35, SD = 10.83) was significantly above the standard value of 38.08 [21], ($t(42) = 5.61$, $p < .001$). At skin closure (M = 33.96, SD = 7.43) and 2 h post surgery (M = 31.11, SD = 7.74) the scores of the present sample were below the standard value (skin closure: $t(44) = -3.72$, $p = .001$; 2 h post surgery: $t(43) = -5.97$, $p < .001$).

Analysis of variance

Three independent repeated measures ANOVAs with *time point* as the within-subject factor and STAI-state, VASA and cortisol respectively as the dependent variables were conducted and showed a significant main effect of *time point* on all three variables (STAI-state: $F(2, 82) = 55.39$, $p < .001$, $\eta p^2 = .575$; VASA: $F(1.60, 55.81) = 42.68$, $p < .001$, $\eta p^2 = .549$; Cortisol: $F(1.40, 35.06) = 34.74$, $p < .001$, $\eta p^2 = .582$). Planned post-hoc paired-sample t-tests for STAI-state and VASA showed that subjective anxiety levels were highest at admission before the caesarean (STAI-state 47.13 [SD = 9.57]; VASA 5.01 cm [SD = 3.14]) and that anxiety levels significantly decreased ($p < .001$ for both measures) from admission to skin suture (STAI-state 33.49 [SD = 7.49]; VASA 1.56 cm [SD = 2.06]). After the caesarean section no further significant reduction of the subjective measures could be revealed ($p > .14$) with STAI-state being 30.54 [SD = 7.05] and VASA 1.21 cm [SD = 1.90] 2 h post caesarean. Cortisol levels showed their peak at skin suture (26.67 μg/L [SD = 10.88]) with a significant increase from admission (12.62 μg/L [SD = 3.85]) to skin suture ($p < .001$) and a significant decrease from skin suture to 2 h post caesarean section (12.97 µg/L [SD = 4.87]; $p < .001$).

Correlation of different measuring methods

A significant positive correlation was found between STAI-state and VASA at all 3 time points (admission: $r = .76$, $p < .001$; skin closure: $r = .60$, $p < .001$; 2 h post caesarean: $r = .65$, $p < .001$). No significant correlations were found between cortisol and the subjective measures at any time point.

Analysis by trait anxiety group

For a more detailed analysis we divided the patients by STAI-trait median into a high anxiety trait group ($N = 20$) and low anxiety trait group ($N = 20$). Three repeated measures ANOVAs with *time point* as the within-subject variable and *STAI-trait group* as the between subject variable were performed for the dependent variables STAI-State, VASA and cortisol respectively. A significant main effect of *STAI-trait group* was found for the VASA ($F(1, 32) = 9.27$, $p = .005$, $\eta p^2 = .225$), no significant main effect for STAI-state ($F(1, 37) = 3.36$, $p = .075$, $\eta p^2 = .083$) and no significant main effect for cortisol ($F(1, 22) = 2.31$, $p = .143$, $\eta p^2 = .095$). Furthermore significant *time point x STAI-trait group* interactions were revealed for STAI-state ($F(2, 74) = 6.78$, $p = .002$, $\eta p^2 = .155$) and VASA ($F(2, 64) = 4.71$, $p = .012$, $\eta p^2 = .128$) and no significant interaction was shown for cortisol ($F(2, 44) = 2.89$, $p = .066$, $\eta p^2 = .116$).

Planned post-hoc independent sample t-tests showed significant differences between the STAI-trait groups for STAI-state at admission ($t\ (37) = 3.58$, $p = .001$), VASA at admission ($t\ (32) = 3.20$, $p = .002$) and cortisol at skin closure ($t\ (22) = 1.89$, $p = .037$), indicating that women with high anxiety trait scores show significantly increased anxiety levels at the peak of the anxiety measures.

Figure 2 demonstrates the course of STAI-state, VASA and cortisol in total and separated by STAI-trait median.

Discussion

The aim of the study was to explore level, course and extent of anxiety in women giving birth by CS by means of subjective and objective measures.

Firstly, the results highlight that subjective anxiety levels were highest before the CS. This finding is in line with studies showing preoperative anxiety in woman expecting a CS [5]. Additionally, the present study examined the course of anxiety levels on the day of the caesarean and revealed that anxiety levels evaluated by subjective measures significantly decrease from admission to skin suture. No further reduction is traceable from skin closure to two hours after the caesarean. This is an important finding as it highlights that the negative psychological impact of CS is present before the surgery and that the most significant decrease of anxiety happens during surgery in a relief like reaction reflected by STAI-state values at the time of skin closure significantly below mean STAI-state values of a normal population. This effect is further consolidated for at least the following two hours where the STAI-state values are still significantly lower in both STAI-trait groups than in a normal population. The interesting finding of anxiety scores being below the mean of the normative data is a new finding which to our knowledge has not been reported in the literature to date. However, this finding is in accordance with a study showing that the feeling of anxiety and fear was predominant before an emergency caesarean section whereas happiness overtook the mothers' emotional state as soon as they saw their newborn baby [22].

Secondly, STAI-state and VASA highly correlated at all time-points suggesting high convergent validity between the measures as well as indicating that both measure subjective anxiety levels during CS to the same degree. This finding proposes that it would be adequate to evaluate subjective anxiety at repeated time points using the VASA in surgical settings which would be time-saving and much more practicable. A study by Davey et al., 2007 measuring anxiety in women awaiting a breast screening could also show a strong correlation between the STAI-state and the VASA suggesting that the VASA could be an adequate and more feasible approach to measure current anxiety [23]. Our results strengthen and extend this finding as we show a strong and robust correlation between these two variables at three different time points during the course of anxiety of a surgical procedure.

Furthermore, the results of the objective measure of saliva cortisol showed peak anxiety at skin suture with a significant increase of anxiety from admission to skin suture and a significant decrease from skin suture to 2 h post CS. This different pattern of anxiety development can be explained by the fact that the cortisol level in saliva samples occurs with a latency of around 30 min after the stressful event [16]. Based on this finding, the cortisol level taken at skin suture may reflect anxiety experienced during the caesarean in which tension of the expectant mother is extremely high. It is worth noting in this respect that it would be desirable for a follow-up study to include another time of measurement immediately before the CS when the woman is already in the operating room evaluating STAI-state and VASA in order to evaluate whether the subjective measures of anxiety reach a further peak at the start of the surgery. Nevertheless, a strength of the study is that three assessment points were included in order to be able to examine the course of anxiety during the day of the CS. Previous studies looking at anxiety in the context of CS measured preoperative anxiety only [4, 5, 24]. These

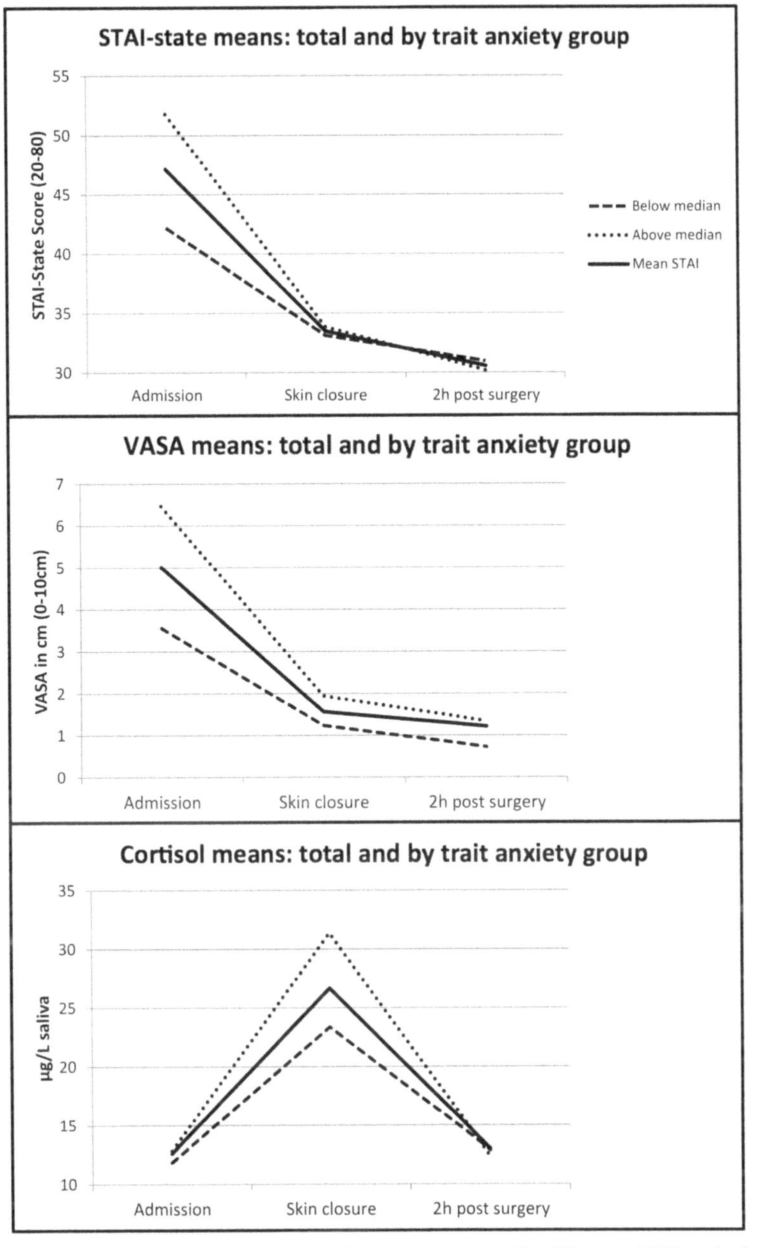

Fig. 2 Anxiety during caesarean section. The course of the mean anxiety levels measured by STAI-state, VASA and saliva cortisol for the whole sample as well as split by Trait-group (above/below the median)

studies are in line with our results showing high anxiety before the caesarean but the present study extends previous findings by showing that women experience a significant anxiety reduction from admission to skin suture. Furthermore, there is one study which used a qualitative approach (i.e. semistructured interviews) as well as the STAI-state questionnaire to evaluate women's expectations and subjective experience of a planned CS which also showed that STAI-state scores (i.e. anxiety) were high before the CS and moderate after the CS which fits well to our results [25].

Additionally, the study depicts that patients with high general anxiety trait scores experience the CS with higher anxiety levels in terms of preoperative STAI-state and VASA values and intraoperative cortisol levels. This suggests that patients with higher general tendencies towards anxiety also experience stronger negative psychological side effects during the CS. It would be desirable to identify these patients at an early stage e.g. when they receive the indication for a CS, in order to provide sufficient counteractions to develop high anxiety towards the CS. As it has been shown that preoperative anxiety correlates positively to postoperative pain [7, 26, 27], the aim should be the reduction of anxiety levels before and during the CS in order to further improve wellbeing of the mothers after the CS.

In this respect, it is worth highlighting that there are interventions before or during the CS that could have a soothing impact on the patients' anxiety levels. Several studies have shown that music before or during various surgical operations can soothe anxiety and pain levels [11, 12, 28, 29]. Referring to the CS, a study showed that music played preoperatively to the CS led to reduced self-reported anxiety and pain levels [30]. Furthermore, acupuncture could be beneficial in order to reduce anxiety levels in women waiting for a CS [31]. Another possible approach is the application of perioperative hypnosis which has been found to effectively reduce anxiety during and after CS [32].

To the best of our knowledge, this study is the first approach investigating the course of anxiety in woman having a CS looking at three assessment points on the day of the surgery and including subjective and objective measurements of anxiety. We believe that the findings of the present study are valuable for clinical implementations as the study highlights that pregnant woman awaiting a CS are extremely anxious before the operation, especially if they have a high general anxiety trait. This emphasizes that intensified attention should be provided to the pregnant women before the CS by the medical staff in order to identify patients who are prone to develop high anxiety levels and therefore requiring appropriate support or interventions.

Nevertheless, a couple of limitations warrant a comment here, which should be considered in future research. It would be desirable to conduct a study comparing the course of anxiety in woman giving birth by different modes (e.g. vaginal birth, delivery with instrumental intervention, CS) in order to examine whether different modes provoke a different development and degree of perceived anxiety. Furthermore, we acknowledge that the sample size in the present study is relatively small but comparable to other studies in the field [12, 28, 30] and according to the prospectively conducted power analysis.

Conclusion

The present study revealed the course of anxiety during a CS by means of subjective (STAI and VASA) measures as well as saliva cortisol. The results highlight that interventions in order to reduce anxiety levels should be applied before or during the surgery and that women with high trait anxiety might benefit more from these interventions.

Ethics approval and consent to participate

The ethics committee of the Heinrich-Heine-University Düsseldorf, Germany, has approved this study (reference number 3625). Written consent has been obtained from all patients included in the study.

Abbreviations

ANOVA: analysis of variance; CS: caesarean section; SD: standard deviation; STAI: State-Trait Anxiety Inventory; VASA: visual analogue scale for anxiety.

Competing interests

The authors declare that they have no competing interests.

Authors' contributions

PH, CH, TF, OW and NKS conceived and designed the study. PH, CH, BB and BJ were in charge of data collection. PH and NKS analyzed the data and wrote a first draft of the paper. All authors revised the manuscript critically for content. All authors read and approved the final version of the manuscript.

Acknowledgements

We thank our patients for taking part in the study. We are very grateful, that we have the honor to do our research with a motivated team of midwives, nurses and colleagues. Special thanks go to Sarah Märthesheimer for her effort and input.

Funding

This study was funded by a grant of the Anton-Betz-Stiftung der Rheinischen Post e.V.; Zülpicher Straße 10; 40196 Düsseldorf; Germany.

Author details

[1]Clinic for Gynecology and Obstetrics, Heinrich-Heine-University, Düsseldorf, Germany. [2]Department of Cognitive Psychology, Institute of Cognitive Neuroscience, Faculty of Psychology, Ruhr-University Bochum, Bochum, Germany. [3]Department of Experimental Psychology, Heinrich-Heine-University, Düsseldorf, Germany. [4]Clinic for Gynecology and Obstetrics, HELIOS Universitätsklinikum Wuppertal, University Witten/Herdecke, Vogelsangstr. 109, 42109 Wuppertal, Germany.

References

1. Statistisches Bundesamt. Mehr Krankenhausentbindungen 2014 bei gleicher Kaiserschnittrate. Statistisches Bundesamt. 2015. https://www.destatis.de/EN/FactsFigures/SocietyState/Health/Hospitals/Tables/TabcaesareanopByLaender.html. Accessed 16 May 2016.
2. Clement S. Psychological aspects of caesarean section. Best Pract Res Clin Obstet. 2001;15:109–26.
3. Edwards GJ, Davies N. Elective caesarean section-the patient's choice? J Obstet Gynaecol (Lahore). 2001;21:128–9.
4. Hobson JA, Slade P, Wrench IJ, Power L. Preoperative anxiety and postoperative satisfaction in women undergoing elective caesarean section. Int J Obstet Anesth. 2006;15:18–23.
5. Wyatt S, Jones D, Peach M, Gurrin L. Anxiety in patients having caesarean section under regional anaesthesia: a questionnaire and pilot study. Int J Obstet Anesth. 2001;10:278–83.
6. Spielberger CD. State-trait anxiety inventory: a comprehensive bibliography. 2nd ed. Palo Alto, CA, USA: Consulting Psychologists Press; 1993.
7. Carr E, Brockbank K, Allen S, Strike P. Patterns and frequency of anxiety in women undergoing gynaecological surgery. J Clin Nurs. 2006;15:341–52.
8. Ventura T, Gomes MC, Carreira T. Cortisol and anxiety response to a relaxing intervention on pregnant women awaiting amniocentesis. Psychoneuroendocrinology. 2011;37:148–56.

9. Koelsch S, Fuermetz J, Sack U, Bauer K, Hohenadel M, Wiegel M, Kaisers UX, Heinke W. Effects of music listening on cortisol levels and propofol consumption during spinal anesthesia. Front Psychol. 2011;2:58.
10. Orbach-Zinger S, Ginosar Y, Sverdlik J, Treitel C, MacKersey K, Bardin R, Peleg D, Eidelman LA. Partner's presence during initiation of epidural labor analgesia does not decrease maternal stress: a prospective randomized controlled trial. Anesth Analg. 2012;114:654–60.
11. Zengin S, Kabul S, Al B, Sarcan E, Doğan M, Yildirim C. Effects of music therapy on pain and anxiety in patients undergoing port catheter placement procedure. Complement Ther Med. 2013;21:689–96.
12. Lai H-L, Hwang M-J, Chen C-J, Chang K-F, Peng T-C, Chang F-M. Randomised controlled trial of music on state anxiety and physiological indices in patients undergoing root canal treatment. J Clin Nurs. 2008;17:2654–60.
13. Kindler CH, Harms C, Amsler F, Ihde-Scholl T, Scheidegger D. The visual analog scale allows effective measurement of preoperative anxiety and detection of patients' anesthetic concerns. Anesth Analg. 2000;90:706–12.
14. Abend R, Dan O, Maoz K, Raz S, Bar-Haim Y. Reliability, validity and sensitivity of a computerized visual analog scale measuring state anxiety. J Behav Ther Exp Psychiatry. 2014;45:447–53.
15. Dedovic K, Duchesne A, Andrews J, Engert V, Pruessner JC. The brain and the stress axis: the neural correlates of cortisol regulation in response to stress. Neuroimage. 2009;47:864–71.
16. Dickerson SS, Kemeny ME. Acute stressors and cortisol responses: a theoretical integration and synthesis of laboratory research. Psychol Bull. 2004;130:355–91.
17. Turpeinen U, Hämäläinen E. Determination of cortisol in serum, saliva and urine. Best Pract Res Clin Endocrinol Metab. 2013;27:795–801.
18. Gatti R, Antonelli G, Prearo M, Spinella P, Cappellin E, De Palo EF. Cortisol assays and diagnostic laboratory procedures in human biological fluids. Clin Biochem. 2009;42:1205–17.
19. Hellhammer DH, Wüst S, Kudielka BM. Salivary cortisol as a biomarker in stress research. Psychoneuroendocrinology. 2009;34:163–71.
20. Faul F, Erdfelder E, Buchner A, Lang A. Statistical power analyses using G* Power 3.1: Tests for correlation and regression analyses. Behav Res Methods. 2009;41: 1149–60.
21. Laux L, Glanzmann P, Schaffner P, Spielberger CD. Das State-Trait-Angstinventar (STAI) (Beltz-Test). Göttingen: Beltz Test GmbH; 1981.
22. Ryding E, Wijma K, Wijma B. Experiences of emergency cesarean section: A phenomenological study of 53 women. Birth. 1998;25:246–51.
23. Davey HM, Barratt AL, Butow PN, Deeks JJ. A one-item question with a Likert or Visual Analog Scale adequately measured current anxiety. J Clin Epidemiol. 2007;60:356–60.
24. Orbach-Zinger S, Ginosar Y, Elliston J, Fadon C, Abu-Lil M, Raz A, Goshen-Gottstein Y, Eidelman LA. Influence of preoperative anxiety on hypotension after spinal anaesthesia in women undergoing Caesarean delivery. Br J Anaesth. 2012;109:943–9.
25. Blüml V. A qualitative approach to examine women's experience of planned cesarean. J Obstet. 2012;41:E82–90.
26. Chieng YJS, Chan WCS, Klainin-Yobas P, He H-G. Perioperative anxiety and postoperative pain in children and adolescents undergoing elective surgical procedures: a quantitative systematic review. J Adv Nurs. 2014;70:243–55.
27. Schupp CJ, Berbaum K, Berbaum M, Lang EV. Pain and anxiety during interventional radiologic procedures: effect of patients' state anxiety at baseline and modulation by nonpharmacologic analgesia adjuncts. J Vasc Interv Radiol. 2005;16:1585–92.
28. Voss JA, Good M, Yates B, Baun MM, Thompson A, Hertzog M. Sedative music reduces anxiety and pain during chair rest after open-heart surgery. Pain. 2004;112:197–203.
29. Smolen D, Topp R, Singer L. The effect of self-selected music during colonoscopy on anxiety, heart rate, and blood pressure. Appl Nurs Res. 2002;15:126–36.
30. Li Y, Dong Y. Preoperative music intervention for patients undergoing cesarean delivery. Int J Gynaecol Obstet. 2012;119:81–3.
31. Bae H, Bae H, Min B-I, Cho S. Efficacy of acupuncture in reducing preoperative anxiety: a meta-analysis. Evid Based Complement Alternat Med. 2014;2014:850367.
32. Slater P. Post-traumatic stress disorder managed successfully with hypnosis and the rewind technique: two cases in obstetric patients. Int J Obstet Anesth. 2015;24:272–5.

21

Caesarean deliveries in China

Xin Wang[1], Susan Hellerstein[2], Lei Hou[1], Liying Zou[1], Yan Ruan[1] and Weiyuan Zhang[1*]

Abstract

Background: The caesarean section rate has risen rapidly in China. The purpose of this retrospective study was to estimate caesarean section rates and indications by hospital facility level in Mainland China to investigate reasons contributing to the high rate.

Methods: This cross-sectional hospital-based study collected data from 39 hospitals in three geographical regions in China, covering 14 different provinces, municipalities, and autonomous regions, including 20 tertiary health hospitals and 19 secondary hospitals. Data from all women who gave birth at these hospitals during 2011 were included.

Results: A total of 112,138 women who gave birth after 24 weeks of gestation were surveyed. Of these pregnancies, 54.5% (61,084 cases) resulted in caesarean section, non-indicated caesarean section accounted for 38.4% of caesarean sections. Overall caesarean section rates were higher at the tertiary level hospitals (55.9%) compared to the secondary level hospitals (50.9%). The secondary level hospitals had higher rates of non-indicated caesarean section (48.9% of caesarean sections) compared to tertiary level hospitals (34.5% of caesarean sections). The rate of caesarean section on maternal request was higher in the secondary hospitals (16.6%) than in the tertiary hospitals (10%) ($P < 0.001$), as well as the caesarean section rate for CPD prior to labour. Operative vaginal deliveries were overall rare (1.2%) with 90.9% (1200/1320 cases) performed in the tertiary hospitals.

Conclusions: Caesarean section on maternal request accounts for a large portion of China's high caesarean section rate, especially in the secondary hospitals. The first step to reduced caesarean section rates is to decrease the number of non-indicated caesarean sections.

Keywords: Caesarean section, Indication, Tertiary level hospital, Secondary level hospital

Background

The caesarean section rate has risen rapidly worldwide in recent decades and is a global concern [1–6]. A World Health Organization (WHO) survey from 2004 to 2008 reported a 25.7% average global caesarean section rate, with 27.3% in Asia, 19.0% in Europe and 29.2% in Latin America [1, 2]. China had the highest overall caesarean section rate (46.2%) of the 24 countries in the survey [1]. Over the past decades, the caesarean section rate in China increased sharply for women in all regions, from all socio-economic groups, and in all levels of hospitals [7]. Huang reported that the caesarean section rate increased from 8.9% in 1993–1994 to 24.8% in 2001–2002 [8]. Feng reported that 64.1% of urban women and 11.3% of women in the poorest rural region gave birth by caesarean section in 2008 [9]. Between 1993 and 2008, the risk of caesarean section increased more than three times in urban areas and more than 15-fold in rural areas in China [9]. A recent study of one region found a caesarean section rate of 80% [10]. The overuse of caesarean section has become an important public health problem in China.

It has been suggested that non-indicated caesarean sections are among the main drivers of the high caesarean section rate [1, 8, 9]. A study of 56,968 caesarean sections in southern China showed that the prevalence of caesarean section during 1993–1995, 1996–2000, and 2001–2005 was 13.1, 28.3, and 50.4%, respectively and that the prevalence of caesarean section on maternal request was 0.6, 3.8, and 12.9%, respectively [7]. In the above mentioned WHO study, the overall proportion of women delivering by non-indicated caesarean section ranged from 0.01 to 2.10%, except in China, where this figure was exceptionally high at 11.6% [1].

* Correspondence: zhangwy9921@hotmail.com
[1]Department of Obstetrics, Beijing Obstetrics and Gynecology Hospital, Capital Medical University, No. 251 YaoJiayuan Road, Chaoyang District, Beijing 100026, China
Full list of author information is available at the end of the article

In China, hospitals are classified into three groups: primary, secondary and tertiary level hospitals according to their service level, size, medical technology, medical equipment, management and medical quality. The tertiary level hospitals provide the highest level of medical service. Primary care facilities include hospitals and community-based health care facilities that provide preventive care, and other basic community services but no delivery care.

Little is known about the actual rate of caesarean section in China. Previous studies have been limited to several hospitals or regions. Information about mode of delivery and indications for caesarean section at secondary and tertiary facilities needs analysis to understand the high caesarean section rates in China. The goal of this study is to compare mode of delivery and indications for caesarean section in secondary and tertiary level hospitals to better understand reasons for China's high caesarean section rate.

Methods

Study design and subjects

In this multi-center cross-sectional study, discharge data were collected from all live births from January 1, 2011 through December 31, 2011in 39 public hospitals from14 provinces of China. All participating facilities are members of an obstetrics cooperative center, with broader medical and academic collaboration.

The hospitals included were all part of the public system, since in 2011 more than 95% of deliveries occurred at public hospitals. The 14 provinces, municipalities, and autonomous regions within China included hospitals from Beijing, Shanghai, Jilin, Liaoning, Jiangsu, Sichuan, Shanxi, Hubei, Guangdong, Hebei, Inner Mongolia, Shandong, Shanxi, and Xinjiang.

There were twenty tertiary care hospitals and nineteen secondary care hospitals from 3 regions: East China, Central China, and West China. In China by 2011 98.7% of deliveries took place in hospitals [11] and in 2012, 94.4% of all inpatients in China were admitted to secondary and tertiary level hospitals [12]. Most primary care hospitals do not have obstetrics departments or neonatal care services and are not equipped to perform caesarean section. Therefore, primary care hospitals were not included in the present study. This study was not able to study urban versus rural patient origin.

All individual-level data obtained from medical records were coded in a de-identified format, thus patient consent was not required. The investigators had no contact with patients. The procedures of this study received approval from the Human Ethics Committees of every participating hospital.

Data collection

All women who had live births in the calendar year 2011 at each hospital site were included in the data collection. There was uniform face-to-face training on data extraction for the physician coordinator at each site. At the end of 2011, the data were extracted from the medical records and discharge summaries by trained medical staff on a standardized coded form for computer-based statistical analysis. The data points included: demographics, maternal data (age, parity, education, medical comorbidities), obstetric factors (gestational age, presentation, gestational diabetes, preeclampsia, premature rupture of membranes, third trimester bleeding), mode of delivery, and indication for caesarean section. The physician-documented indication for caesarean section was recorded. If there was more than one indication the physician designated primary indication was used.

Data analysis

Vaginal birth, operative vaginal birth and overall caesarean section rates were calculated for the total sample and for secondary and tertiary level facilities. Caesarean section was divided into two categories: indicated and non-indicated. The indicated caesarean section category was defined as caesarean section performed based on a recorded medical indication. The indicated categories included: repeat caesarean section, non-reassuring foetal heart tracing (NRFHT), failure to progress or cephalopelvic disproportion (CPD) in labour, and previous uterine surgery. NRFHT criteria were consistent with definitions in Williams Obstetrics (23rd Edition).

Other common indications in China which are not necessarily globally accepted indications for caesarean section such as: preeclampsia/eclampsia/HELLP, oligohydramnios, third trimester bleeding (previa/accrete/abruption placenta), multiple gestation, suspected macrosomia, and others (for indications with low frequencies) were included in the "indicated" category in this study. For these diagnoses there was not sufficient clinical information in the database to determine which of these cases would meet internationally accepted criteria. For example the severity of preeclampsia, the etiology of the third trimester bleeding (placenta previa versus abruption placenta), or details of the multiple gestation, higher order pregnancies, twin presentation and concordance were unknown.

The non-indicated category was defined as a primary caesarean section documented by the physician based solely on maternal request in the absence of any maternal or foetal medical indications or physician documented "indications" that show a provider preference but non-standard indication. These included: diagnosis of cephalopelvic disproportion prior to the onset of labour based on clinical pelvimitry and/ or estimated foetal weight, maternal request for their ages greater than or equal to 35 years old, maternal request for precious foetus, precious foetus defined as in vitro pregnancy or poor obstetric history (i.e. prior foetal death, neonatal death, chromosomal or structural abnormality), isolated premature rupture of membranes without foetal heart rate abnormalities, nuchal cord seen on ultrasound without foetal heart rate abnormalities, severe myopia, request for concomitant myomectomy or ovarian cystectomy, or other (isolated chronic hypertension; gestational hypertension; diabetes mellitus without macrosomia, etc.).

Definition of other terms utilized in the study based on Chinese terms: operative vaginal delivery includes forceps delivery, vacuum extraction delivery and breech extraction. Preterm birth was defined as delivery between 24 and 36 6/7 weeks in gestation. Foetal Growth Restriction refers to a foetus with a birth weight less than the 10th percentile. Previous uterine surgery was defined as previous uterine surgery, such as myomectomy, excluding prior caesarean section; malpresentation includes breech presentation, face presentation, transverse lie, and unstable lie. Gestational Diabetes Mellitus refers to abnormal glucose tolerance occurring or initially found during pregnancy by oral glucose tolerance test with any single blood glucose at or above the fasting,1 and 2 h values of 5.1, 10.0, 8.5 mmol/L (92, 180,153 mg/dl), respectively. Obesity in China is defined as body mass index (BMI) ≥ 28 [13]. Suspected macrosomia defined as an estimated foetal weight >4000 g based on ultrasound or Leopold's maneuvers, regardless of diabetic status. Oligohydramnios represented amniotic fluid index (AFI) ≤5 cm regardless of foetal growth.

Statistics analysis

Statistics were performed using SPSS statistics software version 18.0. Data was presented as percentages or median with inter-quartile range. Mann–Whitney *U* test was used for the comparison of maternal age and maternal education among groups. Pearson's chi-square test of independence was used for comparing other frequencies.

Results

Modes of delivery

A total of 112,414 deliveries occurred during the study period, and 112,138 (99%) deliveries were used for this survey. Two hundred seventy-six participants were excluded because of missing information (11 cases), or giving birth prior to 24-week gestation (265 cases) (Fig. 1). The overall caesarean section rate among the study participants was 54.5%.

The tertiary hospitals comprised 71% (79, 631/ 112,138) of the study deliveries. In the tertiary hospitals, the caesarean section rate was 55.9% (44, 535/79, 631),

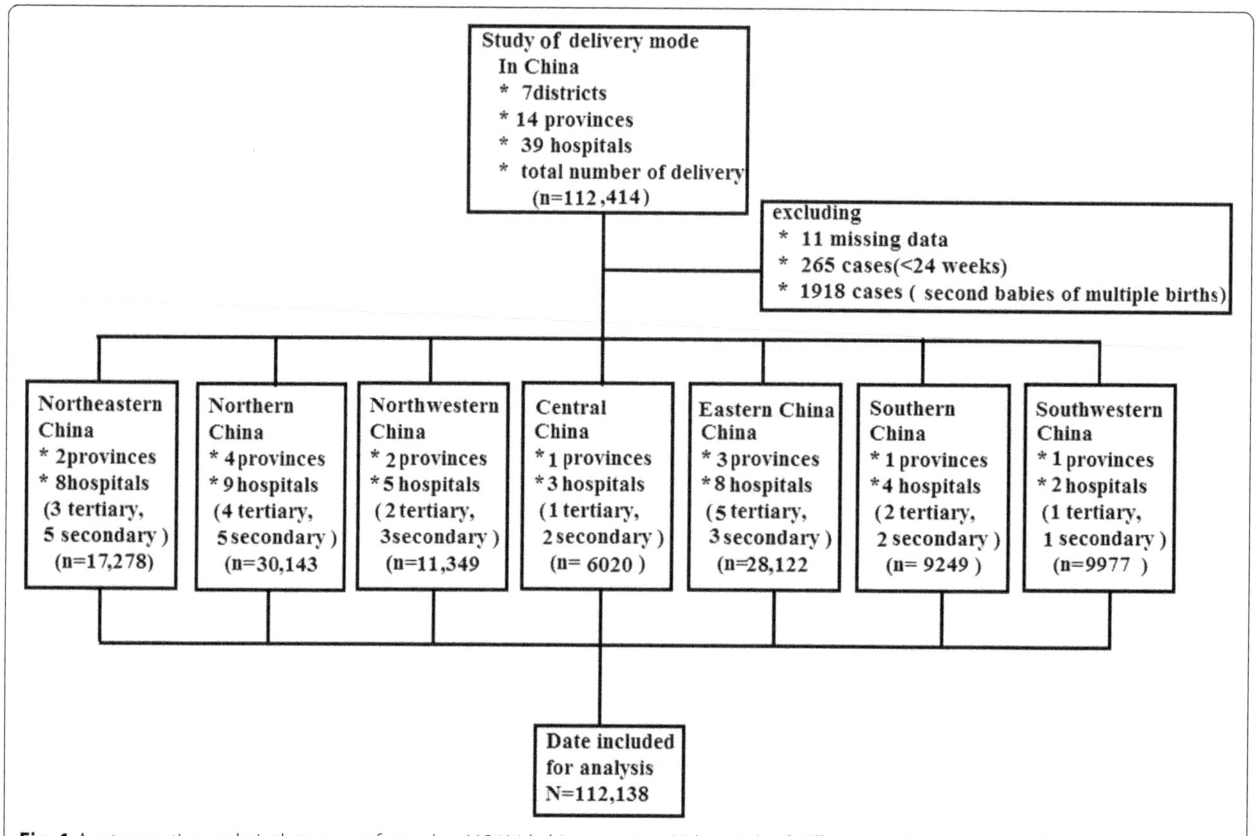

Fig. 1 A retrospective analysis that was performed on112414 babies, covering 39 hospitals of different levels in mainland China

significantly higher than that of the secondary hospitals (50.9%, 16, 549/32, 507). Caesarean section with indications accounted 61.6% of caesarean sections. Non-indicated caesarean section accounted for 20.9% of all deliveries or 38.4% of all caesarean sections. Although the secondary level hospitals had lower overall caesarean section rates, there were more non-indicated caesarean sections (48.9% of caesarean sections (8,092/16, 549)) compared to tertiary care hospitals (34.5% (15,382/44535) (Table 1).

The overall operative vaginal delivery rate was 1.2% with 90.9% (1200/1320) of the operative vaginal deliveries performed in the tertiary level hospitals. The operative vaginal delivery rate in the secondary level hospitals was 0.4% (120/32,507).

Population characteristics

The characteristics of women by the level of hospitals are presented in Table 2. The average age of the parturients was 28 years old. Women delivering in the tertiary hospitals were significantly older than women who delivering in the secondary hospitals ($P < 0.001$). Women who delivered in the tertiary hospitals had a significantly higher level of education than women who delivered in the secondary hospitals ($P < 0.001$). The overall obesity prevalence was 17.4%. Significantly more women in the tertiary hospitals were obese (19.0%), compared to those in the secondary hospitals (13.2%, $P < 0.001$). Overall, 81.1% of all deliveries were women having their first child. There were more primiparous women in the tertiary hospitals (83.9%, 66,827/79,631) than in the secondary hospitals (74.3%, 24,144/32,507). Male infants accounted for 54.7% of all deliveries. The rate of mothers carrying a male-foetus in the tertiary hospitals was lower than that in the secondary hospitals (54.3% vs. 55.8%,$P < 0.001$). Compared to secondary hospitals, pregnancy complications were more likely in women in the tertiary hospitals, including hypertension disorder complicating pregnancy (HDCP), gestational diabetes, PROM, preterm birth, multiple foetus or late pregnancy bleeding.

Indications for caesarean section

Among 61,084 caesarean sections, 7.8% (4,783) were repeat caesarean section and 92.2% (56,301) were primary caesarean section. Analysis of the primary caesarean section showed that 53.7% were with indications and 38.4% were without indications (Table 3). Overall caesarean section on maternal request was the most common reason (22% of all caesarean sections).

In the overall study population, of the top 11 indications for caesarean section, NRFHT was the most common medical indication (12.8% of all caesarean sections), followed by cephalopelvic disproportion/ failure to progress (8.8% of all caesarean sections), and malpresentation (5.7% of all caesarean sections). Other indications included suspected macrosomia (5.6%), preeclampsia/ eclampsia (4.3%), oligohydramnios (3.9%), late pregnancy bleeding (2.7%), prior uterine surgery (2.5%), multiple foetuses (2.1%) and FGR (2.0%) (Table 3).

There were differences in indications for caesarean section between the different level of hospitals. In the tertiary hospitals, of the 79, 631deliveries, there was a higher percent of caesarean section for NRFHT or cephalopelvic disproportion/ failure to progress ($P < 0.001$). The caesarean section rate for pregnancy complications (such as HDCP, malpresentation, oligohydramnios, late pregnancy bleeding, prior uterine surgery and multiple foetuses) in the tertiary hospitals was higher than in the secondary hospitals ($P < 0.001$).

Of the top 7 non-indications for caesarean section, the top three reasons recorded were: maternal request without any reason (56.9% of caesarean sections,13,367/23,474),CPD prior to labour (20.2% of caesarean sections,4756/23,474) and maternal request for age ≥35 years (11.2% of caesarean sections, 2630/23,474) which accounted for 88.4% of the non-indicated caesarean sections, followed by maternal request for precious baby (3.2%), request for myomectomy (2.3%), nuchal cord (1.5%), isolated PROM (1.4%), and severe myopia (1.0%) (Table 4).

The caesarean section rate for maternal request without any reason was much higher in the secondary hospitals than in the tertiary hospitals ($P < 0.001$), as well as the caesarean section rate for CPD prior to labour ($P < 0.001$). The caesarean section rate for other non-indications, such as maternal request for older age or precious baby was higher in the tertiary hospitals than that in the secondary hospitals ($P < 0.001$) (Table 4).

Table 1 Detailed information about the rates of different deliveries at the 39 hospitals across China

Regions	Cesarean delivery		Overall rates of CS (%)	Vaginal Delivery		Number of deliveries (n)	Number of hospitals (n)
	With indications (%)	Without indications (%)		Spontaneous (%)	Operative (%)[a]		
Tertiary hospitals	29153 (36.6)	15382 (19.3)	44535 (55.9)	33896 (42.6)	1200 (1.5)	79631	20
secondary hospitals	8457 (26.0)	8092 (24.9)	16549 (50.9)	15838 (48.7)	120 (0.4)	32507	19
Total	37610 (33.5)	23474 (20.9)	61084 (54.5)	49734 (44.4)	1320 (1.2)	112138	39

[a]Operative vaginal delivery includes forceps delivery, vacuum extraction delivery and breech extraction

Table 2 Characteristics of study populations

Variable	All (n = 112138) n (%)	Tertiary hospital (n = 79631) n (%)	Secondary hospital (n = 32507) n (%)	X^2	p
Maternal age (years)					<0.001
(Years)		29 (26–31)	26 (23–30)		
≤ 24	25734 (23.1)	12950 (16.4)	12784 (39.7)		
25–34	74355 (66.8)	57536 (72.8)	16819 (52.2)		
≥ 35	11197 (10.1)	8583 (10.9)	2614 (8.1)		
Maternal education level					<0.001
College or above	55473 (51.3)	46093 (59.0)	9380 (31.3)		
High school	29935 (27.7)	20411 (26.1)	9524 (31.8)		
Primary school	22468 (20.8)	11442 (14.6)	11026 (36.8)		
Illiteracy	258 (0.2)	214 (0.3)	44 (0.1)		
Residents	77661 (69.3)	56595 (71.1)	21066 (64.8)	425.80	<0.001
Obesity	15980 (17.4)	12512 (19.0)	3468 (13.2)	1584.92	<0.001
Primiparous	90971 (81.1)	66827 (83.9)	24144 (74.3)	1403.10	<0.001
Previous bad obstetric history	1084 (1.0)	952 (1.2)	132 (0.4)	150.28	<0.001
Male infants	61345 (54.7)	43028 (54.3)	18137 (55.8)	28.84	<0.001
Multiple fetus	1918 (1.7)	1771 (2.2)	147 (0.5)	431.05	<0.001
GDM/DM	5344 (4.8)	5024 (6.3)	320 (1.0)	1442.08	<0.001
HDCP	5357 (4.8)	4594 (5.8)	763 (2.3)	594.21	<0.001
Preeclampsia/eclampsia	4137 (3.7)	3650 (4.6)	487 (1.5)	618.52	<0.001
PROM	17078 (15.2)	13965 (17.5)	3113 (9.6)	1133.14	<0.001
Preterm birth	9014 (8.0)	8156 (10.2)	858 (2.6)	1805.02	<0.001
Late pregnancy bleeding	2364 (2.1)	2127 (2.7)	237 (0.7)	421.85	<0.001
oligohydrammios	4200 (3.7)	2938 (3.7)	1262 (1.6)	2.37	0.12
Fetus weight ≥ 4000 g	7366 (6.7)	5075 (6.5)	2291 (7.1)	14.38	<0.001

Quantitative variables of age are expressed as median (25th percentile–75th percentile)
852 missing cases for maternal age; 4004 missing cases for maternal education, 20187 missing cases for maternal BMI;, 2071 missing cases for neonatal weight
IVF-ET In Vitro Fertilization Pre-Embryo Transfer, *PROM* Preterm Rupture Of Membranes, *HDCP* Hypertension Disorder Complicating Pregnancy

Discussion

This study of 112,138 births is one of the largest-scale surveys including indications for delivery conducted in China to date, covering three geographical regions, and focusing on non-indicated caesarean sections. It showed an overall caesarean section rate of 54.5% in 2011 which is substantially higher than the 46.2% found in the 2008 WHO study [1]. As an example, at the Beijing Obstetrics and Gynecology Hospital, the largest tertiary specialty hospital in Beijing, the caesarean section rate steadily increased from 19.5% in 1980–1984, to 25.4% in 1985–1988, then 35.3% in 1989–1992 [14], and the rate was the highest ever recorded at 47.9% in 2011 in this survey. The high caesarean section rate in China is concerning and efforts to analyze caesarean section rates and indications are important first steps in designing programs to decrease these rates.

In this study, 38.4% of all caesarean section were non-indicated, with 85.6% scheduled and performed before labour. Non-indicated caesarean section in this study accounted for 20.9% of deliveries compared to only 11.2% in the 2008 WHO study.

In China as early as 1996, caesarean section on maternal request or caesarean section for social factors received attention from researchers [15]. Previous studies also demonstrated that caesarean section on maternal request or caesarean section for "social factors" accounted for 35.9–46.2% of all caesarean section in certain areas of China [7]. In this study 11.9% of deliveries were caesarean section on maternal request compared to rates estimated at 2.5% in the USA or 1-2% in the United Kingdom. Caesarean section on maternal request was the most common recorded reason for caesarean section in this study. The non-indicated caesarean section rate varied greatly by level of facility and region and was much higher in the secondary level hospitals than in the tertiary level hospitals. This suggested that clinical practice patterns affect the number of caesarean sections performed. In China in 2011, there was

Table 3 The indications for cesarean by regions

Indications	Total (% of 61084)	Total (% of 112138)	Tertiary hospital (% of 79631)	Secondary hospital (% of 32507)	X^2 value	*P* value
Total Cesarean Delivery	100	61084 (54.5)	44535 (55.9)	16549 (50.9)	234.35	<0.001
Repeat Cesarean Delivery	7.8	4783 (4.3)	3640 (4.6)	1143 (3.5)	62.91	<0.001
Primary Cesarean Delivery	92.2	56301 (50.2)	40895 (51.4)	15406 (47.4)	145.00	<0.001
Non-indicated	38.4	23474 (20.9)	15382 (19.3)	8092 (24.9)	433.71	<0.001
Cesarean Delivery on maternal demand	21.9	13367 (11.9)	7957 (10.0)	5410 (16.6)	972.35	<0.001
Other non-indicated Cesarean Delivery	16.5	10107 (9.0)	7425 (9.3)	2682 (8.3)	32.45	<0.001
Indicated Cesarean Delivery	53.7	32827 (29.3)	25513 (32.0)	7314 (22.5)	1014.56	<0.001
NRFHT	12.8	7840 (7.0)	5736 (7.2)	2104 (6.5)	19.00	<0.001
FTP/CPD (in labor)	8.8	5373 (4.8)	4006 (5.0)	1367 (4.2)	34.48	<0.001
Malpresentation	5.7	3500 (3.1)	2811 (3.5)	689 (2.1)	151.88	<0.001
Suspected macrosomia	5.6	3427 (3.1)	2463 (3.1)	964 (3.0)	1.27	0.26
Preeclampsia/ eclampsia	4.3	2650 (2.4)	2356 (3.0)	294 (0.9)	422.18	<0.001
Oligohydrammios	3.9	2393 (2.1)	1807 (2.3)	586 (1.8)	24.06	<0.001
Late pregnancy bleeding	2.7	1637 (1.5)	1476 (1.9)	161 (0.5)	296.05	<0.001
Prior uterine surgery	2.5	1554 (1.4)	1244 (1.6)	310 (1.0)	62.56	<0.001
Multiple fetus	2.1	1280 (1.1)	1178 (1.5)	102 (0.3)	277.90	<0.001
FGR	2.0	1194 (1.1)	629 (0.8)	565 (1.7)	197.01	<0.001
Other medical disease	1.2	727 (0.6)	694 (0.9)	33 (0.1)	211.49	<0.001
Other indications	2.0	1252 (1.1)	1113 (1.4)	139 (0.4)	196.77	<0.001

not a gatekeeper system or a pre-operative view required for caesarean section [16] so if a woman requested a caesarean section, some hospitals were more likely to comply.

Prior studies in China have reported that fear of pain and perceived better health for the child and mother are the main reasons women request caesarean section [17–19]. In China in 2011, most public hospitals were unable to routinely offer pain relief or epidurals in labour making the fear of pain a real concern. Emotional and nursing support for women in labour requires adequate nurse to patient staffing ratios, which may be lacking with the current system.

CPD diagnosed prior to labour was the second most common coded reason for non-indicted caesarean section, accounting for 20% of the non-indicated caesarean section or 4.2% of total deliveries. Even in the tertiary hospitals, CPD prior to labour accounted for 18.9% of the non-indicated caesarean section or 3.6% of total deliveries. In most hospitals in China routine clinical pelvimitry is performed antenatally. Previous Chinese studies classifed this as a medical indication for caesarean section. Despite abandonment of this practice in the USA and UK due to its poor predictive value for failure to progress in labour, in China it

Table 4 The non-indications for cesarean by regions

Indications	Total (% of 23474)	Total ($n = 112138$)	Tertiary hospitals (% of 79631)	Secondary hospital (% of 32507)	X^2 value	*P* value
Maternal request without any reason	56.9	13367 (11.9)	7957	5410	972.35	<0.001
CPD prior to labor	20.2	4756 (4.2)	2904	1852	238.96	<0.001
Maternal request for Age >35 (multip + primip)	11.2	2630 (2.3)	2097	533	99.53	<0.001
Materal request for precious baby	3.2	761 (0.7)	662	99	95.04	<0.001
Maternl request for myomectomy	2.3	540 (0.5)	503	37	129.17	<0.001
Nuchal Cord	1.5	342 (0.3)	306	36	55.80	<0.001
Isolated: PROM	1.4	336 (0.3)	292	44	41.35	<0.001
Severe myopia	1.0	225 (0.2)	221	4	81.09	<0.001
TOTAL	100	23474 (20.9)	15382	8092	433.71	<0.001

is a common physician documented reason for caesarean section.

In China, tertiary level hospitals often provide leadership in clinical teaching, research, and development of clinical guidelines. Physicians from tertiary hospitals may be considered more informed than those at secondary level hospitals, but this study suggests a wide gap between the tertiary level physician practice and international guidelines. The development of standardized evidence-based guidelines in obstetrics may help obstetricians decrease the number of non-indicated caesarean section.

In China, high risk pregnant women delivered more often in the tertiary hospitals. The higher overall caesarean section rate in tertiary level hospitals compared to secondary level hospitals may be partially explained by the higher risk patient mix at the tertiary level hospitals.

In this study 33.5% of deliveries were caesarean section with documented indications, with 29.3% of primary caesarean section with indications. Among the indicated caesarean sections, the most common diagnosis was NRFHRT or foetal distress (12.8% of all caesarean section, 7.0% of all deliveries). This is consistent with a previous study of teaching hospitals in China [20] and is higher than that in the United States (4.0-5.9%) [21, 22]. The rate for this indication was much higher in the tertiary hospitals than in the secondary hospitals in this study. NRFHT can be a relatively subjective indication for caesarean section [22, 23]. In this study NRFHT was diagnosed before labour 36.0% (2824/7840) of the time. This finding may be partially explained by the common overuse of technology in low risk pregnancies in China. For example, in many hospitals, the standard of care is to perform weekly non-stress tests (NSTs) in all healthy pregnant women in the third trimester. The positive predictive value of these tests is poor when used in low risk populations. Isolated abnormal umbilical cord dopplers or nonspecific electronic foetal monitor findings may result in unnecessary caesarean section for "foetal distress".

The non-indicated caesarean section rate would be even higher if some diagnoses that we included in the "indicated" category such as preeclampsia/eclampsia/HELLP, oligohydramnios, third trimester bleeding (previa/accrete/abruption placenta), multiple gestation, and suspected macrosomia were further analyzed and recategorized since they are not globally accepted and evidence based indications for caesarean section. In this analysis we were unable, for example, to discern which pregnancies had placenta previa (an accepted caesarean section indication) versus an abruptio placenta without intrauterine foetal death (not a caesarean section indication) or which multiple gestation cases had a non-vertex presenting twin, higher order multiples or non-concordant breech second twins (all accepted caesarean section indications). Thus with rigorous auditing of the "indicated" category of cases, many would be reclassified as "non-indicated", raising the overall non-indicated caesarean section rate.

Isolated oligohydramnios is also not an evidence based indication for caesarean section.

Consistent with previous research in China, our study showed that isolated oligohydramnios was one of the major indications for caesarean section in China, accounting for 3.9% of all caesarean section. A prior study involving 2326 women of rural eastern China showed that, during antenatal care, 46.8% women received at least 3 ultrasound scans and the maximum number reached 11 [8]. It showed a statistically significant association between the number of antenatal ultrasound scans and caesarean section rates. A growing body of evidence demonstrates that isolated oligohydramnios in the absence of other maternal or foetal risk factors is not associated with adverse perinatal outcomes [24]. Caesarean section for preeclampsia could also be reassigned to non-indicated caesarean section if we were able to analyze the cases with more clinical information.

In this study, the overall operative vaginal delivery rate was very low at 1.2% and even lower in the secondary hospitals. This is consistent with Wang's report, which surveyed 887 health facilities in the year 2002 and reported a national caesarean section rate of 38.0% and an extremely low operative vaginal delivery rate (5.5%) [25]. Low operative vaginal delivery rates may be due to pressure on the caregivers to practice "defensive medicine" and lack of training and experience with the techniques. Caesarean section for malpresentation accounted for 3.2% of all deliveries. Perhaps due to the same pressures few hospitals offer external cephalic versions.

Numerous studies of caesarean section have shown a strong association between increased maternal education, older maternal age and low parity and an increased risk of caesarean section [6, 15, 16]. In China, tertiary hospitals are located in big cities, treating mainly urban patients or rural patients referred from secondary and primary hospitals. Secondary and primary hospitals are usually in moderate or small cities, treating patients from towns or rural areas. In this study, the tertiary level hospital parturients were older, more educated, more likely to be having their first child later, pregnancy complications and indicated caesarean section.

The major strength of this study is that it is one of the largest-scale surveys conducted in China to date, covering three geographical regions, and focusing on non-indicated caesarean section in China. The biggest limitation of this study is that the facilities were not randomly selected, which may have introduced selection bias. Thus the caesarean section rates should not be regarded as representative for the entire country, nor for all the regions.

Furthermore, our survey included only the secondary and tertiary hospitals, so our results cannot be generalized to smaller facilities. Second, prior studies show an association between insurance coverage and caesarean section but this cannot be analyzed since insurance data was not recorded in our survey. Third, we have no data on labour management including: induction of labour, augmentation of labour, or the availability of anesthesia. Furthermore, In the paper based on the same database, which we published in Chinese in 2014 [26], we put the indictions, such as cephalopelvic disproportion prior to labor, Age >35,etc. into indicated caesarean section as we used to do, it showed that the non-indicated caesarean section rate was 24.553%, was lower than that of this article, we have corrected in this article. Even so, there is some misclassification bias given that many of the caesarean section classified as "indicated" would likely be "non-indicated" if we had more clinical data on the cases. This suggests that we have underestimated the number of non-indicated caesarean sections.

The ideal caesarean section rate is not known. One ecological study using longitudinal data in 159 countries showed caesarean section rates higher than around 10% at the population level are not associated with decreases in maternal and neonatal mortality rate [27]. Another suggested that rates up to approximately 19% were associated with lower maternal and neonatal mortality rates in WHO member states [28]. Regardless, the caesarean section rate in China in this study of 54.5% is well above accepted target rates with at least 38% that were non-indicated. The motivations for providers are to perform caesarean sections for non-medical, vague or subjective indications is a complex issue. A broader perception of caesarean section as safe has been raised as a possibility. The use of globally recognized indications that are evidence- based to create clinical obstetric guidelines could standardize diagnosis and treatment in pregnancy and result in fewer unnecessary caesarean section at tertiary and secondary level hospitals. Additionally, medical malpractice reform and focus on the birth experience may be a way to reduce caesarean section rates. Analysis of maternal and perinatal outcomes associated with mode of delivery in China needs further study. With the end of the One Child policy, as of January 2016, the risks associated with non-indicated caesarean section will likely increase as more women are allowed and choose to have a second child. This makes it imperative to reduce the number of unnecessary primary caesarean sections.

Conclusions

Caesarean section on maternal request accounts for a large portion of China's high caesarean section rate, especially in the secondary hospitals. More guidelines and bulletins are urgently needed to standardize the diagnosis and treatment of diseases nationally among different level of hospitals. On the other side, legislation to protecting doctors to do the appropriate treatment rather than defense treatment is still the important things to do.

Abbreviations

AFI: Amniotic fluid index; BMI: Body mass index; CI: Confidence intervals; CPD: Cephalopelvic disproportion; DM: Preexisting diabetes mellitus; FGR: Foetal growth restriction; GDM: Gestational diabetes mellitus; HDCP: Hypertension disorder complicating pregnancy; IVF-ET: In vitro fertilization pre-embryo transfer; NRFHT: Non-reassuring foetal heart tracing; OR: Odds ratios; PROM: Preterm Rupture Of Membranes; WHO: World Health Organization

Acknowledgments

We thank the subjects for their participation and medical staffs involved in this survey at the following hospitals: Capital Medical University Beijing Obstetrics and Gynecology
Hospital, Capital Medical University Friendship Hospital (Li Lin), Obstetrics and Gynecology Hospital of Fudan University (Xiaotian Li), First Affiliated Hospital of Medical College of Xi'an Jiaotong University (Wenli Gou), Nanjing Drum Tower Hospital (Yali Hu), Shandong Provincial Hospital (Xietong Wang), the Second Affiliated Hospital of West China Hospital (Xinghui Liu), Shengjing Hospital of China Medical University (Caixia Liu), Nanfang Hospital of Nanfang Medical University (Yanhong Yu), the Second Hospital of Jilin University (Yanhui Zhao), the First Affiliated Hospital of Xinjiang Medical University (Qiming Zhu), Hebei Changzhou Central Hospital (Junfeng Zhang), the First Affiliated Hospital of Inner Shandong Provincial Hospital. We thank Maynard S. Clark for his reviews and suggestions (Department of Global Health and Population, Harvard School of Public Health, Boston).

Funding

This project was supported by "Health industry special funds for Public Benefit Research Foundation" from the Ministry of Health, People's Republic of China (Grant number 201002013).

Authors' contributions

XW did the initial data interpretation, and wrote an early draft of the manuscript. SH reviewed and extensively rewrote the manuscript and guided the analysis. LH analysis of the data and edit the manuscript. ZL and YR mainly carried out data collection and analysis. WZ initially set up the study design, conceived of creating this dataset and supervised the data collection training and logistics. All authors have seen and approved the final version of this abstract for publication.

Competing interests

The authors declare that they have no competing interests.

Author details

[1]Department of Obstetrics, Beijing Obstetrics and Gynecology Hospital, Capital Medical University, No. 251 YaoJiayuan Road, Chaoyang District, Beijing 100026, China. [2]Department of Obstetrics and Gynecology, Brigham and Women's Hospital, Harvard Medical School, Boston, MA 01210, USA.

References

1. Lumbiganon P, Laopaiboon M, Gülmezoglu AM, Souza JP, Taneepanichskul S, Ruyan P, et al. World Health Organization Global Survey on Maternal and Perinatal Health Research Group: Method of delivery and pregnancy outcomes in Asia: the WHO global survey on maternal and perinatal health 2007–08. Lancet. 2010;375:490–8.

2. Villar J, Valladares E, Wojdyla D, Zavaleta N, Carroli G, Velazco A, et al. WHO 2005 Global Survey on Maternal and Perinatal Health Research Group: Caesarean delivery rates and pregnancy outcomes: the 2005 WHO global survey on maternal and perinatal health in Latin America. Lancet. 2006;367:1819–29.
3. Laws PJ, Sullivan EA. Australia's mothers and babies 2002. Perinatal Statistics Series No. 15. Sydney: National Perinatal Statistics Unit; 2004.
4. Tranquilli AL, Giannubilo SR. Cesarean delivery on maternal request in Italy. Int J Gynaecol Obstet. 2004;84:169–70.
5. Caesarean sections. Post note No.184. London: Parliamentary Office of Science and Technology; 2002.
6. Dobson R. Caesarean section rate in England and Wales hits 21%. BMJ. 2001;323:951.
7. Cui HS, Li HT, Zhu LP, Li ZW, Zhou YB, Liu JM. Secular trends in cesarean delivery and cesarean delivery on maternal request among multiparous women who delivered a full-term singleton in Southern China during 1993–2005. Beijing Da Xue Xue Bao. 2013;45:422–6. Chinese.
8. Huang K, Tao F, Bogg L, Tang S. Impact of alternative reimbursement strategies in the new cooperative medical scheme on caesarean delivery rates a mixed-method study in rural China. BMC Health Serv Res. 2012;12:217.
9. Feng XL, Xu L, Guo Y, Ronsmans C. Factors influencing rising caesarean section rates in China between 1988 and 2008. Bull World Health Organ. 2012;90(1):30–9.
10. Long Q, Klemetti R, Wang Y, Tao F, Yan H, Hemminki E. HighCaesarean section rate in rural China: is it related to health insurance (New Co-operative Medical Scheme)? Soc Sci Med. 2012;75:733–7.
11. National Bureau of Statistics of China. China heath statistical yearbook 2010. Available at: http://www.nhfpc.gov.cn/htmlfiles/zwgkzt/ptjnj/year2012/index2012.html. Accessed 2 Feb 2017.
12. National Bureau of Statistics of China. China heath statistical yearbook 2013. Available at: http://www.nhfpc.gov.cn/htmlfiles/zwgkzt/ptjnj/year2013/index2013.html . Accessed 2 Feb 2017.
13. Cooperative Meta-analysis Group of China Obesity Task Force. Predictive values of body mass index and waist circumference to risk factors of related diseases in Chinese adult population. Chinese J Epidemiol. 2002;23:5–10.
14. Huang X. What are we thinking when facing the cesarean section nowadays? Chinese. J Practical Gynecol Obstet. 2003;19(7):385. Chinese.
15. Zheng P, Huang X, Wang S. The changing trend of cesarean section rates in 35 years. Zhonghua Fu Chan KeZaZhi. 1996;31(3):142–5. Chinese.
16. Wu WL. CD in Shantou, China: a retrospective analysis of 1922 women. Birth. 2000;27:6–90.
17. Fu L, Cui M, Cheng J. Analysis of the factors affecting cesarean section rates and indications. Chin J Pract Chin Gynecol Obstet. 2003;19:405–7.
18. Lin Y, Wen A, Zhang X. Analysis on the 10-year changes of rates and indications of cesareansection. Guangdong Med J. 2000;21:477–8. Chinese.
19. Zhang J, Liu Y, Meikle S, Zheng J, Sun W, Li Z. Cesarean delivery on maternal request in southeast China. Obstet Gynecol. 2008;111:1077–82.
20. Gao Y, Xue Q, Chen G, Stone P, Zhao M, Chen Q. An analysis of the indications for cesarean section in a teaching hospital in China. Eur J Obstet Gynecol Reprod Biol. 2013;170:414–8.
21. Leeman L, Leeman R. A Native American Community with a 7% CD Rate: Does Case Mix, Ethnicity, or Labor Management Explain the Low Rate? Ann Fam Med. 2003;1:36–43.
22. Barber EL, Lundsberg LS, Belanger K, Pettker CM, Funai EF, Illuzzi JL. Contributing indications to the rising cesarean delivery rate. Obstet Gynecol. 2011;118(1):29–38.
23. Boyle A, Reddy UM, Landy HJ, Huang CC, Driggers RW, Laughon SK. Primarycesarean delivery in the United States. Obstet Gynecol. 2013;122:33–40.
24. Zhang J, Landy HR, Branch DW, Burkman R, Haberman S, Gregory KD, et al. Contemporary patterns of spontaneous labor with normal neonatal outcome. Consortium on Safe Labor. Obstet Gynecol. 2010;116:1281–7.
25. Wang B, Shi Q, Wang Y, Li N, Shi L. National survey on midwifery practice in health facilities in China. Zhonghua Fu Chan Ke Za Zhi. 2007;42(5):305–8.
26. Hou L, Li G, Zou L, Li C, Chen Y, Yuan Y, Wang X, et al. Cesarean delivery rate and indications in mainland China: a cross sectional study in 2011. Zhong hua Fu Chan Ke Za Zhi. 2014;49:728–35.
27. Ye J, Zhang, Mikolajczyk R, Torloni MR, Gülmezoglu AM, Betran AP. Association between rates of caesarean sectionand maternal and neonatal mortality in the 21st century: a worldwide population-based ecological study with longitudinal data. BJOG. 2015;123:745–53.
28. Molina G, Weiser T, Lipsitz R, Haynes A. Relationship between cesarean delivery rate and maternal and neonatal mortality. JAMA. 2015;314(21):2263–79.

Chewing gum for intestinal function recovery after caesarean section

Zunjia Wen[1,2†], Meifen Shen[1,2*†], Chao Wu[1†], Jianping Ding[2] and Binbin Mei[2]

Abstract

Background: Gum chewing has been reported to enhance the intestinal function recovery after caesarean section, current perspectives and practice guidelines vary widely on the use of gum chewing, more studies on the role of gum chewing after caesarean section are needed.

Methods: We performed a comprehensive, systematic meta-analysis of randomized controlled trials (RCTs) on the efficacy of gum chewing after caesarean section. Studies were identified by searching EMBASE et al database (until June 30, 2016). Summary odd ratios or weighted mean differences with 95% confidence intervals were calculated for each outcome with fixed- or random-effects model.

Results: Ten RCTs with a total of 1659 women were included in our meta-analysis. Gum chewing provided significant benefits in reducing the time to first passage of flatus, first defecation, first bowel sound, first bowel movement and the length of hospital stay, but not in the time to first feeling of hunger.

Conclusions: Gun chewing hastens the intestinal function recovery after caesarean section and offers a safe and inexpensive option. High-quality and larger-scale RCTs are still warranted to clarify the role of gum chewing in intestinal function recovery after caesarean section.

Keywords: Caesarean, Gum, Intestinal function, Meta-Analysis, Recovery, Review

Background

With the development of medical care and policy supports, the caesarean delivery, a most commonly seen operation, has increased worldwide over the past decades [1]. However, it may lead to many complications such as postoperative ileus with a mean incidence of 10–15% [2, 3], result in longer hospital stay, increased postoperative morbidity and excessive medical costs [4].

Promoting intestinal function recovery after caesarean section is on the top of research agenda of healthcare providers. Traditionally, physicians forbid oral feeding with concern to the risks of intestinal fistula, re-bleeding and aspiration mistakenly [5], but recent studies have supported that early postoperative feeding can stimulate bowel motility and shorten hospital stay [6, 7], however, patients may not tolerate the early feeding regimen [8]. Several methods have been proposed to accelerate the return of gastrointestinal motility after caesarean section, including early oral hydration, ambulation and gum chewing.

Gum chewing as a kind of sham feeding was introduced in hope that it may hasten the intestinal function recovery in recent years, by means of stimulating the cephalic vagal reflex, the hormones secretion may increase [9]. The efficacy of gum chewing have been fully elucidated in the intestinal function recovery in patients after colorectal surgery and it can provide various benefits [10, 11], yet the efficacy of chewing gum after caesarean section remain inconsistent. Several previous meta-analysis [12–17] including randomized controlled trials (RCTs) on the gum using after caesarean have been conducted, but the included data are rather limited. Up to date, no guideline has officially support the use of chewing gum for intestinal

* Correspondence: smf8165@126.com
†Equal contributors
[1]The First Affiliated Hospital of Soochow University, No. 188 Shizi Street, Gusu district, Su Zhou, Jiangsu province, China
[2]Nursing School of Soochow University, Su Zhou, China

function recovery in obstetrics and gynaecology, more evidences of higher quality on this issue are warranted.

Given the recently emerging evidence on the role of gum chewing after caesarean section, we performed this systematic review and meta-analysis of RCTs with the following objectives: (1) to review and sum up the current evidence on the influence of gum chewing in intestinal function after caesarean section; (2) to compare the efficacy of chewing gum and standard care in intestinal function recovery after caesarean section; and (3) to analyze and conclude the appropriateness of gum chewing in patients after caesarean section.

Methods

Search strategy

We tried to plan, perform and report this meta-analysis in comply with PRISMA guideline [18]. Related articles either published in English or Chinese were identified and selected by searching PUBMED, EMBASE, Science Direct, Cochrane Central Register of Controlled Trials, China National Knowledge Infrastructure (CNKI) and Wanfang Database (until June 30, 2016) using the following search terms including "gum-chewing", "chewing-gum", "sham-feeding", "'caesarean section"', "caesarean", "caesarean delivery", we combined these terms in accordance to the instructions of the database. In addition, the reference lists of the retrieved studies and pervious reviews and meta-analyses were reviewed and manually searched, and we made no attempt to identify unpublished reports.

Study selection

Study selection was made based on a first screen of identified titles or abstracts and on a second check-up of full-text articles. Studies were considered to be eligible if the criteria below were met: (1) RCT design; (2) study subjects had receiving caesarean section; (3) included the comparison groups of added gum chewing and standard nursing care post caesarean delivery; and (4) the relative outcome data (the time to first passage of flatus after operation, et al) were reported. Studies were excluded if: (1) it's not RCT design, which may produce more heterogeneity for data analysis; (2)the study subjects had not received caesarean section; (3) the relative outcome data were not accessible for data synthesis.

Data extraction

The following data information were extracted by two reviewers independently: first author, year of publication, country, patient population, participants, methods of gum chewing, other concurrent interventions, main outcomes and study results. The studies selection and data extraction were conducted by two authors independently, any disagreement was resolved by further discussion.

The outcomes we collected for data analysis included: (1) the time to first passage of flatus; (2) the time to first defecation; (3) the time to first bowel movement; (4) the length of hospital stay; (5) time to first feeling of hunger; (6) the time to first bowel sound; (7)postoperative complications such as nausea, abdominal distension, vomiting et al.

Assessment of the quality of the included studies

The Cochrane Collaboration's "risk of bias" tool was adopted for evaluating the methodological quality and risk of bias of included RCTs, seven specific domains were examined and measured in this tool: sequence generation, allocation concealment, blinding of participants and personnel, blinding of outcome assessment, incomplete outcome data, selective outcome reporting, and "other" issues. Every domain could be classified as "low risk of bias", "high risk of bias" or "unclear risk of bias" under the guidance of judgment criteria (Cochrane Handbook for Systematic Reviews of Intervention. Part 2: 8.5).

Data synthesis and analysis

All the extracted data were processed in a freeware program Review Manager (RevMan) Version 5.3. Binary outcomes (i.e., VAP and mortality) were presented as Mantel-Haenszel style odd ratios (ORs) with 95% confidence intervals, and continuous outcomes were reported as inverse variance weighted mean differences (WMDs). A fixed-effect model was adopted in cases of homogeneity (p value of $\chi 2$ test >0.10 and $I^2 < 50\%$), while a random-effects model was used in cases of obvious heterogeneity (p value of $\chi 2$ test >0.10 and $I^2 > 50\%$). Publication bias was evaluated by the demonstration of funnel plots, and asymmetry was assessed by means of the Egger regression test (p-value < 0.1 was considered to be significant of funnel plot asymmetry).

Results

Literature search

A sum of 528 relevant publications were yielded by the comprehensive search, and the first screen of titles and abstracts excluded 473 papers, and 55 potentially related studies were included for further full-text review, participants and interventions not meeting the including criteria were the main concern for further consideration, eventually, 10 RCTs [19–28] were included for data analyses (Fig. 1).

Study characteristics

The basic characteristics of 10 included studies are shown in Table 1. In brief, a total of 1659 patients were involved, specifically with 835 patients for gum chewing

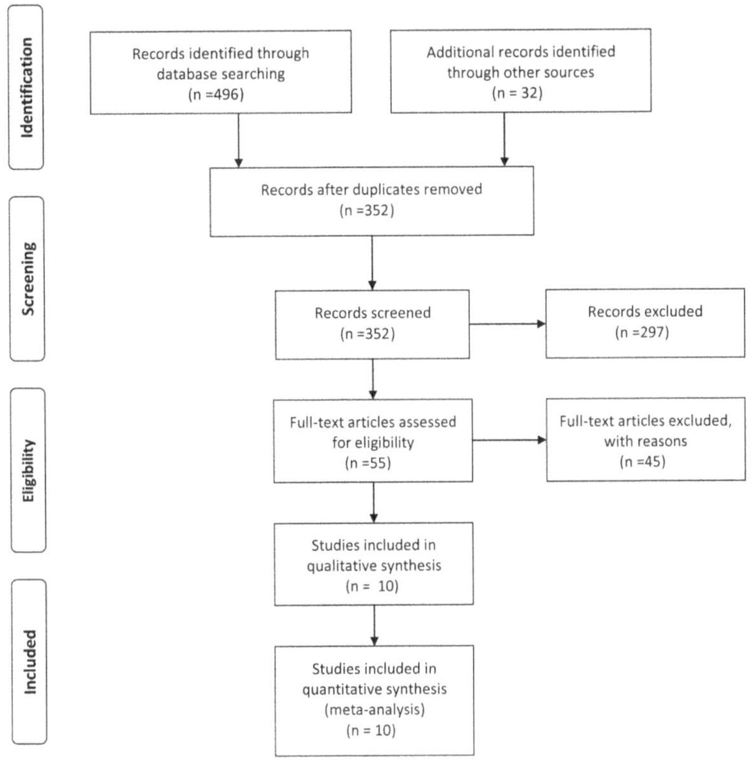

Fig. 1 Flow diagram of study selection

intervention, and 824 for standard postoperative care, the countries of included studies ranged from Egypt, Nigeria, Thailand, Turkey, Iran, Philippines to China, and four RCTs were conducted in China, the numbers of included participants among studies differed from 50 to 386. It's noteworthy that one study was reported as conference paper, although the structure and data were relatively complete, the details on how study conduct remain unclear, we attempted to contact the original authors for more information, yet no response was achieved, therefore, we still included this study for data analysis, but we put more cautions on the quality of study details. All studies have reported no statistical significant differences in the baseline characteristics between intervention and control groups. Meanwhile, some differences among studies were found in the gum chewing interventions, including the timing of initiation and frequency of gum chewing, one study [24] also compared the efficacy of xylitol-containing and xylitol-free gum chewing with standard postoperative care protocol, in our study we only extracted the data in xylitol-free gum chewing and control groups. Interestingly, all the results favored the usage of gum chewing after caesarean sections.

Methodological quality and risk of bias

Figure 2a illustrates all of the bias classifications in a way of cross-tabulation for the included RCTs, and the summary of qualitative methodological quality abiding by the bias classification ("Low risk", "High risk", "Unclear risk") is presented in Fig. 2b. Briefly, all included RCTs mentioned that the randomization was adopted in their studies, yet three RCTs [25, 26, 28] made no reports on the methods for random sequence generation, only two studies reported the strategies to achieve allocation concealment and then were marked as low bias of risk. Considering that it's hard to blind patients and care providers on the gum chewing intervention, most RCTs adopted single-blind or no blind study design instead of a double-blind study design, all RCTs made no blind study design on participants and personnel then were classified as high risks of bias, and only two [19, 27] adopted the blind design on outcome assessment. Except for the details lack of Zaroma' study [28],all the other RCTs have provided the necessary data and outcomes for selective reporting and other bias evaluations.

Main analysis

The WMDs for each study on the time to first passage of flatus, the time to first defecation, the time to first bowel sound, the length of hospital stay, the time to first bowel movement, time to first feeling of hunger are shown in Fig. 3.

Table 1 The characteristics of included studies

Author(year)	Country	Numbers of participants(GC/NGC)	Gum intervention	Main outcomes	Results
Abd-El-Maeboud 2009 [19]	Egypt	200(93/107)	Started from 2 h after surgery, lasted for 15 min every 2 h in the daytime but not in the night, until the passage of flatus	①,②,④,⑤	Gum chewing after CS is safe, well tolerated, and associated with rapid resumption of intestinal motility and shorter hospital stay
Ajuzieogu 2014 [20]	Nigeria	180(90/90)	Started from the first day after operation for 5 consecutive days, 3 times daily, 30 min for every time.	①,②,④,⑤	Gum chewing has a beneficial effect on early return of bowel function following cesarean section and should be included in the postoperative management protocol
Jakkaew 2013 [21]	Thailand	50(25/25)	Started since the regain of consciousness after operation, 4 times a day (morning, noon, evening, and before bed time), 30 min for every time, until the first passage of flatus	①,⑤,⑥,⑦	Gum chewing is associated with faster recovery of bowel function following cesarean section
Kafali 2010 [22]	Turkey	150(74/76)	Started from 2 h after surgery, 3 times daily in the morning, afternoon, and evening, each episode of gum chewing lasted 1 h except the initial one which lasted 15 min	①,④,⑤	Gum chewing provides a simple method for early recovery of bowel function after cesarean section
Ledari 2012 [23]	Iran	100(50/50)	Chewing gum for at least 1 h, three times daily from 6 h after surgery (after recovery from anesthesia) until being discharged	①,④,⑥	chewing is acceptable and inexpensive physiologic method for decreasing the time to the passage of flatus, bowel movements, and feeling of hunger in patients undergoing cesarean section
Lee 2016 [24]	China	120(40/40/40)	Chewing xylitol-free or xylitol-containing gum started from 2 h after surgery, repeated every 2 h between 9 a.m. and 8 p.m, 15 min for every time, until the first passage of flatus	①,②,④	After cesarean section, chewing gum increased participants' return of bowel activity and xylitol-containing gum may be superior to xylitol-free gum
Liang 2007 [25]	China	120(60/60)	Started after recovery from anesthesia, repeated every 2 h for 15 min every time	①,②,⑦,⑧	Chewing gum can promote gastrointestinal motility recovery after cesarean section, and the method is simple, convenient, safe
Luo 2010 [26]	China	300(150/150)	Started from 2 h after surgery, 4 times daily in the morning, afternoon, and evening, each episode of gum chewing lasted 10-15min	①,②,④,⑦,⑨	Chewing gum can promote the recovery of gastrointestinal function after cesarean section
Shang 2010 [27]	China	386(195/191)	Chew gum for at least half an hour, three times per day after returning to the ward	①,②,④,⑤,⑩	Gum chewing is an inexpensive, convenient, and physiological method in enhancing the recovery of bowel function
Zamora 2012 [28]	Philippines	53(18/35)	Gum chewing involved chewing two pellets of sugarless gum at 12 h post operation for 15 min then advanced to sips of clear liquids at 16 h post operation	①,③,⑤,⑩	Postoperative gum chewing stimulates the earlier return of bowel motility after cesarean delivery

Notes: ①, the time to first passage of flatus; ②, the time to first defecation; ③, the time to first bowel movement; ④, the time to first bowel sound; ⑤, the length of hospital stay; ⑥, time to first feeling of hunger; ⑦, abdominal distension; ⑧, vomiting; ⑨, post operation incision pain; ⑩, postoperative ileus(POI)

The time to first passage of flatus All included studies have reported the time to the first passage of flatus, The summary WMDs on the time to first passage of flatus (hours) was -5.91(95% CI: -7.08– -4.73), with evidence of heterogeneity ($P = 0.005$, $I^2 = 61\%$) (Fig. 3a).

The time to first defecation Seven studies [19, 20, 23–27] have reported the time to the first passage of flatus, The summary WMDs on the time to first defecation (hours) was -7.91(95% CI: -11.14– -4.67), with evidence of heterogeneity ($P < 0.001$, $I^2 = 93\%$) (Fig. 3b).

The time to first bowel sound Six studies [19, 20, 22–24, 26] have reported the time to first bowel sound, The summary WMDs on the time to first bowel sound

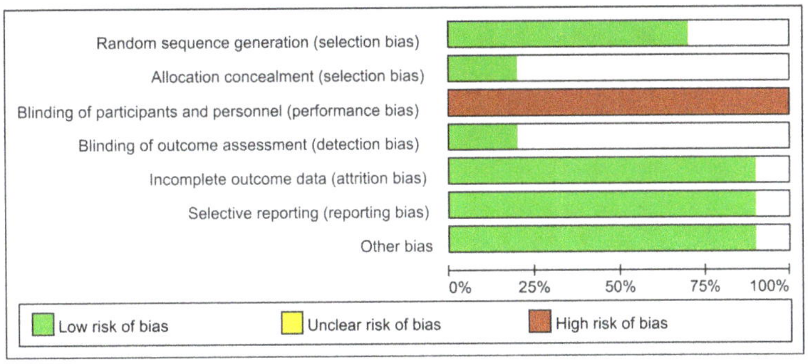

A Risk of bias graph

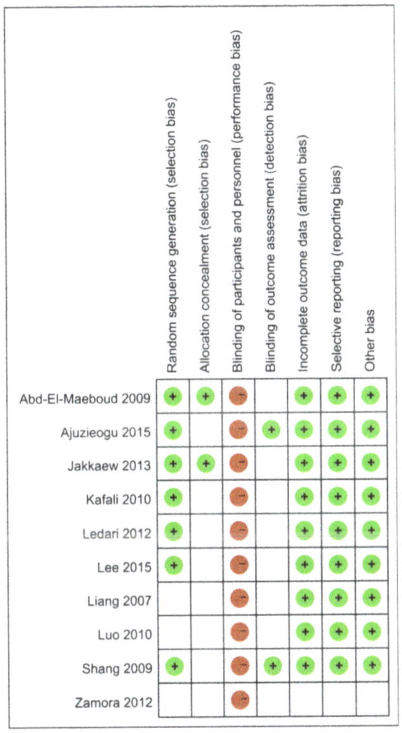

B Risk of bias summary

Fig. 2 Methodological quality and risk of bias of the included studies

(hours) was -4.19(95% CI: -6.41– -1.97), with evidence of heterogeneity ($P < 0.001$, $I^2 = 97\%$) (Fig. 3c).

The length of hospital stay Six studies [19–22, 27, 28] have reported the length of hospital stay, The summary WMDs on the length of hospital stay (days) was -0.30(95% CI: -0.46– -0.14), with evidence of heterogeneity ($P = 0.28$, $I^2 = 80\%$) (Fig. 3d).

The time to first bowel movement Two studies [27, 28] have reported the time to first bowel movement, The summary WMDs on the time to first bowel movement(hours) was -5.38(95% CI: -7.39– -3.38), with no evidence of heterogeneity ($P < 0.001$, $I^2 = 13\%$) (Fig. 3e).

Time to first feeling of hunger Three studies [21, 23, 28] have reported time to first feeling of hunger, The summary WMDs on time to first feeling of hunger (hours) was -0.70(95% CI: -2.97– 1.57), with no evidence of heterogeneity ($P = 0.32$, $I^2 = 13\%$) (Fig. 3f).

Publication bias analysis

Funnel plot, a simple scatter plot of the intervention effect estimates from every studies, is plotted against some measure of each study's size or precision (Cochrane Handbook for Systematic Reviews of Intervention. Part 2:8.5). Ten or more studies are required for the significant evidence of funnel plot. In our studies, due to the limitation of included data, we only performed funnel plot analysis on the time to first passage of flatus. As presented in Fig. 4, the distribution of study estimates in the funnel plot was symmetrical and well-proportioned, no significant publication bias have been found.

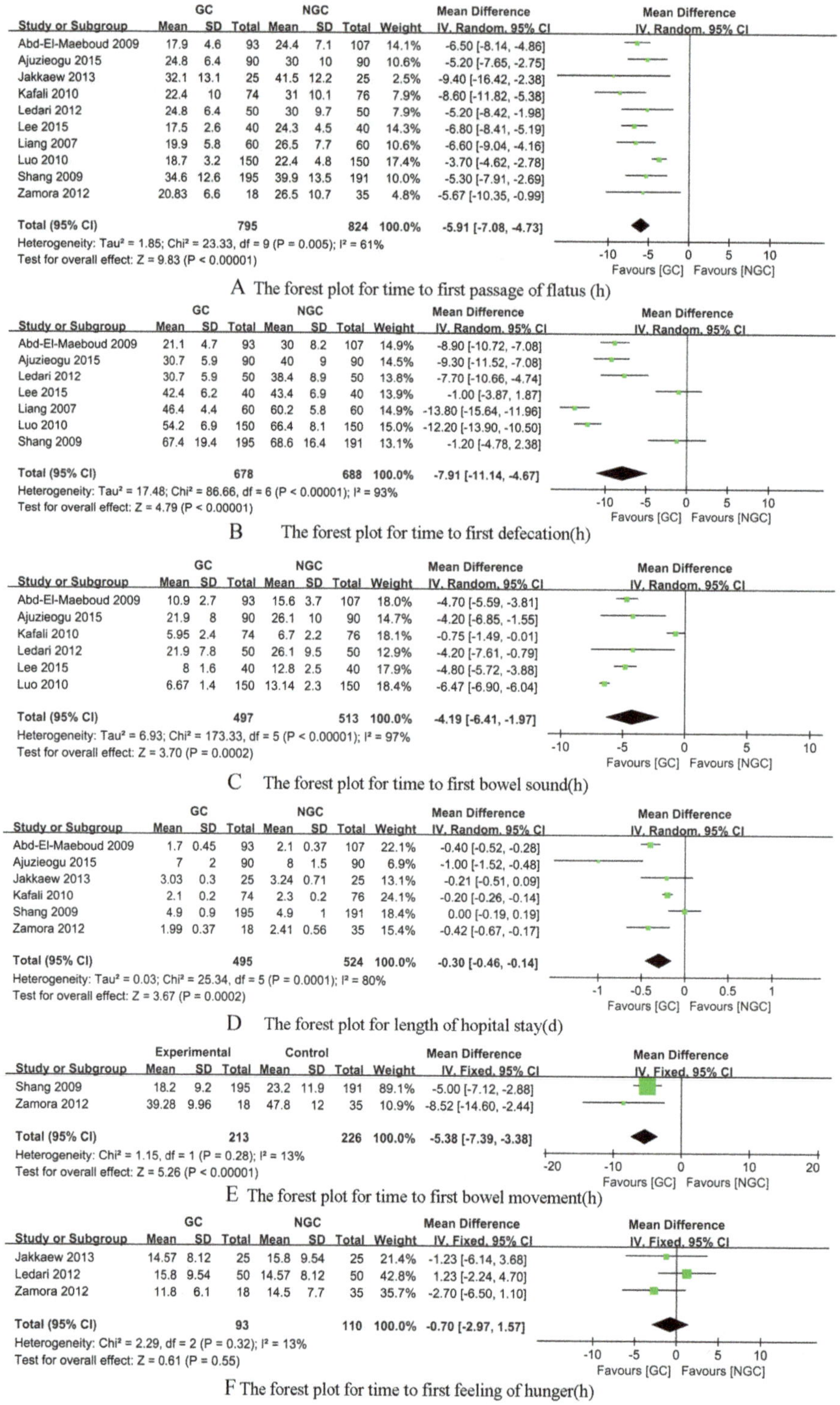

Fig. 3 The forest plots for different outcomes

Subgroup and sensitivity analyses

No subgroup analyses were made in this study. Sensitivity analyses which investigate the impact of a single study on the overall risk estimate by abandoning one study in each turn. In the process of sensitivity analyses, we found that the results of time to first bowel movement changed when we neglected the study conducted by Shang [27], yet the data on this outcome still quite

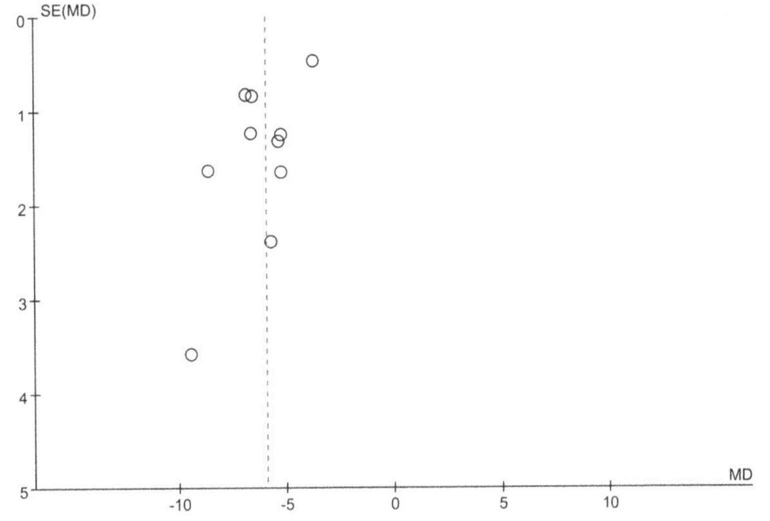

Fig. 4 The funnel plot for the time to first passage of flatus

limiting. For other outcomes, no significant change of the overall risk estimates by abandoning any single study was found.

Discussion

The results of our meta-analysis have indicated gum chewing after caesarean section can significantly promote the intestinal function recovery by accelerating the time to first passage of flatus, first defecation, first bowel sound, first bowel movement and shortening the length of hospital stay. The gum-chewing groups' faster recovery of gastrointestinal tract motility may result from stimulating intestinal motility by strengthening the cephalic-vagal reflex and increasing the gastrointestinal hormones secretion associated with bowel motility [9]. However, we did not find benefits of gum chewing on the time to first feeling of hunger, one possible explanation is that the chewing movement cause a feeding feedback to the brain, making a full feeling for our central nerve systems, additionally, the early feeding program employed in some studies can further enhance the hunger stimulus, previous study [10] has concluded that sham feeding confers no advantage if patients are placed on a rapid postoperative feeding regimen. Also, all the included studies have reported no side effects of gum chewing intervention in patients after caesarean section, therefore, gum chewing may be a safe and feasible intervention for accelerating the intestinal function recovery in patients after caesarean section.

Similar to other meta-analyses, our study has upheld the use of gum chewing in the early stage after caesarean section to accelerate the intestinal function recovery. A recent meta-analysis by Huang [12] included only five RCTs involving 882 patients, the sample size and number of included studies were small. An earlier meta-analysis by Hochner [15] also included five RCTs with a total of 846 participants, the process for meta-analysis was rather strict, yet the publication bias could not be evaluated quantitatively by a funnel plot due to the small number of studies available, the other meta-analyses [14, 16, 17] also had problems in this area. Another comprehensive Cochrane meta-analysis [13] identified 81 studies involving 9072 participants to investigate whether the chewing gum after surgery hasten the return of gastrointestinal function after abdominal surgery, come to the finding that gum chewing showed a beneficial impact on the major outcomes of digestive system activation, including bowel sound, flatus passage and bowel movement, yet the including studies were rather heterogeneous. Different from previous meta-analysis, with more related RCTs published, our study has included more RCTs for synthesized analysis, which may have more advantages in reducing publication bias.

Several previous meta-analyses [10, 29] focused on the influence of chewing gum after colorectal cancer surgery, come the finding that it might promote the recovery of intestinal function. A meta-analysis [30] including12 RCTs focused on chewing gum and postoperative ileus in adults, found that chewing gum provided small benefit in reducing time to flatus, and time to bowel motion, but not in the length of stay or the incidence of complications, it's noteworthy that this studies included patients receiving either colorectal surgery or cesarean sections, in which lots of heterogeneities might exist, it should be emphasized that the surgery differences may lead to different injuries to the intestinal function, and gum chewing may offer different effects on the recovery process, specific intervention details(-starting time, frequency et al.) of gum chewing for different surgeries remain further investigation.

Although early oral intake has been promoted as standard care after caesarean section [31], only one RCT [22] adopted oral intake within six hours postpartum in both groups, still, when early oral intake was standardized in each group, the gum chewing added more benefits to the intestinal function recovery. A recent study [32] compared the effect of gum chewing, early oral hydration, and early mobilization on intestinal motility after cesarean birth, concluded that all of the three different interventions increased intestinal motility, and should be recommended during postoperative routine care to shorten hospital stay and prevent postoperative ileus, future research needs to further clarify the roles of those three interventions. Notably, one included RCT [24] also evaluated the effects of xylitol-containing and xylitol-free gum chewing on gastrointestinal recovery after cesarean section, the results indicated that xylitol-containing gum might be superior to xylitol-free gum, while the most included RCTs adopted the sugar-free gum in their interventions. The sugar ingredients in sugar free gum (e.g., sorbitol and xylitol) may stimulate bowel mobility and exert a laxative effect, yet the evidence on whether sugar substitutes in sugar-free gum affect bowel function remain conflicting [33, 34], more researches in this area are also warranted.

Several limitations in this meta-analysis should be considered. First, there are some differences in gum chewing interventions (e.g., initiation, ingredients and frequency) among included RCTs, this is most likely accountable for the heterogeneity observed, however, due to the data limitations, we did not perform meta-regression analyses on patient population characteristics. Second, the quality of the included studies was not rather high, most included RCTs made no report on the randomization concealment and blinding, due to the nature of gum chew intervention, it's rather difficult to blind the participants in this study setting, but blinding the observers is achievable and might reduce the bias, future studies should put more attentions on the RCT design. Third, limited by study data, we did not perform subgroup analysis and funnel plot in some outcomes, still, it's possible that the end point susceptible to missing data from studies that were not published due to an overall null effect.

Conclusions

In conclusion, our study has further supported that gum chewing is associated with early recovery of intestinal function after caesarean section, which may be helpful to reduce the time to first passage of flatus, first defecation, first bowel sound, first bowel movement and shorten the length of hospital stay. Gum chewing offers a safe, simple and inexpensive for hastening the recovery of intestinal function after caesarean section, which is worthy of promotion for clinical use.

Abbreviations

CNKI: China National Knowledge Infrastructure; ORs: Odd ratios; RCTs: Randomized controlled trials; WMDs: Weighted mean differences

Acknowledgments

None.

Funding

This research have received no specific grant from any funding agency in the public, commercial, or not-for-profit sectors.

Authors' contributions

SMF and WZJ contributed to the conception and design of the research; WZJ, SMF DJP, MBB and WC contributed to the collection and analysis of the data; WZJ, SMF and WC contributed to the analysis and interpretation of the data; and WZJ wrote the first draft of manuscript. All authors have critically revised the manuscript, agreed to be fully accountable for ensuring the integrity and accuracy of the work, and read and approved the final manuscript.

Competing interests

The authors declare that they have no competing interests.

References

1. Degani N, Sikich N. Caesarean delivery rate review: an evidence-based analysis. Ont Health Technol Assess Ser. 2015;15(9):1–58.
2. Whitehead WE, Bradley CS, Brown MB, Brubaker L, Gutman RE, Varner RE, Visco AG, Weber AM, Zyczynski H, Pelvic Floor N. Gastrointestinal complications following abdominal sacrocolpopexy for advanced pelvic organ prolapse. Am J Obstet Gynecol. 2007;197(1):78 e71–77.
3. Allen AM, Antosh DD, Grimes CL, Crisp CC, Smith AL, Friedman S, McFadden BL, Gutman RE, Rogers RG. Management of ileus and small-bowel obstruction following benign gynecologic surgery. Int J Gynaecol Obstet. 2013;121(1):56–9.
4. Doorly MG, Senagore AJ. Pathogenesis and clinical and economic consequences of postoperative ileus. Surg Clin North Am. 2012;92(2):259–72. viii.
5. Stewart D, Waxman K. Management of postoperative ileus. Dis Mon. 2010;56(4):204–14.
6. Selby LV, Rifkin MB, Yoon SS, Ariyan CE, Strong VE. Decreased length of stay and earlier oral feeding associated with standardized postoperative clinical care for total gastrectomies at a cancer center. Surgery. 2016; 160(3):607–12.
7. Aydin Y, Altunyurt S, Oge T, Sahin F. Early versus delayed oral feeding after cesarean delivery under different anesthetic methods–a randomized controlled trial anesthesia, feeding in cesarean delivery. Ginekol Pol. 2014;85(11):815–22.
8. Hasler WL. Pharmacotherapy for intestinal motor and sensory disorders. Gastroenterol Clin North Am. 2003;32(2):707–32. viii-ix.
9. Lunding JA, Nordstrom LM, Haukelid AO, Gilja OH, Berstad A, Hausken T. Vagal activation by sham feeding improves gastric motility in functional dyspepsia. Neurogastroenterol Motil. 2008;20(6):618–24.
10. Ho YM, Smith SR, Pockney P, Lim P, Attia J. A meta-analysis on the effect of sham feeding following colectomy: should gum chewing be included in enhanced recovery after surgery protocols? Dis Colon Rectum. 2014;57(1):115–26.
11. Su'a BU, Pollock TT, Lemanu DP, MacCormick AD, Connolly AB, Hill AG. Chewing gum and postoperative ileus in adults: a systematic literature review and meta-analysis. Int J Surg. 2015;14:49–55.
12. Huang HP, He M. Usefulness of chewing gum for recovering intestinal function after cesarean delivery: A systematic review and meta-analysis of randomized controlled trials. Taiwan J Obstet Gynecol. 2015;54(2):116–21.
13. Short V, Herbert G, Perry R, Atkinson C, Ness AR, Penfold C, Thomas S, Andersen HK, Lewis SJ. Chewing gum for postoperative recovery of gastrointestinal function. Cochrane Database Syst Rev. 2015;2:CD006506.

14. Zhu YP, Wang WJ, Zhang SL, Dai B, Ye DW. Effects of gum chewing on postoperative bowel motility after caesarean section: a meta-analysis of randomised controlled trials. BJOG. 2014;121(7):787–92.
15. Hochner H, Tenfelde SM, Abu Ahmad W, Liebergall-Wischnitzer M. Gum chewing and gastrointestinal function following caesarean delivery: a systematic review and meta-analysis. J Clin Nurs. 2015;24(13-14):1795–804.
16. Craciunas L, Sajid MS, Ahmed AS. Chewing gum in preventing postoperative ileus in women undergoing caesarean section: a systematic review and meta-analysis of randomised controlled trials. BJOG. 2014;121(7):793–9. discussion 799.
17. Yuan Y, Zhao H, He J, Gong X. Chewing gum in promoting bowel recovery after cesarean section: a systematic review. Chin J Evid Based Med. 2011;11(4):6.
18. Liberati A, Altman DG, Tetzlaff J, Mulrow C, Gotzsche PC, Ioannidis JP, Clarke M, Devereaux PJ, Kleijnen J, Moher D. The PRISMA statement for reporting systematic reviews and meta-analyses of studies that evaluate health care interventions: explanation and elaboration. PLoS Med. 2009;6(7):e1000100.
19. Abd-El-Maeboud KH, Ibrahim MI, Shalaby DA, Fikry MF. Gum chewing stimulates early return of bowel motility after caesarean section. BJOG. 2009;116(10):1334–9.
20. Ajuzieogu OV, Amucheazi A, Ezike HA, Achi J, Abam DS. The efficacy of chewing gum on postoperative ileus following cesarean section in Enugu, South East Nigeria: A randomized controlled clinical trial. Niger J Clin Pract. 2014;17(6):739–42.
21. Jakkaew B, Charoenkwan K. Effects of gum chewing on recovery of bowel function following cesarean section: a randomized controlled trial. Arch Gynecol Obstet. 2013;288(2):255–60.
22. Kafali H, Duvan CI, Gozdemir E, Simavli S, Onaran Y, Keskin E. Influence of gum chewing on postoperative bowel activity after cesarean section. Gynecol Obstet Invest. 2010;69(2):84–7.
23. Ledari FM, Barat S, Delavar MA. Chewing gums has stimulatory effects on bowel function in patients undergoing cesarean section: a randomized controlled trial. Bosn J Basic Med Sci. 2012;12(4):265–8.
24. Lee JT, Hsieh MH, Cheng PJ, Lin JR. The role of xylitol gum chewing in restoring postoperative bowel activity after cesarean section. Biol Res Nurs. 2016;18(2):167–72.
25. Liang J, Gao Z, Han W, Zhang G, Liu S, Dai Q. The clinical observation of enhancing recovery of gastrointestinal function after cesarean section by gum chewing. J Tongji Univ (Med Sci). 2007;28(2):3.
26. Luo S, Wu C, Yang X, Lei L, Deng H, Li H. Effect of chewing gum afar cesarean section Oll restoration of gastrointestinal function. J Mod Nurs. 2010;16(24):2.
27. Shang H, Yang Y, Tong X, Zhang L, Fang A, Hong L. Gum chewing slightly enhances early recovery from postoperative ileus after cesarean section: results of a prospective, randomized, controlled trial. Am J Perinatol. 2010;27(5):387–91.
28. Zamora BBB, Kalalo RE. Abstracts of XX FIGO World congress of gynecology and obstetricsO752 GUM chewing versus traditional feeding on the early return of bowel motility after cesarean delivery: a prospective randomized controlled trial. Int J Gynecol Obstet. 2012;119:S525.
29. Purkayastha S, Tilney HS, Darzi AW, Tekkis PP. Meta-analysis of randomized studies evaluating chewing gum to enhance postoperative recovery following colectomy. Arch Surg. 2008;143(8):788–93.
30. Noble EJ, Harris R, Hosie KB, Thomas S, Lewis SJ. Gum chewing reduces postoperative ileus? a systematic review and meta-analysis. Int J Surg. 2009;7(2):100–5.
31. Millen KR, Kuo K, Zhao L, Gecsi K. Evidence-based guidelines in labor management. Obstet Gynecol Surv. 2014;69(4):209–17.
32. Sahin E, Terzioglu F. The effect of gum chewing, early oral hydration, and early mobilization on intestinal motility after cesarean birth. Worldviews Evid Based Nurs. 2015;12(6):380–8.
33. Storey D, Lee A, Bornet F, Brouns F. Gastrointestinal tolerance of erythritol and xylitol ingested in a liquid. Eur J Clin Nutr. 2007;61(3):349–54.
34. Tandeter H. Hypothesis: hexitols in chewing gum may play a role in reducing postoperative ileus. Med Hypotheses. 2009;72(1):39–40.

23

Identification of barriers and facilitators for optimal cesarean section care: perspective of professionals

Sonja Melman[1*], Rachel Hellen Petra Schreurs[2], Carmen Desiree Dirksen[3], Anneke Kwee[4], Jan Gerrit Nijhuis[1], Nicol Anna Cornelia Smeets[2], Hubertina Catharina Johanna Scheepers[1] and Rosella Petronella Maria Gemma Hermens[5]

Abstract

Background: The cesarean section (CS) rate has increased over recent decades with poor guideline adherence as a possible cause. The objective of this study was to explore barriers and facilitators for delivering optimal care as described in clinical practice guidelines.

Methods: Key recommendations from evidence-based guidelines were used as a base to explore barriers and facilitators for delivering optimal CS care in The Netherlands. Both focus group and telephone interviews among 29 different obstetrical professionals were performed. Transcripts from the interviews were analysed. Barriers and facilitators were identified and categorised in six domains according to the framework developed by Grol: the guideline recommendations (I), the professional (II), the patient (III), the social context (IV), the organizational context (V) and the financial/legislation context (VI).

Results: Most barriers were found in the professional and organizational domain. Barriers mentioned by healthcare professionals were disagreement with specific guideline recommendations, and hesitation to allow women to be part of the decision making process. Other barriers are lack of adequately trained personal staff, lack of collaboration between professionals, and lack of technical equipment.

Conclusions: Clear facilitators and barriers for guideline adherence were identified in all domains. Several barriers may be addressed by using decision aids on mode of birth or prediction models to individualise care in women in whom both planned vaginal birth and CS are equal options. In women with an intended vaginal birth, adequate staffing and the availability of both fetal blood sampling and epidural analgesia are important.

Keywords: Barriers, Facilitators, Guidelines, Cesarean section, Professionals

Background

The cesarean section (CS) rate has increased over recent decades in both developed and developing countries. The World Health Organization has targeted the CS rate to be 10% to 15%, although this low rate has recently been questioned [1, 2]. In The Netherlands, the CS rate has increased steadily over the past decade from 10.8% in 1999 to 16.5% in 2014 [3, 4]. In absolute numbers, the most impressive rise was documented among healthy women with a singleton in vertex position between 37 and 42 weeks gestation [5]. Furthermore, in The Netherlands in 2013, a large variation in vaginal birth rates per hospital were observed in the nulliparous term singleton vertex group, with rates ranging from 45.1–73.2% [6].

This worldwide increasing CS rate is a cause for concern since this will lead to increased maternal and neonatal complications, increased risks for future pregnancies, and increased healthcare costs [7–10]. Literature mainly focusses on individual-level explanations for the CS rise, including increased maternal age, technological innovation, women's choice or clinical risk factors such as obesity and

* Correspondence: s_melman@hotmail.com
[1]Department of Obstetrics and Gynaecology, GROW- School for Oncology and Developmental Biology, Maastricht University Medical Centre, Maastricht, The Netherlands
Full list of author information is available at the end of the article

previous CS. However, these explanations do not account for the majority of the variation observed [11].

In order to optimize CS practice, the Royal College of Obstetricians and Gynecologists (RCOG) developed an evidence-based guideline with clear recommendations that have a direct effect on the decision to perform a CS [12]. In the CS implementation study (SIMPLE), a RAND-modified Delphi procedure resulted in 27 quality indicators describing optimal CS care based on international guidelines and literature [13]. The adherence to CS quality indicators was measured in 21 hospitals in The Netherlands in order to gain insight into current obstetrical care.

Besides insight into optimal and current care, insight into facilitators and barriers among all professionals involved in CS decision-making is essential. This insight can support the development of a tailored strategy to overcome barriers and improve guideline implementation. The present qualitative study explored facilitators and barriers for optimal CS care among midwives, obstetrical residents and obstetricians.

Methods

Design

A qualitative study was conducted to determine facilitators and barriers that influence the decision to perform a CS from a healthcare professional's perspective. Two separate focus group interviews were performed; one with obstetricians and one with obstetrical residents from different regions and different types of hospitals in The Netherlands. Due to organizational difficulties, a focus group among independent midwives could not be arranged. Therefore, we conducted telephone interviews among nine midwives until data saturation was reached (the last interview did not reveal any new information).

Setting

Currently in The Netherlands, pregnant women without medical complications are supervised by a registered midwife (primary care) and have the possibility to choose where to give birth (at home or in an outpatient hospital setting). If medical complications exist or develop during pregnancy or birth, the attending midwife refers the pregnant woman to an obstetrician in a hospital (secondary care). Certain obstetric situations may lead to the advice to deliver by planned CS, whereas others may lead to the need for counselling on risks and benefits of a planned vaginal birth opposed to a planned CS. Mode of birth counselling is mostly performed by obstetricians and residents. Therefore, all situations that may lead to a planned CS are the responsibility of secondary care. However, referring midwives may provide their opinion before referral and are often consulted by the women for a second opinion and are therefore an influencing factor.

Study population

Thirty obstetricians and residents from university and non-university hospitals in different regions of The Netherlands were invited to participate in focus group interviews. The obstetricians and residents were all members of the Dutch Society of Obstetrics and Gynaecology (NVOG). The midwives were invited based on recommendations from the Royal Dutch National Association of Midwifery (KNOV) and worked in primary or secondary care.

Development interview guide and data collection

Quality indicators from the SIMPLE study were used as a base for exploration of barriers and facilitators (Table 1) [13].

These quality indicators were based on key recommendations on CS care, abstracted from guidelines of the RCOG, the American Congress of Obstetricians and Gynaecologists, the Dutch Society of Obstetrics and Gynaecology and the Society of Obstetricians and Gynaecologists of Canada. The indicators considered mode of birth counselling, planned CS and prevention of (emergency) CS, and were discussed separately during the interviews. Facilitators and barriers were explored at different domains, based on the model developed by Grol [14, 15] concerning the guideline recommendations itself (domain I), the professional (domain II), the patient (domain III), the social domain (domain IV), the organizational domain (domain V) and the financial/legislation domain (domain VI). The focus group interview among obstetricians was moderated by a project member (obstetrician). The focus group interview among residents was moderated by another project member (resident). Individual telephone interviews among midwives were conducted by the same resident.

Data analysis

The interviews were fully transcribed and analysed using the qualitative analysis tool of ATLAS.ti GmbH Version 7 (Berlin, Germany). Two reviewers (SM and RS) independently read the interviews and coded facilitators and barriers for each of the recommendations and transcripts. The identified factors were assigned to the appropriate domains. Disagreements were resolved by discussion between the reviewers. If there was no consensus, a third independent reviewer was consulted (RH).

Results

The obstetricians worked at non-university non-teaching hospitals (N = 6) or non-university teaching hospitals

Table 1 Quality indicators in caesarean section care

1) Quality indicators on planned CS
a) General counseling, CS is not mentioned (vaginal birth is the normal conduct)
1. Twin pregnancy and first child cephalic position
2. Fetal macrosomia (<4.5 kg in maternal diabetes, <5 kg no maternal diabetes)
3. Preterm labour, cephalic position
4. Small for gestational age without fetal distress
5. Previous shoulder dystocia without impaired perinatal outcome
b) Counseling directed at vaginal birth (vaginal birth and CS are options, vaginal birth is preferred)
6. Position of the placenta at 1-2 cm of the internal os
Request for CS without medical grounds:
7. Explore reason for request
8. Discuss (dis)advantages to CS birth
9. In case of extreme fear: offer psychological counselling
10. Preterm breech birth (frank, complete breech)
c) Counseling mentioning both vaginal birth and CS as equal options
11. Breech presentation at term
Previous CS (inform on risks and chance of successful vaginal birth after cesarean)
12. Inform on low risk of uterine rupture
13. Inform on high chance of successful vaginal birth after cesarean
14. Inform on increased risk and lower success rate in case of need for labour induction
d) Prevention of planned CS
15. Offer external cephalic version in case of non-cephalic position
16. Use of internal audit on CS
2) Quality indicators on emergency CS
17. In case of suspected fetal distress use ST analysis or micro blood analysis
In case of non-progressive labour first stage:
18. Rupture of membranes,
19. Urinary catheterization,
20. Use of pain medication, preferably epidural analgesia,
21. Adequate contractions or augmentation of labour
In case of non-progressive labour second stage in nulliparous women:
22. Active pushing recommended,
23. Adequate contractions recommended,
24. Consider vacuum extraction if the head is <1/5th palpable per
Abdomen
25. Continuous support during labour for women with or without prior training
26. Use of partogram
27. Involvement of consultant obstetrician in decision making for CS

(N = 4). Five residents from a non-university hospital and five residents from a university hospital were included. The midwives worked either in a private practice (N = 5) (rural and urban areas), non-university hospital (N = 3) or university hospital (N = 2).

The quotations were categorised, resulting in a total of 38 barriers and 11 facilitators which mainly concerned the professional and organizational domain. These are described in detail hereinafter (Table 2).

Domain I: The CS guideline recommendations

All types of professionals mentioned that guidelines do not adequately consider individual patient characteristics that might influence guideline adherence. As one of the obstetricians described:

> *'If the woman is nulliparous, pregnant with a child that is expected to be large for gestational age and with a fetal head not engaged at term, it depends on her characteristics whether or not I will discuss a CS'.*

This barrier mainly applies to guidelines aiming at vaginal birth in specific situations, such as fetal macrosomia, labour dystocia, breech presentation and previous shoulder dystocia. Furthermore, obstetricians mentioned that guidelines were not easily available on the professional website, whereas residents noted that local protocols were not always recently updated.

Furthermore, not all professionals agreed with guideline recommendations. Almost all types of professionals disagreed with the recommendation: 'A CS should not be mentioned in case of a previously experienced shoulder dystocia if there is no residual neonatal damage'. The decision to offer a CS mainly depends on the severity of the previous shoulder dystocia, and not on residual neonatal damage alone. A midwife describes:

> *'It depends on the client whether or not I would discuss a CS or induction of labour. If the shoulder dystocia was severe, I would not risk to experience that again.'*

Domain II: The professional domain

Obstetricians and residents mentioned unclear documentation on previous deliveries, including advice on mode of birth in future pregnancies, as an important barrier for guideline adherence. Furthermore, they stated that incomplete counselling or unclear documentation of the decision making process for mode of birth in the current pregnancy, is an important factor for acting in line with the agreed mode of birth. For example:

> *You have planned a CS for a woman with a history of fetal macrosomia (4500 grams) and shoulder dystocia.*

Table 2 Professionals' perceived barriers and facilitators for adherence to CS guidelines

Most important influencing factors per domain:

Domain I Guideline itself	Domain II Professionals	Domain II Professionals	Domain IV Social	Domain V Organizational
Design • The guidelines are designed for an average patient, instead of an individual	Clinical characteristics • Non-adherence to the guidelines due to patient characteristics	Information by others • Negative experience of friends/family (eg with external cephalic version)	Hampering collaboration • Between obstetricians and anesthesiologists regarding epidural analgesia • Between midwives and obstetricians/residents	No agreements regarding • Responsibility for counseling: the midwife or obstetrician • Variation in standard policy between hospitals (regarding e.g. fetal scalp blood sampling, breech deliveries) • Indications for CS
Availability • Guidelines are not easy available • Local protocols are not up to date	Counseling • No or too late agreement regarding the possibility of a preterm birth	Patients' view • Patients do not accept any risks for the fetus. • Refusal of external cephalic version.	Variation in policy • Between different obstetricians	
	Documentation • Unclear documentation on mode of birth counselling • Unclear documentation on previous births		Strict hierarchy • Preventing adequate feedback	Staffing • Appropriate staff not present at the discussion regarding obstetrical decisions • Inadequate staffing and allocation of tasks • Midwives are not invited for audits
	Knowledge and skills Insufficient experience or expertise regarding: • Breech deliveries • Foley catheter induction in case of previous CS • Estimation of fetal weight • Fetal scalp blood sampling • External cephalic version			Availability of staff • Obstetricians • Anesthesiologists • Inadequate to provide 1-on- 1 support to women in labour
	Attitude • Policy depends on time (day/night) • Fetal scalp blood sampling is time consuming			Availability of diagnostics • Partogram • Fetal scalp blood sampling
	Disagreement with guidelines • Behaviour therapy in case of fear for pain is not always strictly necessary • Epidural analgesia is not strictly necessary in case of failure to progress in labor • Don't use a partogram in case of rapid labour progression ▪ CS should be mentioned in case of severe shoulder dystocia in previous pregnancies, even if there is no residual damage ▪ Assessment by an obstetrician in case of failure to progress before performing a CS depends on a residents' experience			

If labour starts prematurely, you might advise her to undergo a vaginal birth, since the expected fetal weight is probably less than 4000 grams'.

Lack of experience regarding clinical skills in daily practice was also mentioned among all types of professionals to affect guideline adherence, mainly concerning vaginal breech deliveries, fetal scalp blood sampling and external cephalic version. A midwife adds:

'The mode of delivery in case of a breech presentation depends on the expertise of the obstetrician in attendance'.

One of the obstetricians describes:

'I believe that we perform a fetal scalp blood sampling about 5 times a year'.... 'I think this is probably due to insufficient expertise among some of the obstetricians'.

Another barrier mentioned by the residents regarding the use of fetal scalp blood sampling is the large variation in policy between obstetricians as well as between hospitals. Some obstetricians favour a vacuum extraction when full dilatation of the cervix is reached, whereas others would perform fetal scalp blood sampling in order to, possibly, avoid an operational vaginal birth.

Obstetricians mentioned that the ability to evaluate a cardiotocogram during delivery on any computer as facilitator for optimal care. This improves communication between the obstetrician on call and the resident without the necessity to be present at the delivery ward.

Domain III: The patient context

A barrier mentioned by obstetricians and residents is mode of birth advice by friends or family of a pregnant woman. Particularly negative experiences regarding the outcome of the neonate are perceived to be cause of anxiety and reduced cooperation of a pregnant woman, which can complicate communication between a pregnant woman and her caregiver. An example: *'You can never ignore the information a patient receives from a neighbour or a niece. That sometimes seems more important than the medical information you provide.'*

Another barrier mentioned by obstetricians is that they feel it might be difficult for women to adequately balance current and future fetal risks, next to maternal risks and benefits in choosing mode of birth.

'Counselling in pregnancy is fundamentally different, since it concerns the mother but also her child. Women seem more concerned for their current child than for a possible future pregnancy. Sometimes weighing the risks of a vaginal birth after previous CS and taking consequences for future pregnancies into account, is difficult even for healthcare providers'.

Domain IV: The social context

All types of professionals mentioned troublesome collaboration as a barrier. Some residents might hesitate to call the anaesthesiologist to provide epidural anaesthesia, especially at night. This might reduce the number of women with adequate pain relief. As one of the residents described:

'In our hospital, the residents are not allowed to independently consult the anaesthesiologist at night. We first have to call the obstetrician, and he or she has to consult the anaesthesiologist. It is a barrier for providing epidural anaesthesia at night.'

Clear agreements on availability of epidural analgesia are mentioned to be a facilitator in this situation.

The residents and midwives mentioned the presence of a strict hierarchy and wide variation in obstetrical policy between obstetricians as barriers for collaboration. The hierarchy causes some residents and midwives to be reluctant in providing feedback on a decision. An open attitude is essential in an obstetrical team. Residents add that the decision to perform a CS for non-progressing labour might also depend on the time (evening or night).

Domain V: The organizational context

Some barriers are specifically related to the Dutch obstetrical care system. All types of professionals mentioned there are no general agreements on the responsibility for mode of birth counselling. Some obstetricians feel they should be responsible for mode of birth counselling. One of the midwives described:

'Obstetricians are sometimes even angry that we already performed the mode of birth counselling and that the pregnant woman chose her mode of birth..'

In women with a previous CS, obstetricians and residents stated that, although a consultation in secondary care is preferred before 20 weeks of pregnancy, the current habit of referral to secondary care at 36 weeks of pregnancy seems too late for an adequate shared decision making process on mode of birth. Women are often already fully focussed on a particular mode of birth, which makes counselling by an obstetrician more difficult. Protocols for cooperation between first and secondary care, considering mode of birth counselling, as well as timing of referral, would facilitate optimal care.

Considering the use of additional diagnostics for evaluating the fetal condition during labour, prior to performing a CS for suspected fetal distress, there are several barriers perceived by residents and midwives. Fetal scalp blood sampling might be limited due to technical limitations during sample collection or sample assessment in laboratories. The procedure seems time consuming and often needs to be repeated. One of the residents adds:

> *'At first, we had to send the collected blood samples to the laboratory. After they bought a new device, approximately 3 out of 4 samples could not be analysed. You do not wish to experience that.'*

Domain VI: The financial/ legislation domain

Finally, almost all professionals mentioned that there is insufficient staffing and monetary compensation in order to provide continuous support to women during labour. One of the obstetricians mentions:

> *'In our hospital improved support during labour could reduce CS rates. However, we know upfront that an increase in staffing is not an option.'*

Discussion

Main findings

In order to improve CS care, and possibly lower the rate of unnecessary CS, a high level of adherence to evidence based clinical guidelines is required. We conducted a qualitative study to determine which factors influence the adherence to recommendations that have a direct effect on the decision to perform a CS. Among professionals, we identified 11 main facilitators and 38 main barriers for optimal care to previously developed quality indicators on mode of birth counselling, planned CS and prevention of (emergency) CS [13].

In our previous study on actual care, four groups of women with highest expected impact on improvement of care were identified: 1.women with a previous CS, 2. nulliparous women without continuous support during labour, 3.nulliparous women with an unplanned CS performed for suspected fetal distress without applying additional diagnostics (ST-analysis or fetal scalp blood sampling), and 4. nulliparous women with an unplanned CS performed for non-progressing labour without adequate waiting period (2–4 h) [13]. The barriers and facilitators will be discussed with regard to these target groups in order to apply these factors in an implementation strategy.

Regarding counselling women with a previous CS, professionals hesitate to allow women to be part of the decision making process, since they fear women are not equipped to decide on mode of birth when balancing risks and benefits for both their own health, that of their baby and a possible future pregnancy. A main facilitator for obstetricians and residents was detailed mode of birth counselling and clear documentation of the decision making process for mode of birth. This emphasizes the importance of adequately describing the counselling process and also to discuss exceptions or conditions to the agreed mode of birth. Structured counselling using decision aids can help to address women's anxiety. When the content of this counselling is agreed upon by both first and second line healthcare providers, variation in care between different healthcare providers is likely to reduce. The use of prediction models may help to individualise care.

Insufficient staffing due to lack of monetary compensation is mentioned as the main barrier to provide continuous support to women during labour. Although the Dutch ministry of Health encourages continuous support during labour, this is not realized in the majority of cases.

The main barriers mentioned for applying additional diagnostics prior to performing a CS for suspected fetal distress were a lack of technical skills, but also technical limitations during sample collection or sample assessment in laboratories. A structured training programme might improve care and technical skills. Furthermore, the failure rate during sample assessment might improve with the introduction of fetal scalp lactate sampling [16].

Several barriers and facilitators were mentioned regarding nulliparous women with an unplanned CS performed for non-progressing labour. For example, 24/7 availability of epidural analgesia is agreed upon, however this is not always implemented. Clear agreements on availability of epidural analgesia is mentioned to be a facilitator and might improve the number of women with adequate pain relief. The remarks stating that timing of a CS is partially based on the time of day suggests that availability of different healthcare providers is a clear barrier.

Interpretation

The present study is, to our knowledge, the first to analyse facilitators and barriers for optimal CS care with international guidelines as a basis. Chaillet et al. studied the implementation of guidelines on vaginal birth after CS in Quebec, Canada. They concluded that adoption of guidelines may be improved if local healthcare professionals' perceptions are considered [17]. In line with our study, others identified availability of equipment and staff, skill levels, acceptance of guidelines and women's motivations to be of influence [17, 18].

There are however, some factors that can be explained by cultural differences or local habits, for example economical, political or medico-legal concerns. In the study by Chaillet et al., obstetricians mentioned medico-legal concerns on several occasions as a barrier for optimal care [16]. This is not in line with our findings, probably due to differences in medico-legal habits. The study of Yazdizadeh et al., revealed several barriers regarding the economic and political domain, which may be explained by a differently regulated healthcare system in Iran [18].

The unique structure of the Dutch obstetrical care system entails several challenges for health care providers in terms of continuity of care, referral of pregnant women and responsibility of care. When considering the Dutch healthcare system, improved collaboration between midwives and obstetricians seems an important step in improvement of care.

Although evidence based guidelines are the basis of our obstetric management, the obstetrical healthcare professional is faced with multiple factors in a single patient. There is no clear protocol for a woman with multiple problems during birth, for example macrosomia and a prior CS in combination with suspected fetal distress during labour. That is starting point for discussing the concept of mindlines, first described by Gabbay et al. Mindlines are collectively reinforced, internalised tacid guidelines. These guidelines are based on personal experience, experience of colleagues, as well as interactions with colleagues, opinion leaders and patients and are often developed in early training. These mindlines can be modified e.g. based on brief reading or interaction with colleagues and individual patients. Protocols that are easily accessible as well as up to date are required to initially set and maintain mindlines. In order to change mindlines and keep them up to date, (local) opinion leaders might play an important role [19, 20]. In the current study we did not evaluate these mindlines. However, when considering CS in complex cases, one can imagine the importance of CS audits. An audit can promote the development and modification of mindlines, based on the discussion with colleagues.

Strengths and limitations

As framework for the interviews (Additional file 1), we used recommendations derived from evidence based guidelines on CS care, as described in the SIMPLE study [13]. Barriers and facilitators were explored for those factors that are considered as most important for measuring optimal CS care.

We invited different types of obstetric healthcare providers that might have an influence on the offered CS care to participate to this qualitative study: obstetricians, residents and midwives, respectively. Professionals from different types of hospitals and private practices from different Dutch regions participated to this study, thereby representing all different elements of Dutch obstetrical care. The different types of healthcare providers were interviewed separately, in order to let them speak without restraint. The main barriers and facilitators were frequently mentioned among all different types of professionals, suggesting that the identified barriers are useful for the development of a new implementation strategy.

Although a standardized method for the identification of barriers and facilitators was used, there are some limitations to this study. First, the analysis of the interviews is prone to interpretation bias. In order to reduce this bias, all interviews were interpreted by two independent reviewers, based on the theoretical model by Grol [14, 15].

Since the influencing factors were identified using a qualitative, explorative method, no quantitative conclusions can be justified by this method. Finally, this study is performed in a national setting. The interviews were based on previously developed quality indicators, derived from national and international guidelines. We identified some facilitators and barriers that are typical for the Dutch system, concerning the collaboration between first and secondary care: for example the responsibility for mode of birth counselling and barriers relating to the timing of referral from midwife to obstetrician. It is, however, in line with literature that there are barriers specific to regional habits and practice [17, 18]. With international guidelines as a basis, we consider most results to be potentially relevant for international use, since our results describe the availability of equipment and staff, acceptance of guidelines and women's motivations to be of influence in line with literature.

Conclusions

In light of the rising CS rate, clear facilitators and barriers for guideline adherence were identified at all domains, yet particularly on professional and organizational domain. Professionals should be aware of the identified barriers and facilitators and take these into account when implementing CS guidelines into daily practice.

Abbreviations

CS: Cesarean section; KNOV: Royal Dutch National Association of Midwifery; NVOG: Dutch Society of Obstetrics and Gynaecology; RCOG: Royal College of Obstetricians and Gynecologists; SIMPLE: Caesarean Section IMPLEmentation study

Acknowledgements

Not applicable.

Funding

This study was funded by zonMW (No 17100.3006). ZonMW had no influence on the design of the study, data collection, data analysis, data interpretation or the content of this manuscript.

Authors' contributions

All authors participated in the study design (SM, RS,CD,AK,JN, NS,HS,RH). SM, RS, HS and RH were responsible for drafting the manuscript. SM, RS, HS and

RH were responsible for the acquisition, analysis and interpretation of the data. All authors read and edited earlier versions of the manuscript and approved of the final version (SM, RS,CD,AK,JN, NS,HS,RH).

Authors' information

Not applicable.

Competing interests

All authors declare that they have no competing interests.

Author details

[1]Department of Obstetrics and Gynaecology, GROW- School for Oncology and Developmental Biology, Maastricht University Medical Centre, Maastricht, The Netherlands. [2]Department of Obstetrics and Gynaecology, Zuyderland Medical Centre, Heerlen, The Netherlands. [3]Department of Clinical Epidemiology and Medical Technology Assessment (KEMTA), CAPHRI- School for Public Health and Primary Care, Maastricht University Medical Centre, Maastricht, The Netherlands. [4]Department of Obstetrics and Gynaecology, University Medical Hospital Utrecht, Utrecht, The Netherlands. [5]Scientific Institute for Quality of Healthcare (IQ healthcare), Radboud University Nijmegen Medical Centre, Nijmegen, The Netherlands.

References

1. World Health Organization. Appropriate technology for birth. Lancet. 1985;2: 436–7.
2. D'Alton ME, Hehir MP. Cesarean delivery rates revisiting a 3-decades-old dogma. JAMA. 2015;314:2238–40.
3. Years perinatal registration in The Netherlands, 1999–2008. Utrecht: Foundation Perined The Netherlands; 2011.
4. Perinatal care in The Netherlands 2014. Utrecht: Foundation Perined The Netherlands, 2013.
5. The result counts hospitals. 2012. Health Care Inspectorate (IGZ) Netherlands. Ministry of Health, Welfare and Sport.
6. Kwee A, Elferink-Stinkens PM, Reuwer PJ, Bruinse HW. Trends in obstetric interventions in the Dutch obstetrical care system in the period 1993-2002. Eur J Obstet Gynecol Reprod Biol. 2007;132:70–5.
7. Deneux-Tharaux C, Carmona E, Bouvier-Colle MH, Breart G. Postpartum maternal mortality and cesarean delivery. Obstet Gynecol. 2006;108:541–8.
8. Shorten A. Maternal and neonatal effects of caesarean section. BMJ. 2007; 335:1003–4.
9. Yang Q, Wen SW, Oppenheimer L, Chen XK, Black D, Gao J, et al. Association of caesarean delivery for first birth with placenta praevia and placental abruption in second pregnancy. BJOG. 2007;114:609–13.
10. Heer IM, Kahlert S, Rummel S, Kumper C, Jonat W, Strauss A. Hospital treatment - is it affordable? A structured cost analysis of vaginal deliveries and planned caesarean sections. Eur J Med Res. 2009;14:502–6.
11. Bragg F, Cromwell DA, Edozien LC, Gurol-Urganci I, Mahmood TA, Templeton A, et al. Variation in rates of caesarean section among English NHS trusts after accounting for maternal and clinical risk: cross sectional study. BMJ. 2010;341:c5065.
12. NICE Clinical Guideline: Caesarean section. CG132. 23-11-2011.
13. Melman S, Schoorel ECN, De Boer K, Burggraaf H, Derks JB, Van Dijk D, et al. Development and measurement of guidelines-based quality indicators of caesarean section care in the Netherlands: a RAND-modified Delphi procedure and retrospective medical chart review. PloS One. 2016;11: e0145771. doi:10.1371/journal.pone.0145771.
14. Grol R. Beliefs and evidence in changing clinical practice. BMJ. 1997;315: 418–21.
15. Grol R. Improving the quality of medical care: building bridges among professional pride, payer profit, and patient satisfaction. JAMA. 2001;286: 2578 85.
16. East CE, Leader LR, Sheehan P, Henshall NE, Colditz PB, Lau R. Intrapartum fetal scalp lactate sampling for fetal assessment in the presence of a non-reassuring fetal heart rate trace. Cochrane Database Syst Rev. 2015;5: CD006174.
17. Chaillet N, Dube E, Dugas M, Francoeur D, Dube J, Gagnon S, et al. Identifying barriers and facilitators towards implementing guidelines to reduce caesarean section rates in Quebec. Bull World Health Organ. 2007;85: 791–7.
18. Yazdizadeh B, Nedjat S, Mohammad K, Rashidian A, Changizi N, Majdzadeh R. Cesarean section rate in Iran, multidimensional approaches for behavioral change of providers: a qualitative study. BMC Health Serv Res. 2011;11:159.
19. Gabbay J, le May A. Evidence based guidelines or collectively constructed "mindlines?" ethnographic study of knowledge management in primary care. BMJ. 2004;329:1013.
20. Wieringa S, Greenhalgh T. 10 years of mindlines: a systematic review and commentary. Implement Sci. 2015;10:45.

24

Clinicians' views of factors of importance for improving the rate of VBAC (vaginal birth after caesarean section): a study from countries with low VBAC rates

Ingela Lundgren[1*], Patricia Healy[2], Margaret Carroll[3], Cecily Begley[3], Andrea Matterne[4], Mechthild M. Gross[4], Susanne Grylka-Baeschlin[4], Jane Nicoletti[5], Sandra Morano[6], Christina Nilsson[1] and Joan Lalor[3]

Abstract

Background: Caesarean section (CS) rates are increasing worldwide and the most common reason is repeat CS following previous CS. For most women a vaginal birth after a previous CS (VBAC) is a safe option. However, the rate of VBAC differs in an international perspective. Obtaining deeper knowledge of clinicians' views on VBAC can help in understanding the factors of importance for increasing VBAC rates. Focus group interviews with clinicians and women in three countries with high VBAC rates (Finland, Sweden and the Netherlands) and three countries with low VBAC rates (Ireland, Italy and Germany) are part of "OptiBIRTH", an ongoing research project. The study reported here aims to explore the views of clinicians from countries with low VBAC rates on factors of importance for improving VBAC rates.

Methods: Focus group interviews were held in Ireland, Italy and Germany. In total 71 clinicians participated in nine focus group interviews. Five central questions about VBAC were used and interviews were analysed using content analysis. The analysis was performed in each country in the native language and then translated into English. All data were then analysed together and final categories were validated in each country.

Results: The findings are presented in four main categories with several sub-categories: 1) "prameters for VBAC", including the importance of the obstetric history, present obstetric factors, a positive attitude among those who are centrally involved, early follow-up after CS and antenatal classes; 2) "organisational support and resources for women undergoing a VBAC", meaning a successful VBAC requires clinical expertise and resources during labour; 3) "fear as a key inhibitor of successful VBAC", including understanding women's fear of childbirth, clinicians' fear of VBAC and the ways that clinicians' fear can be transferred to women; and 4) "shared decision making – rapport, knowledge and confidence", meaning ensuring consistent, realistic and unbiased information and developing trust within the clinician–woman relationship.

Conclusions: The findings indicate that increasing the VBAC rate depends on organisational factors, the care offered during pregnancy and childbirth, the decision-making process and the strategies employed to reduce fear in all involved.

Keywords: VBAC, CS, Clinicians, Focus groups, Qualitative study, Content analysis, Midwifery

* Correspondence: ingela.lundgren@gu.se
[1]Institute of Health and Care Sciences, Sahlgrenska Academy, University of Gothenburg, Box 457SE-405 30 Gothenburg, Sweden
Full list of author information is available at the end of the article

Background

Caesarean section (CS) rates are increasing in both resource-intense and resource-poor countries [1]; however, of concern is the variation in CS rates internationally. For example, in Europe, the Netherlands, Slovenia, Finland, Sweden, Iceland and Norway have rates below 20 %, whereas Italy and Cyprus have national CS rates of 38 and 52 % respectively [2].

As intervention rates continue to rise, concerns have emerged regarding the associated procedure-related risks in terms of maternal morbidity and mortality [3, 4]. In the absence of a robust justification of these increasing rates, an exploration of clinicians' attitudes to CS as a mode of birth is required [2, 5–7], since an understanding of the non-medical factors associated with the decision to perform a CS are becoming more important. These factors include maternal requests [8] and provider attitudes [9].

Also of interest is the variation in rates of the mode of birth such as elective repeat CS emergency CS in labour, and vaginal birth after previous CS (VBAC) following one previous CS. VBAC is an important mechanism for reducing the CS rate [10, 11] given that CS rates in nulliparous women are rising steadily. Based on a limited number of randomised trials comparing outcomes for women planning a repeat elective CS with those planning a vaginal birth [12], current evidence supports VBAC as a reasonable and safe option for most women [13]. VBAC is associated with a lower incidence of maternal mortality and a reduction in overall morbidities for mothers and babies [13]. Although evidence exists that for most women a VBAC is safe, practice varies significantly, with as few as 29–36 % of women in Ireland, Italy and Germany experiencing a VBAC compared with 45–55 % of women in Finland, Sweden and the Netherlands [14].

However, few studies about clinicians' views of VBAC have been done. According to clinicians in countries with high VBAC rates, the important factors for improving the VBAC rate are related to the structure of the maternity care system in the country, the cooperation between midwives and obstetricians, and the care offered during pregnancy and birth [15].

Given the concern that exists regarding increasing CS rates worldwide, and the limited evidence available on clinicians' views of VBAC, this study was designed to explore the views of clinicians from countries with low VBAC rates on factors of importance for improving VBAC rates.

Methods

As part of the ongoing OptiBIRTH study, which aims to increase VBAC rates [16], an exploration of clinicians' views of VBAC in three countries with low rates of VBAC was undertaken. A qualitative approach was employed, which is useful when little is known about the phenomenon of interest [17]. One method of collecting qualitative data is the focus group interview, which has its roots in social science and psychology. It is an efficient way to gather data from a group of individuals about their values and attitudes and the complex phenomena that originate from social interaction [18]. As the purpose of this phase of the study was to inform the development of an intervention to increase VBAC rates in countries with low rates, agreement was reached within the research team that the following five questions (which were generated by consensus) would be asked in the same order, in each site and in each country: What factors are important for VBAC? What are the barriers to VBAC? What is important to you as a professional? What are your views on shared decision making with women? How can women be supported to be confident with VBAC?

Settings

Data were collected using focus group interviews in nine sites – three in Ireland, Germany and Italy respectively – from both rural and urban locations. Although the countries differ in some respects with regard to how maternity care is provided, there are many similarities. For example, all countries provide maternity care free at the point of use through the public health care system; however, private models of maternity care also run in parallel. The key features of note are that the publicly funded model of care is predominantly medically led and that the women give birth in a hospital setting. These factors are important when considering the national CS rate for any country, since significant variations in CS rates have been identified at the unit level, depending on whether the woman attends the public system or utilises health insurance to attend an obstetrician privately [5].

In each country, women following one CS are required to attend an antenatal appointment with a consultant obstetrician to discuss the options for birth in the hospital where the birth is planned to take place.

Data collection and participants

Focus group interviews with clinicians were conducted during 2012–2013. In total, 71 clinicians participated; see Table 1. Clinicians were eligible for inclusion if they were involved in discussing VBAC and supporting women and their partners regarding the optimal mode of birth following previous CS. Clinicians who met the eligibility criteria – commonly midwives, obstetricians and neonatologists – were approached by researchers in each country (initials PH, AM, JN, MG), and if the clinicians expressed interest in participating in the study, they were offered an information leaflet and consent

Table 1 Characteristics of participants

Ireland	FGI 1 (rural)	11 (4 midwives, 4 consultant obstetricians, 1 neonatologist, 2 non-consultant hospital doctors)
	FGI 2 (urban)	8 (4 midwives, 2 consultant obstetricians, 2 non-consultant hospital doctors)
	FGI 3 (rural)	12 (7 midwives, 3 consultant obstetricians, 2 non-consultant hospital doctors)
Italy	FG 1 (urban)	9 (4 midwives, 5 obstetricians)
	FG 2 (urban)	7 (5 midwives, 2 obstetricians)
	FG 3 (urban)	7 (3 midwives, 4 obstetricians)
Germany	FGI 1 (urban)	6 (2 midwives, 4 obstetricians)
	FGI 2 (urban)	3 (1 midwife, 2 obstetricians)
	FGI 3 (urban)	8 (5 midwives, 3 obstetricians)

FGI (Focus group interviews)

form. The focus group interviews were held at a local site for the convenience of the participants.

Data analysis

When analysing the focus groups interviews, the authors were influenced by inductive conventional content analysis [19, 20]. In qualitative content analysis, the aim is to build a model to describe a phenomenon in a conceptual form, derived from the data [20]. Content analysis is a flexible, pragmatic method for developing and extending knowledge of the human experience of health and illness [19].

The focus group interviews were transcribed verbatim in the participants' native language. The following steps were used during analysis: selecting the units of analysis; making sense of the data as whole; conducting open coding; using coding sheets; and grouping, categorising and abstracting the data [20]. The units of analysis were the sections of the interview texts that answered the five questions. Each participating researcher (PH, JL, AM, MG, JN, SM) in the three countries did open coding in their native language, resulting in 5–10 subcategories per question. In order to ensure consistency, two researchers in each country coded the data independently and clarified any remaining inconsistencies. At this point, each country forwarded their preliminary analysis in English to the first author (IL) and CN for the datasets to be synthesised. This synthesis allowed for similarities between countries to be identified and equally for context-specific findings to be noted for the implementation phase of the OptiBIRTH trial. Again, to ensure consistency and accuracy of interpretation (a critical step in forwards and backwards translation) the research team held several Skype meetings in English to discuss the coding and the findings. Rigour was maintained through "peer debriefing" and repeated validation of the findings by all team members as the data analysis proceeded and the findings emerged. In order to identify the quotations by country of origin, the following identifiers are added: Ireland (IR), Germany (G) and Italy (IT).

Results

The findings are presented in four main categories: "parameters for VBAC", "organisational support and resources for women undergoing a VBAC", "fear as a key inhibitor of successful VBAC", and "shared decision making – rapport, knowledge and confidence". Each category contains a number of subcategories.

Parameters for VBAC

Successful VBAC depends on several factors, not least a careful consideration of the previous obstetric history, the present obstetric factors, a positive attitude in all who are centrally involved, and strategies such as early follow-up after the first CS and antenatal classes.

The importance of the obstetric history

A key theme that emerged is that not all women are suitable candidates for VBAC – hence the importance of the obstetric history (in particular, progress in a previous labour) and consideration of potential risk factors in the selection process. Of interest, clinicians in Ireland and Italy considered obesity to be a factor that militates against offering a VBAC.

> *A good history, I think, is very important, so that one really knows in preparation of the birth why the first was a CS, and discussions can take place at that point.* (G)

Clinicians in Ireland were also concerned as to whether the previous CS was planned or was an emergency procedure.

> *If you look at the outcomes ... the morbidity from an emergency CS is three times that of an elective one. So ... there isn't any massive benefit clinically in terms of*

> *reducing risk. Then you have the big risk of a very bad outcome [with a VBAC] hanging over you, which you don't get with an elective CS.* (IR)

Present obstetric circumstances

Even when a VBAC is planned early in pregnancy, the plan is often reviewed again as the woman approaches term and, in particular, if the pregnancy extends beyond the expected date of delivery. Although opinions varied on whether women should or should not be offered an induction of labour once the pregnancy is prolonged, clinicians expressed increasing concern about the associated risk of uterine rupture. Clinicians highlighted that even when a decision to induce labour is made, a level of uncertainty exists as to the best time to undertake the procedure.

> *I am happy to induce; are we happy to induce? I am in my own practice. I would prefer to induce them at T + 3 or 4 rather than let them go to T + 10 personally. ... I look at these women who have had one previous CS as normal, so I don't think about doing anything until they were postdates, as if they were normal.* (IR)

Although there was some discussion regarding the potential of a maternal request for VBAC, not all clinicians thought that the women should have an automatic right to choose their preferred option without consideration of the associated obstetric risks involved.

> *I think that women shouldn't have a right to choose a vaginal birth after CS. The decision should be the result of an overall evaluation, which can't exclude vaginal birth. A process of assessment of suitability is necessary, leaving flexibility for the clinician.* (IT)

A positive attitude to VBAC in all who are centrally involved

Clinicians indicated that for VBAC to be successful, the woman must be motivated and willing to consider the options. Clinicians in Ireland were keen to stress that even when a woman has an open mind towards VBAC, the final decision on the mode of birth cannot be made until late in the pregnancy. Clinicians in Italy suggested careful evaluation of the woman's suitability for VBAC is required. Clinicians in Ireland indicated they were positively disposed to supporting a woman to have a VBAC if they had laboured previously, and were enthusiastic about supporting these women to labour.

> *At the first visit, I always put down are they open minded about it or are they keen for CS. And if they are keen for another CS, I put down: "Not un-keen on another CS". ... If they are open minded, you can play along with them, like if they come in spontaneous labour.* (IR)

Clinicians indicated that the impact of a negative attitude towards VBAC among their colleagues should not be underestimated as a potential barrier to increasing the rate of VBAC. This was particularly the case for those working alongside clinicians in private practice. In addition to hospital-based colleagues, clinicians in Ireland found the support, or lack thereof, from the family doctor, known as the GP (general practitioner), as crucial in achieving a successful VBAC.

> *The GP is vital because there are some GPs who will send the women in and say: "She had a CS last time and I really feel she needs a CS this time" at 6 weeks of gestation. They are not always a barrier. There are some who are very supportive and some who are extremely negative. If the GP will support you, then you are in business.* (IR)

Supporting women to have a VBAC requires a positive attitude, good teamwork and sufficient experienced staff available to ensure success. Clinicians commented that the obstetric and midwifery staff must be convinced that it is possible for carefully selected women to give birth vaginally after a previous CS, and must cooperate with each other in supporting these women to achieve success. If this is not the case, then the woman may lose confidence in her ability to give birth vaginally.

> *A woman was sure she wanted to give birth with a VBAC, but the obstetrician wanted her to sign an informed consent where he wrote that, despite his having explained all the risks of VBAC, the woman wanted to deliver vaginally and that he was available for CS any time during labour. The woman's husband was shocked. After all this, the woman started saying: "Perhaps a CS would be better!" Everything went well, but the woman spent the whole time wondering if she was doing the right thing.* (IT)

The family and the social environment are also influential in the decision-making process. Women are influenced by family members and require a level of determination to achieve a VBAC. Hence, clinicians in Germany reported that it is important to know that the woman herself is motivated to achieve a VBAC.

> *Yes, quite clearly also the motivation of the partner, the woman's attending gynaecologist, the motivation of the midwife who leads the antenatal class, the motivation of female friends who have had a CS, who say that a spontaneous delivery was possible and somehow went well.* (G)

Early follow-up and antenatal classes

The topic of the potential for a VBAC in the future should be raised soon after the first CS birth (including information about why the CS was required), to "sow the seeds" and increase a woman's confidence for giving birth vaginally next time.

> *Well, actually, you would have to begin in prenatal care because that is when you have the first contact with the woman, perhaps even after the first CS. That you somehow make it clear to her that it does not mean that your second child also needs to come into the world by CS; you can also give birth naturally.* (G)

Clinicians in Ireland and Italy also commented that focused antenatal education classes, targeted at encouraging VBAC as an option, would offer the opportunity to provide women with consistent evidence-based information. It was suggested that these classes might include the participation of women who have already experienced a VBAC, either face to face or through sharing a recorded interview, in order to inspire the other women and reawaken a confidence in their potential to give birth vaginally.

Organisational support and resources for women undergoing a VBAC

A successful VBAC requires clinical expertise and resources during labour.

VBAC requires clinical expertise

The staff must also have the requisite clinical experience in caring for women labouring after a previous caesarean section. Clinicians in Italy raised concerns that changes to obstetric training in the past decade have led to more clinicians choosing to sub-specialise in areas other than labour ward management, such as fertility and endoscopic surgery. Maintaining an appropriate level of competence in managing VBAC in a culture that favours sub-specialisation may be problematic in the future.

> *Nobody can tell what will happen during a trial of labour (TOL), so we should say that a TOL is possible, but only if we have staff who are not overworked and exhausted.* (IT)

Obstetricians in Italy reported that in the past few decades, many have left the field of obstetrics in favour of other specialities with fewer unsocial working hours and higher remuneration packages. They indicated that lack of training due to the very low VBAC rates has an impact on clinical competence and consequently on the potential to increase VBAC rates.

> *Nowadays we can see how the culture has affected the training of residents [junior obstetricians]. For residents, a previous CS means another CS. They have to be told that a woman can have a VBAC.* (IT)

However, clinicians in Italy emphasised that it is critical that VBACs are undertaken in a unit with expertise to support these women in labour. If that proficiency or experience is not available, then it is safer to repeat the CS.

> *The patient shouldn't get to a hospital where she'll find a negative attitude to VBAC.* (IT)

VBAC requires resources during labour

Clinicians' attitudes to and confidence in caring for women having a VBAC do vary, but appropriate staffing of birthing suites by those with relevant expertise was considered essential by the Irish and German clinicians.

> *If you come on duty and you know you have someone who is having a trial of labour and there is another midwife who is very confident at that too, that is reassuring for you too. ... And it goes back to staffing levels and to managers on the labour ward.* (IR)

In Ireland, it was suggested that specific expertise in managing VBAC is required. This could be achieved through the provision and staffing of a dedicated area to monitor these women in labour. In addition, such an area must have speedy access to an operating theatre in case a repeat CS is required.

> *We need a place for the group of VBAC women, something between the labour ward and the antenatal ward.* (IR)

Fear as a key inhibitor of successful VBAC

Understanding women's fear of labour and vaginal birth is a key component in successful VBAC. Fear in clinicians may also be transferred to the women and may influence the outcome.

Understanding women's fear of childbirth

Clinicians reported that fear of childbirth after a previously traumatic birth experience is a key component, and it is important to understand the basis of that fear when discussing VBAC with women.

> *You have to think about what the fear is really about. Is the fear about pain or is the fear about having a labour, getting to 8 cm, getting stuck and then having an emergency section?* (IR)

A previous negative or traumatic birth experience is highly influential, and following up after the first birth is therefore critical. A previous negative childbirth experience with a long labour that ended up in an emergency CS was considered to be a barrier by clinicians in Italy. The clinicians in Germany stated that if women have a negative or traumatic first birth experience (for example, emergency CS or a baby born in poor condition), in an effort to avoid a repeat of this experience some women ask for an elective CS with the next pregnancy.

> *I find the idea to reflect on the first birth quite good. .... If I know that the woman had a traumatic birth experience, I would tell her: "Listen, go home. I would like to see you in 6 weeks and again in 3 months." Time enough to process the first birth. And when she is pregnant again, the issue must be revisited, simply to process it.* (G)

However, as a woman approaches term, clinicians indicated that, in their experience, the woman's resolve may weaken as she acquiesces to outside influences such as family and information sources on the Internet.

> *Sometimes it is not even us; it is not the mother. Sometimes it is the mother's mother and her sister and all that out there [general agreement], and they come in with all the baggage into the clinic. They are all set up for a VBAC and they come into the clinic at 37 weeks freaking out, even though they are all set up for a VBAC and you are really in trouble then. It is very, very difficult to handle that "I am afraid, I am reading this". And it is the Internet, it's Dr. Google.* (IR)

Understanding clinicians' fear of VBAC

The reassurance that VBAC is possible requires that the treating clinician also believes that this is the case and adopts an evidence-based approach to care planning and delivery. Despite a personal belief in the value of increasing VBAC rates, clinicians in Ireland and Italy also feared the consequences (personally) of a poor neonatal outcome.

> *The medico-legal issues in Ireland are probably adverse compared with Sweden, where there is absolutely no chance of you being sued over a VBAC. ... A high VBAC rate with a poor neonatal outcome is not acceptable. We live in a small community. ... Your reputation is important. If you have a serious event, everyone knows and keeps talking about it for about 6 months ... no one will give you a gold medal for a VBAC rate of 95 % if you make one mistake. It's a cultural issue; the culture in Ireland is they [women in the community] keep talking and keep talking, and if the mother requests a planned CS, it's very hard to refuse.* (IR)

Therefore, shared decision making between the clinician and the woman is a critical factor in achieving a VBAC, and having a fearful mother and a reluctant clinician will not bode well for success. If women are informed of the evidence indicating that VBAC is a safe option and are included in the decision, then it is harder for them to think of suing the obstetrician following an adverse outcome.

> *Fear is very negative during labour. The obstetrician's anxiety is transferred to the woman in labour, who hasn't got the will she had before labour ... after being in labour for a long time, the woman goes in the operating theatre and she hasn't achieved her goal.* (IT)

Clinicians' fear can be transferred to women

Clinicians in Germany indicated that their personal attitude to and motivation for VBAC are important, in both public and private practice settings. The clinicians in Germany were of the opinion that clinicians' self-confidence is important because if the clinicians are confident, they will transfer this feeling to the women. Furthermore, if obstetricians are not authentic in their support for VBAC, the clinicians also believed that women sense that too.

> *Whereas I do believe that they are sensitive to our personal attitudes. They are very sensitive and know: "She is quite confident" and "That is okay", or if they themselves think: "Oh, they are all standing there". That creates, I think, uncertainty. ... And I think that it transfers quite quickly, before you know it yourself. Maybe a wrinkled nose; they already get the impression ... before we are actually aware of it. So I think that our personal attitude is not to be underestimated as we approach the women. I believe that being genuine is still very important.* (G)

Clinicians in Ireland expressed concern as to who was fearful of VBAC – the woman or the clinician. Clinicians in Italy mentioned that clinicians should aim to control their anxiety. If not, midwives, for instance, may be called on to manage "triple anxiety": their own, the obstetrician's and the woman's.

> *A midwife is the link between the woman and the doctor, and if [the midwife] often normally is a little bit anxious, you can imagine if the woman has had a previous CS. The anxiety of the midwife is double; the*

obstetrician will enter the room and ask: "Is there progress? Only 1 cm?" It is a kind of anxiety that is difficult to manage: it is difficult to work impartially while dealing with the woman's anxiety, the obstetrician's anxiety and your own anxiety! (IT)

Shared decision making between women and clinicians – rapport, knowledge and confidence

Shared decision making requires consistent, realistic and unbiased information, and trust within the clinician–woman relationship.

Providing consistent, realistic and unbiased information

For women to make an informed choice, the information they receive must be factually correct and readily accessible. While all the clinicians agreed that women should be made aware that VBAC is an option, it is also important to address the risks and to highlight that a repeat CS is also a potential outcome.

These women must be informed about everything – what being in labour involves after a CS, what is involved in a repeat CS – because it wouldn't be fair if we only talked about the risks [of VBAC] and not about what will happen with a repeat CS. (IT)

However, clinicians in Ireland thought that having faith in her obstetrician was highly influential in the woman's decision-making process.

The presence of her own personal obstetrician [is important]. I think it is an issue certainly with the small number of patients who are private ... they want to know that you are going to be there. I think if you are transferring a patient to your colleague and they have only met you during the visits: "Oh look, just do a CS on the Thursday before you go on holidays". ... I think the barrier is the uncertainty about who is going to be looking after them. (IR)

Trust within the clinician–woman relationship

Clinicians in Ireland and Germany suggested that giving information early in the pregnancy helps to build a woman's confidence that she can achieve a VBAC. It can also help her to view VBAC as the "norm", which is vital.

Not many of them will make a decision at the first point of contact. They will want to go home and have a think about it. If we don't start the discussion at the booking. ... The idea is to have the decision taken before 36 weeks. (IR)

Consequently, a relationship between the woman and the clinician that is based on trust is important to success, and a high level of continuity of carer is essential if this relationship is to be maintained. In the Italian context, a woman who would like a VBAC should be looked after by either her obstetrician or a pro-VBAC obstetrician when she is in labour. If the obstetrician in charge on the day is not pro-VBAC, the likelihood of success is diminished.

Continuity of care is of fundamental importance. If a colleague and I believe in VBAC, when a woman wants to have a VBAC, we have to be on duty when that woman is in labour; otherwise, it will be a total failure. (IT)

Therefore, when continuity of carer is not feasible, the clinicians suggested that a plan for the birth needs to be clearly documented in the woman's case notes.

It is very important that the plan that is made between woman and clinician is documented because of different people [on duty], different consultants, different registrars ... as we do not cover the labour ward over 24 hours with the same person/consultant. (IR)

There was much debate within the focus groups as to whether the woman should ultimately have the choice to request a VBAC or indeed a repeat CS given the risks associated with both options. Ultimately there was agreement that a shared decision was in the best interest of all concerned. It was also suggested that midwives and partners should be part of the process, to maximise support for the woman in labour.

Discussion

Strengths and limitations

Using a qualitative approach can result in a deep understanding of the phenomenon being explored. This method is preferable when little is known beforehand about the topic [20]. The qualitative approach selected meant that we were able to generate a dataset across three countries with a range of professionals for comparison. However, when seeking depth, the researcher often has to sacrifice on achieving a large sample size, thereby limiting the generalisability of the findings. As for all qualitative studies, the findings must be interpreted in relation to the study's context [21]. To facilitate transferability to other contexts, the researcher should clearly describe the context, selection and characteristics of the participants, the method or methods of data collection and the process of analysis [20, 21], which we sought to do.

A limitation with a focus group is that some participants may be invisible as a result of others wielding more influence in the group. In contrast, individual interviews permit all participants to take part in the same way [18]. However, in this study, since the participants had volunteered to take part because of their interest in the subject, all of them actively contributed to the discussion.

Interpretation

Parameters for consideration for VBAC include a careful consideration of the previous obstetric history and present obstetric circumstances, both factors identified as being of critical importance. Clinicians acknowledged that not all women are suitable for VBAC, and in certain circumstances such as limited VBAC experience among available staff, the option to undertake a repeat elective CS is preferred. The extent to which maternal requests for CS for non-medical reasons impact on CS rates is a contentious issue [22], with comparison across studies posing a challenge owing to the wide variations in what is understood by the term "maternal request" [23]. Clinicians indicated that maternal requests for elective CS were often due to a lack of robust information on VBAC combined with a woman's fear of childbirth. The solutions suggested by clinicians are to address the knowledge deficit, to instigate routine debriefing around the previous birth and to encourage women to keep an open mind around the mode of birth. Clinicians spoke about the value of evidence in making decisions about the mode of birth, but were very clear that they took into account many other factors in their decision-making process. Studies have found that significant variations in the rates of attempted VBAC [24] suggest that the decision-making process around the birth mode after a previous CS is complicated and multidimensional for both women and care providers, and this certainly was the case for the clinicians in this study. According to a meta-synthesis of the views of women, they need evidence-based information on both the risks and the positive aspects of VBAC [25]. Some of the findings in our study highlight that an understanding of the impact of personal opinion and the consequent variation in practice is critical for clinicians when interpreting CS and VBAC rates, since this understanding is likely to influence the guidance women receive when exploring their options for birth.

A number of the clinicians indicated that the decision-making process should begin immediately following the first CS. Without some discussion around the birth and the necessity for the CS, women may develop a fear of childbirth and may be more likely to request a CS in a subsequent pregnancy. However, evidence to support the practice of early processing of previous birth experiences is yet to be generated. Previous traumatic birth experiences are related to future fear of childbirth [26, 27], and clinicians in this study spoke of the need to understand this fear by offering women opportunities to tell their birth story; in this way, the women have a way to share, understand and integrate their fears, concerns or feelings of disappointment, and missing pieces of information [28].

Our findings highlight that organisational support and resources for women undergoing VBAC are of importance, including both the clinical expertise and the resources for monitoring these women during labour. Definitions of one-to-one support in labour differ [29], but continuous support in labour has been shown to reduce CS and instrumental vaginal births [30]. Clinicians in this study cautioned that women labouring with a previously scarred uterus have a unique set of risks and therefore do require close one-to-one support and supervision in labour. Previous studies agree with the general consensus of opinion among participating clinicians in this study that women planning a VBAC should be cared for in a suitably staffed and equipped delivery suite, with readily available recourse to facilities for a CS and neonatal resuscitation should the need arise in line with professional guidance [31–33]. However, some clinicians reported that due to sub-specialisation in obstetric training, the availability of expertise in this area of labour management is in decline.

According to the present study, fear around VBAC may not just be an issue for women, but may also be a concern for clinicians. A study showed that the likelihood of undergoing a VBAC was increased in women cared for by obstetricians with low levels of anxiety [9]. Dahlen [34] emphasised that an important part of professional competence is achieving the balance between a fear of complications and a faith in the birthing process. Our data indicate that part of maintaining that balance is establishing who is fearful of VBAC (the woman or the clinician) and why. Such understanding could be promoted in maternity units by giving clinicians the time and the opportunity for mutual reflection on their clinical practice and for debriefing after adverse events.

Fear of litigation and increasing risk aversion have become common issues affecting clinical decision making [3, 35]. The participants spoke repeatedly about safety as a central issue around the mode of birth choices after previous CS, without perhaps appreciating fully all the dangers of repeat CS [13]. Participating clinicians would only support increasing VBAC rates if the risks of maternal and neonatal morbidity were acceptable in their eyes.

Good relationships and shared decision making between women and clinicians were vital when making decisions around VBAC. Women have consistently cited care providers as having significant external influence on the decisions they make during pregnancy [36, 37].

However, there is a growing body of evidence to suggest that clinicians and women conceptualise and interpret risk differently, with each bringing their own experiences and biases to the discussion [38–41]. Goodall et al. [40] have described similar variations between what women want to know and what health professionals believe that they should know. These variations can lead to challenges, with the lack of concordance between the expectations and preferences of women and those of clinicians potentially impacting negatively on building a trusting relationship.

Women require evidence-based information about the positive aspects of VBAC and their body's ability to birth normally [42] if they are to be supported in making truly informed decisions regarding the mode of birth following CS. Clinicians should be sensitive to the fact that in addition to appraising hard data based on risk, women are frequently influenced by the obstetrician's personal values, attitudes, experiences and expectations of birth when making decisions. Women are also influenced by the relationships they have with friends, family and other sources of maternity information, and the impact of these influences on the decision-making process should not be underestimated.

Conclusion

According to clinicians in low VBAC countries, in seeking to improve the VBAC rate, careful consideration of the parameters for VBAC is of importance. A careful obstetric history, a positive attitude by all centrally involved and strategies such as early follow-up after the first CS require attention. If VBAC rates are to increase, organisational support and resources for women undergoing VBAC, including clinical expertise and resources during labour, are central to achieving a successful outcome. Fear is a key inhibitor of successful VBAC; therefore, understanding both women's and clinicians' fear is critical. Shared decision making requires the availability of consistent, realistic and unbiased information, as well as a trusting relationship between the woman and her clinician. Some of these findings are in line with a similar study with clinicians in high VBAC countries [15] – for example, trust in the clinician–woman relationship, a positive attitude of all centrally involved, early follow-up and fear reduction [15]. However, according to the study from the high VBAC countries, adopting a common approach, ensuring good cooperation between midwives and obstetricians, having the final decision on the mode of delivery made by obstetricians while still involving women, and strengthening women's trust in VBAC are aspects that promote VBAC [15], but these aspects were not mentioned by the clinicians in the present study. These factors indicate a major difference between the views and attitudes of clinicians in countries with low VBAC rates and the views and attitudes of clinicians in high VBAC countries, a difference that would warrant consideration.

Acknowledgements

We would like to thank the clinicians who took part in these interviews, and the whole of the OptiBIRTH team.

Funding

We are grateful to the European Commission for funding this study under the European Union's Seventh Framework Programme (FP7/2007-2013) through grant agreement no. 305208. The opinions expressed here are those of the study team and are not necessarily those of the European Commission.

Authors' contributions

PH, MC and JL conducted the interviews in Ireland; SM and JN in Italy; and AM and MG in Germany. PH, MC, JL, SM, JN, AM and MG transcribed the interviews in their native language and analysed up to the first step. IL and CN did the analysis after this point, and then verified the analysis with PH, MC, JL, SM, JN, AM, SG-B, MG and CB. IL and JL drafted the manuscript. All authors commented on and agreed on the final version.

Competing interests

The authors declare that they have no competing interests.

Author details

[1]Institute of Health and Care Sciences, Sahlgrenska Academy, University of Gothenburg, Box 457SE-405 30 Gothenburg, Sweden. [2]School of Nursing and Midwifery, National University of Ireland, Upper Newcastle Road, Galway, Ireland. [3]School of Nursing and Midwifery, Trinity College Dublin, 24 D'Olier Street, Dublin 2, Ireland. [4]Midwifery Research and Education Unit, Hannover Medical School, Carl-Neuberg-Str. 1, 30625 Hannover, Germany. [5]Universita Degli Studi di Genova, Via Balbi 5, 16126 Genova, Italy. [6]IRCCS Azienda Ospedaliera Universitaria S. Martino IST, Largo R. Benzi, 10 16132 Genova, Italy.

References

1. World Health Organization. WHO statement of caesarean section rates. Geneva. 2015. http://who.int/reproductivehealth/publications/maternal_perinatal_health/cs-statement/en. Accessed 10 Aug 2016.
2. EURO-PERISTAT. European perinatal health report: health and care of pregnant women and babies in Europe in 2010. Paris. 2013. http://www.europeristat.com/reports/european-perinatal-health-report-2010.html. Accessed 10 Aug 2016.
3. Fuglenes D, Øian P, Kristiansen IS. Obstetricians' choice of cesarean delivery in ambiguous cases: is it influenced by risk attitude or fear of complaints and litigation? Am J Obstet Gynecol. 2009;200(48):e1–8.
4. Lutomski J, Murphy M, Devane D, Meaney S, Greene R. Private health care coverage and increased risk of obstetric intervention. BMC Pregnancy Childbirth. 2014;14:13.
5. Gross MM, Matterne A, Berlage S, Kaiser A, Lack N, Macher-Heidrich S, et al. Interinstitutional variations in mode of birth after a previous caesarean section: a cross-sectional study in six German hospitals. J Perinat Med. 2015; 43(2):177–84.
6. Hanley GE, Janssen PA, Greyson D. Regional variation in the caesarean delivery and assisted vaginal delivery rates. Obstet Gynecol. 2010;115(6):1201–8.
7. Monari F, Di Mario S, Facchinetti F, Basevi V. Obstetricians' and midwives' attitudes towards caesarean section. Birth. 2008;35(2):129–35.

8. Dweik D, Girasek E, Mészáros G, Töreki A, Keresztúri A, Pál A. Non-medical determinants of cesarean section in a medically dominated maternity system. Acta Obstet Gynecol Scand. 2014;93(10):1025–33.
9. Yee LM, Liu LY, Grobman WA. Relationship between obstetricians' cognitive and affective traits and delivery outcomes among women with a prior cesarean. Am J Obstet Gynecol. 2015;213(3):413. e1–7.
10. Sabol B, Denman MA, Guise JM. Vaginal birth after cesarean: an effective method to reduce cesarean. Clin Obstet Gynecol. 2015;58(2):309–19.
11. Cheng Y, Eden K, Marshall P, Pereira L, Caughey A, Guise J-M. Delivery after prior caesarean: maternal morbidity and mortality. Clin Perinatol. 2011;38(2):297–309.
12. Dodd JM, Crowther CA, Huertas E, Guise JM, Horey D. Planned elective repeat caesarean section versus planned vaginal birth for women with a previous caesarean birth. Cochrane Database Syst Rev. 2013;12:CD004224.
13. Guise J-M, Eden K, Emeis C, Denman MA, Marshall N, Fu R, et al. Vaginal birth after cesarean: new insights. Evidence reports/technology assessment No. 191. Rockville: Agency for Healthcare Research and Quality; 2010.
14. EURO-PERISTAT. European perinatal health report. Paris. 2008. http://www.europeristat.com/reports/european-perinatal-health-report2004.html. Accessed 10 Aug 2016.
15. Lundgren I, van Limbeek E, Vehvilainen-Julkunen K, Nilsson C. Clinicians' views of factors of importance for improving the rate of VBAC (vaginal birth after caesarean section): a qualitative study from countries with high VBAC rates. BMC Pregnancy Childbirth. 2015;15:196.
16. Clarke M, Savage G, Smith V, Daly D, Devane D, Gross M, et al. Improving the organisation of maternal health service delivery and optimising childbirth by increasing vaginal birth after caesarean section through enhanced women-centred care (OptiBIRTH trial): study protocol for a randomised controlled trial (ISRCTN10612254). Trials. 2015;16:542.
17. Morse JM, Field PA. Nursing research: the application of qualitative approaches. 2nd ed. Cheltenham: Nelson Thornes; 2002.
18. Barbour R. Focus groups. In: Bourgeault I, Dingwall R, de Vries R, editors. Qualitative methods in health research. London: Sage; 2010. p. 327–52.
19. Hsieh H-F, Shannon S. Three approaches to qualitative content analysis. Qual Health Res. 2005;15:1277–88.
20. Elo S, Kynga H. The qualitative content analysis process. J Adv Nurs. 2011; 62(1):107–15.
21. Graneheim UH, Lundman B. Qualitative content analysis in nursing research: concepts, procedures and measures to achieve trustworthiness. Nurse Educ Today. 2004;24:105–12.
22. Lavender T, Hofmeyr J, Neilson J, Kingdon C, Gyte G. Caesarean section for non-medical reasons at term. Cochrane Database Syst Rev. 2012;3:CD004660.
23. D'Souza R. Caesarean section on maternal request for non-medical reasons: putting the UK national institute of health and clinical excellence guidelines in perspective. Best Pract Res Clin Obstet Gynaecol. 2013;27:165–77.
24. Lundgren I, Begely C, Gross M, Bondas T. "Groping through the fog": VBAC (vaginal birth after casearean section) – a meta synthesis about women's experiences. BMC Pregnancy Childbirth. 2012;12:85.
25. Macfarlane AJ, Blondel B, Mohangoo AD, Cuttini M, Nijhuis J, Novak Z, et al. Wide differences in mode of delivery within Europe: risk-stratified analyses of aggregated routine data from the euro-peristat study. BJOG. 2015;123(4):559–68. doi:10.1111/1471-0528.13284.
26. Størksen H, Garthus-Niegel S, Vangen S, Eberhard-Gran M. The impact of previous birth experiences on maternal fear of childbirth. Acta Obstet Gynecol Scand. 2013;92(3):318–24.
27. Nilsson C. The delivery room: is it a safe place? a hermeneutic analysis of women's negative birth experiences. Sex Reprod Healthc. 2014;5(4):199–204.
28. Callister LC. Making meaning: women's birth narratives. J Obstet Gynecol Neonatal Nurs. 2004;33(4):508–18.
29. Sosa G, Crozier K, Robinson J. What is meant by one-to-one support in labour: analysing the concept. Midwifery. 2012;28(4):451–7.
30. Hodnett ED, Gates S, Hofmeyr GJ, Sakala C. Continuous support for women during childbirth. Cochrane Database Syst Rev. 2012;10:CD003766.
31. Lieberman E, Ernst EK, Rooks JP, Stapleton S, Flamm B. Results of the national study of vaginal birth after cesarean in birth centers. Obstet Gynecol. 2004;104(5):933–42.
32. American College of Obstetricians & Gynecologists. Vaginal birth after previous caesarean delivery. Obstet Gynecol. 2004;104(1):203–11.
33. Royal College of Obstetricians & Gynaecologists. Birth after previous caesarean birth. In: Green-top guideline no. 45. 1st ed. London: RCOG Press; 2007.
34. Dahlen H. Undone by fear? deluded by trust? Midwifery. 2010;26(2):156–62.
35. Hopkins K. Are Brazilian women really choosing caesarean section? Soc Sci Med. 2000;51:725–40.
36. Eden K, Hashima J, Osterweil P, Nygren P, Guise JM. Childbirth preferences after caesarean birth: a review of the evidence. Birth. 2004;31:46–60.
37. Emmett C, Shaw A, Montgomery A, Murphy DJ, DiAMOND Study Group. Women's experience of decision making about mode of delivery after a previous caesarean section: the role of health professionals and information about health risks. BJOG. 2006;113:1438–45.
38. Edwards A, Elwyn G, Mulley A. Explaining risks: turning numerical data into meaningful pictures. BMJ. 2002;324:827–30.
39. Fagerlin A, Wang C, Ubel P. Reducing the influence of anecdotal reasoning on people's healthcare decisions: is a picture worth a thousand statistics? Med Decis Making. 2005;25:398–405.
40. Goodhall K, McVittie C, Magill M. Birth choice following primary caesarean section: mothers' perceptions of the influence of health professionals on decision-making. J Reprod Infant Psychol. 2009;27(1):4–114.
41. Kaimal A, Kupperman M. Understanding risk, patient and provider preferences, and obstetrical decision making: approach to delivery after cesarean. Semin Perinatol. 2010;34(5):331–6.
42. Nilsson C, Lundgren I, Smith V, Vehvilinen-Julkunen K, Nicoletti J, Devane D, et al. Women-centred interventions to increase vaginal birth after caesarean section (VBAC): a systematic review. Midwifery. 2015;31:657–63.

Permissions

All chapters in this book were first published in P&C, by BioMed Central; hereby published with permission under the Creative Commons Attribution License or equivalent. Every chapter published in this book has been scrutinized by our experts. Their significance has been extensively debated. The topics covered herein carry significant findings which will fuel the growth of the discipline. They may even be implemented as practical applications or may be referred to as a beginning point for another development.

The contributors of this book come from diverse backgrounds, making this book a truly international effort. This book will bring forth new frontiers with its revolutionizing research information and detailed analysis of the nascent developments around the world.

We would like to thank all the contributing authors for lending their expertise to make the book truly unique. They have played a crucial role in the development of this book. Without their invaluable contributions this book wouldn't have been possible. They have made vital efforts to compile up to date information on the varied aspects of this subject to make this book a valuable addition to the collection of many professionals and students.

This book was conceptualized with the vision of imparting up-to-date information and advanced data in this field. To ensure the same, a matchless editorial board was set up. Every individual on the board went through rigorous rounds of assessment to prove their worth. After which they invested a large part of their time researching and compiling the most relevant data for our readers.

The editorial board has been involved in producing this book since its inception. They have spent rigorous hours researching and exploring the diverse topics which have resulted in the successful publishing of this book. They have passed on their knowledge of decades through this book. To expedite this challenging task, the publisher supported the team at every step. A small team of assistant editors was also appointed to further simplify the editing procedure and attain best results for the readers.

Apart from the editorial board, the designing team has also invested a significant amount of their time in understanding the subject and creating the most relevant covers. They scrutinized every image to scout for the most suitable representation of the subject and create an appropriate cover for the book.

The publishing team has been an ardent support to the editorial, designing and production team. Their endless efforts to recruit the best for this project, has resulted in the accomplishment of this book. They are a veteran in the field of academics and their pool of knowledge is as vast as their experience in printing. Their expertise and guidance has proved useful at every step. Their uncompromising quality standards have made this book an exceptional effort. Their encouragement from time to time has been an inspiration for everyone.

The publisher and the editorial board hope that this book will prove to be a valuable piece of knowledge for researchers, students, practitioners and scholars across the globe.

List of Contributors

Amy J. Hobbs
Cumming School of Medicine, Department of Community Health Sciences, University of Calgary, TRW Building 3rd Floor, 3280 Hospital Drive NW, Calgary, Alberta T2N 4Z6, Canada

Cynthia A. Mannion and Meredith Brockway
Faculty of Nursing, University of Calgary, 2800 University Way NW, Calgary, AB T2N1N4, Canada

Sheila W. McDonald
Cumming School of Medicine, Department of Paediatrics, University of Calgary, 2888 Shaganappi Trail NW, Calgary, Alberta T3B 6A8, Canada

Suzanne C. Tough
Cumming School of Medicine, Department of Community Health Sciences, University of Calgary, TRW Building 3rd Floor, 3280 Hospital Drive NW, Calgary, Alberta T2N 4Z6, Canada
Cumming School of Medicine, Department of Paediatrics, University of Calgary, 2888 Shaganappi Trail NW, Calgary, Alberta T3B 6A8, Canada

C. Nilsson
Faculty of Caring Science, Work Life and Social Welfare, University of Borås, S-501 90 Borås, Sweden
Institute of Health and Care Sciences, The Sahlgrenska Academy at University of Gothenburg, Gothenburg, SE, Sweden

A. Dencker, E. Jangsten, M. Mollberg, H. Patel, C. Sparud-Lundin and H. Wigert
Institute of Health and Care Sciences, The Sahlgrenska Academy at University of Gothenburg, Gothenburg, SE, Sweden

E. Hessman and H. Sjöblom
Biomedical Library, Gothenburg University Library at University of Gothenburg, Gothenburg, SE, Sweden

C. Begley
Institute of Health and Care Sciences, The Sahlgrenska Academy at University of Gothenburg, Gothenburg, SE, Sweden
Chair of Nursing and Midwifery, School of Nursing and Midwifery,Trinity College Dublin, 24, D'Olier St. Dublin 2, Dublin, Ireland

Shu-Wen Chen
Deakin University, Faculty of Health, School of Nursing and Midwifery, Geelong, Australia
National Taipei University of Nursing and Health Science, School of Nursing, Taipei, Taiwan

Alison M. Hutchinson
Deakin University, Faculty of Health, School of Nursing and Midwifery, Geelong, Australia
Centre for Quality and Patient Safety Research-Monash Health Partnership, Clayton, Australia

Cate Nagle
James Cook University & Townsville Hospital and Health Service, School of Nursing and Midwifery, Townsville, Australia

Tracey K. Bucknall
Deakin University, Faculty of Health, School of Nursing and Midwifery, Geelong, Australia
Centre for Quality and Patient Safety Research-Alfred Health Partnership, Melbourne, Australia

Frank Chimbwandira
Department of HIV and AIDS, Ministry of Health, Lilongwe, Malawi

Lyson Tenthani
Department of HIV and AIDS, Ministry of Health, Lilongwe, Malawi
Institute of Social and Preventive Medicine, University of Bern, Bern, Switzerland
International Training and Education Center for Health, Lilongwe 3, Malawi

Joep J. van Oosterhout
Dignitas International, Zomba, Malawi
Department of Medicine, College of Medicine, Blantyre, Malawi

Andreas D. Haas and Kali Tal
Institute of Social and Preventive Medicine, University of Bern, Bern, Switzerland

Malango Msukwa and Nozgechi Phiri
The Baobab Health Trust, Lilongwe, Malawi
Institute of Global Health, University of Geneva, Geneva, Switzerland

Karoline Aebi-Popp
Department of Infectious Diseases, University Hospital Bern, Bern, Switzerland

Janne Estill
Institute of Social and Preventive Medicine, University of Bern, Bern, Switzerland
Institute of Global Health, University of Geneva, Geneva, Switzerland
Institute of Mathematical Statistics and Actuarial Science, University of Bern, Bern, Switzerland

Olivia Keiser
Institute of Social and Preventive Medicine, University of Bern, Bern, Switzerland
Institute of Global Health, University of Geneva, Geneva, Switzerland

Aaisha Amjad, Uzair Amjad, Rubeena Zakar, Ahmed Usman, Muhammad Zakria and Zakar
Institute of Social and Cultural Studies, University of the Punjab, Lahore, Pakistan

Florian Fischer
Department of Public Health Medicine, School of Public Health, Bielefeld University, Bielefeld, Germany

John Horogo
Department of Obstetrics and Gynaecology, St. Francis Referral Hospital, Ifakara, Tanzania

Jos van Roosmalen
Department of Obstetrics, Leiden University Medical Centre, Leiden, The Netherlands

Luuk Dekker and Tessa Houtzager
Department of Obstetrics and Gynaecology, St. Francis Referral Hospital, Ifakara, Tanzania
Department of Obstetrics, Leiden University Medical Centre, Leiden, The Netherlands

Omary Kilume and Angelo Sadock Nyamtema
Department of Obstetrics and Gynaecology, St. Francis Referral Hospital, Ifakara, Tanzania
St. Francis University College of Health and Allied Sciences, Ifakara, Tanzania

Sunday Dominico, Nguke Mwakatundu and Mkambu Kasanga
Thamini Uhai, Kigoma, Tanzania

Patricia E. Bailey
Pittsboro, USA

Jos van Roosmalen
Department of Obstetrics, Leiden University Medical Center and Athena Institute, VU University, de Boelelaan 1105, 1081 HV Amsterdam, The Netherlands

Sheng Wang, Rajluxmee Beejadhursing, Xiangyi Ma and Ya Li
Department of Obstetrics and Gynecology, Tongji Hospital, Tongji Medical College, Huazhong University of Science and Technology, Wuhan 430030, People's Republic of China

Nirmala Chandrasekaran, Leanne R De Souza and Howard Berger
Department of Maternal and Fetal Medicine, St Michaels Hospital, 30 Bond street, Toronto, ON M5B 1W8, Canada

Marcelo L Urquia
Li Ka Shing Knowledge Institute, St Michael's Hospital, Toronto, Canada

Beverley Young
Perinatal Mental Health Program, Mount Sinai Hospital, Toronto, Canada

Anne Mcleod
Sunnybrook Health Sciences, Toronto, Canada

Rory Windrim
Mt Sinai Hospital, Toronto, Canada

Markus Fleisch
Clinic for Gynecology and Obstetrics, Helios University Hospital Wuppertal, University Witten/ Herdecke, Heusnerstr 40, 42283 Wuppertal, Germany

Percy Balan, Tanja Fehm, Carsten Hagenbeck and Julius Gilles
Clinic for Gynecology and Obstetrics, Heinrich-Heine-University, Düsseldorf, Germany

Philip Hepp
Clinic for Gynecology and Obstetrics, Helios University Hospital Wuppertal, University Witten/ Herdecke, Heusnerstr 40, 42283 Wuppertal, Germany
Clinic for Gynecology and Obstetrics, Heinrich-Heine-University, Düsseldorf, Germany

Oliver T. Wolf
Department of Cognitive Psychology, Institute of Cognitive Neuroscience, Faculty of Psychology, Ruhr-University Bochum, Bochum, Germany

Wolfram Goertz
Musikerambulanz, Heinrich-Heine-University, Düsseldorf, Germany

Wolfgang Janni
Clinic for Gynecology and Obstetrics, University Hospital Ulm, Ulm, Germany

Nora K. Schaal
Department of Experimental Psychology, Heinrich-Heine-University, Düsseldorf, Germany

Tsehaynesh Aslake Wendmagegn, Gerezgiher Buruh Abera, Weyzer Tilahun Tsehaye, Kibrom Brhanu Gebresslasie and Berhe Girmay Tella
School of Nursing, College of Health Sciences, Mekelle University, Mekelle, Ethiopia

Alison Peel
London School of Hygiene and Tropical Medicine, London, UK

Abhishek Bhartia
Sitaram Bhartia Institute of Science and Research, New Delhi, India

Neil Spicer and Meenakshi Gautham
Department of Global Health and Development, Faculty of Public Health and Policy, London School of Hygiene and Tropical Medicine, London, UK

Misgav Rottenstreich, Hen Y. Sela, Ori Shen, Rachel Michaelson-Cohen, Arnon Samueloff and Orna Reichman
Department of Obstetrics and Gynecology, Shaare Zedek Medical Center, Hebrew University, Jerusalem, Israel

Joseph Niyitegeka and Paulin Banguti
Department of Anesthesia, Critical Care and Emergency Medicine, School of Medicine and Pharmacy, College of Medicine and Health Sciences, University of Rwanda, Kigali, Rwanda

Georges Nshimirimana and Regis Habimana
Ministry of Health, Kigali, Rwanda

Allison Silverstein
Program in Global Surgery and Social Change, Harvard Medical School, Boston, MA, USA
Miller School of Medicine, University of Miami, Miami, FL, USA

Jackline Odhiambo
Partners In Health, Boston, MA, USA

Yihan Lin
Program in Global Surgery and Social Change, Harvard Medical School, Boston, MA, USA
Department of Surgery, University of Colorado Hospital, Aurora, CO, USA

Theoneste Nkurunziza
Partners In Health / Inshuti Mu Buzima, Kigali, Rwanda

Robert Riviello
Program in Global Surgery and Social Change, Harvard Medical School, Boston, MA, USA
Department of Surgery, Brigham and Women's Hospital, Boston, MA, USA

Stephen Rulisa
School of Medicine and Pharmacy, College of Medicine and Health Sciences, University of Rwanda, Kigali, Rwanda

Martin Macharia
Partners In Health / Inshuti Mu Buzima, Kigali, Rwanda

Hema Magge
Partners In Health / Inshuti Mu Buzima, Kigali, Rwanda
Division of Global Health Equity, Brigham and Women's Hospital, Boston, MA, USA
Division of General Pediatrics, Boston Children's Hospital, Boston, MA, USA

Bethany Hedt-Gauthier
Partners In Health / Inshuti Mu Buzima, Kigali, Rwanda
Department of Global Health and Social Medicine, Harvard Medical School, Boston, MA, USA

Louise Möller, Ann Josefsson, Marie Bladh, Caroline Lilliecreutz and G. Sydsjö
Department of Obstetrics and Gynaecology, and Department of Clinical and Experimental Medicine, Linköping University, SE-581 85 Linköping, Sweden

Ellika Andolf
Division of Obstetrics and Gynaecology, Department of Clinical Sciences, Karolinska Institutet, Danderyd Hospital, Stockholm, Sweden

Kandice A. Kapinos
RAND Corporation, 1200 South Hayes, Arlington, VA 22202, USA

Olga Yakusheva
University of Michigan, School of Nursing and School of Public Health, 400 North Ingalls Building, Ann Arbor, MI 48109-5482, USA

Marianne Weiss
Marquette University College of Nursing, 530 N 16th St, Milwaukee, WI 53233, USA

Karin Bischoff, Britta Lang, Joerg Meerpohl and Christine Schmucker
Cochrane Germany, Medical Center - University of Freiburg, Faculty of Medicine, University of Freiburg, Freiburg, Germany

Monika Nothacker
AWMF-Institute for Medical Knowledge Management (IMWi), Karl-von-Frisch-Street 1, 35043 Marburg, Germany

Cornelius Lehane
Department of Anesthesiology and Critical Care, University Heart Center Freiburg-Bad Krozingen, Medical Center - University of Freiburg, Freiburg, Germany

Eileen Wang
Institute for Global Health, School of Public Health, Zhejiang University, 866 Yuhangtang Lu, Hangzhou 310058, China

Therese Hesketh
Institute for Global Health, School of Public Health, Zhejiang University, 866 Yuhangtang Lu, Hangzhou 310058, China
Institute for Global Health, University College London, 30 Guilford St., London, UK

Birjna A. Hirani
Kilimanjaro Christian Medical University College, Moshi, Tanzania

Bariki L. Mchome and Nicholaus S. Mazuguni
Department of Obstetrics and Gynecology, Kilimanjaro Christian Medical Centre, Moshi, Tanzania
Kilimanjaro Christian Medical University College, Moshi, Tanzania

Michael J. Mahande
Department of Epidemiology & Biostatistics, Institute of Public Health, Kilimanjaro Christian Medical University College, Moshi, Tanzania
Kilimanjaro Christian Medical University College, Moshi, Tanzania

Carsten Hagenbeck, Bettina Burghardt, Bernadette Jaeger and Tanja Fehm
Clinic for Gynecology and Obstetrics, Heinrich-Heine-University, Düsseldorf, Germany

Philip Hepp
Clinic for Gynecology and Obstetrics, Heinrich-Heine-University, Düsseldorf, Germany
Clinic for Gynecology and Obstetrics, HELIOS Universitätsklinikum Wuppertal, University Witten / Herdecke, Vogelsangstr. 109, 42109 Wuppertal, Germany

Oliver T. Wolf
Department of Cognitive Psychology, Institute of Cognitive Neuroscience, Faculty of Psychology, Ruhr-University Bochum, Bochum, Germany

Nora K. Schaal
Department of Experimental Psychology, Heinrich-Heine-University, Düsseldorf, Germany

Xin Wang, Lei Hou, Liying Zou, Yan Ruan and Weiyuan Zhang
Department of Obstetrics, Beijing Obstetrics and Gynecology Hospital, Capital Medical University, No. 251 YaoJiayuan Road, Chaoyang District, Beijing 100026, China

Susan Hellerstein
Department of Obstetrics and Gynecology, Brigham and Women's Hospital, Harvard Medical School, Boston, MA 01210, USA

Chao Wu
The First Affiliated Hospital of Soochow University, No. 188 Shizi Street, Gusu district, Su Zhou, Jiangsu province, China

Jianping Ding and Binbin Mei
Nursing School of Soochow University, Su Zhou, China

Zunjia Wen and Meifen Shen
The First Affiliated Hospital of Soochow University, No. 188 Shizi Street, Gusu district, Su Zhou, Jiangsu province, China
Nursing School of Soochow University, Su Zhou, China

Sonja Melman, Jan Gerrit Nijhuis and Hubertina Catharina Johanna Scheepers
Department of Obstetrics and Gynaecology, GROW-School for Oncology and Developmental Biology, Maastricht University Medical Centre, Maastricht, The Netherlands

Rachel Hellen Petra Schreurs and Nicol Anna Cornelia Smeets
Department of Obstetrics and Gynaecology, Zuyderland Medical Centre, Heerlen, The Netherlands

Carmen Desiree Dirksen
Department of Clinical Epidemiology and Medical Technology Assessment (KEMTA), CAPHRI-School for Public Health and Primary Care, Maastricht University Medical Centre, Maastricht, The Netherlands

Anneke Kwee
Department of Obstetrics and Gynaecology, University Medical Hospital Utrecht, Utrecht, The Netherlands

Rosella Petronella Maria Gemma Hermens
Scientific Institute for Quality of Healthcare (IQ healthcare), Radboud University Nijmegen Medical Centre, Nijmegen, The Netherlands

Ingela Lundgren and Christina Nilsson
Institute of Health and Care Sciences, Sahlgrenska Academy, University of Gothenburg, Gothenburg, Sweden

Patricia Healy
School of Nursing and Midwifery, National University of Ireland, Upper Newcastle Road, Galway, Ireland

Margaret Carroll, Cecily Begley and Joan Lalor
School of Nursing and Midwifery, Trinity College Dublin, 24 D'Olier Street, Dublin 2, Ireland

Andrea Matterne, Mechthild M. Gross and Susanne Grylka-Baeschlin
Midwifery Research and Education Unit, Hannover Medical School, Carl-Neuberg-Str. 1, 30625 Hannover, Germany

Jane Nicoletti
Universita Degli Studi di Genova, Via Balbi 5, 16126 Genova, Italy

Sandra Morano
IRCCS Azienda Ospedaliera Universitaria S. Martino IST, Largo R. Benzi, 10 16132 Genova, Italy

Index

www.ingramcontent.com/pod-product-compliance
Lightning Source LLC
LaVergne TN
LVHW080657210926
848485LV00003B/388

* 9 7 8 1 6 3 9 2 7 1 5 1 1 *